Sensory Research
Multimodal Perspectives

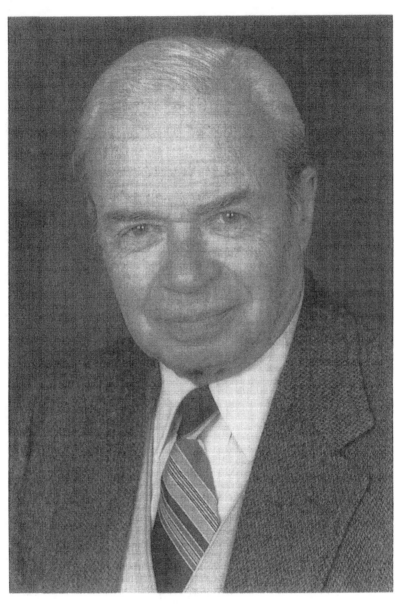

Jozef J. Zwislocki

Sensory Research
Multimodal Perspectives

Edited by
Ronald T. Verrillo
Institute for Sensory Research, Syracuse University

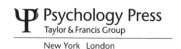

Ψ Psychology Press
Taylor & Francis Group

New York London

First Published by
Lawrence Erlbaum Associates, Inc., Publishers
365 Broadway
Hillsdale, New Jersey 07642

Transferred to Digital Printing 2009 by Psychology Press
270 Madison Ave, New York NY 10016
27 Church Road, Hove, East Sussex, BN3 2FA

Library of Congress Cataloging-in-Publication Data

Sensory research : multimodal perspectives / edited by
Ronald T. Verrilllo.
    p. cm.
Includes bibliographical references and index.
ISBN 0-8058-1342-X
1. Senses and sensation—Congresses. 2. Zwislocki, Jozef J.,
1922–Congresses. I. Verrillo, Ronald T. II. Zwislocki, Jozef
J., 1922-   .
QP431.S456 1993
599'.0182—dc20   93-22160
                                                   CIP

Publisher's Note
The publisher has gone to great lengths to ensure the quality of this reprint
but points out that some imperfections in the original may be apparent.

Dedicated to the fond memory of
Sylvia (Sunny) Zwislocki

Contents

viii   CONTENTS

Preface

This volume is a record of the proceedings of a Festspiel held in honor of Jozef J. Zwislocki at the Sheraton University Inn and Conference Center on the campus of Syracuse University on August 21 and 22, 1992. Professor Zwislocki, upon his retirement, was recognized for his outstanding contributions to science and to Syracuse University.

The participants included former students who received their training and academic degrees from the Syracuse University Doctoral Program in Neuroscience (created by Professor Zwislocki), former colleagues in research, and current members, students, and staff of the Institute for Sensory Research. Although the purpose of the conference was to recognize the many achievements of Professor Zwislocki, the spirit of the participants was to honor him in a manner that best characterized his lifetime dedication to research, that is, to report the results of their own work. Consequently, this volume is first and foremost a compilation of scientific papers in the area of sensory research. Some are reports of recent experiments and some present an overview of research efforts extending from the past to ongoing work. Professor Zwislocki's influence can be recognized in all of the contributions and some contributors explicitly describe the ties between their own work and the germinal ideas planted by him.

—Ronald T. Verrillo

Acknowledgments

The authors gratefully acknowledge the following persons whose generous support has made this conference and volume possible:

William F. Allyn
Gerhard M. Baule
Joanne Covo
Louis M. DiCarlo
Jerome R. Gerber
Robert H. McCaffrey

Syracuse University
Office of the Dean of the L. C. Smith College
  of Engineering and Computer Science
Office of the Vice President for Research
  and Computing

In addition to all the participants and invited guests, we wish to thank the other members of the planning committee, Rhona Hellman, Dr. Stanley Bolanowski and Dr. Robert Smith. We also extend our deep appreciation for the support of the many people who assisted us in so many ways during the preparation of the meeting and of this volume. These include: Shannon Flanagan, Michael Garver, Susan Gingeleski, Jennifer McCarthy, Anne Quesada, Sabina Redington, Michael Schechter, and Patricia Swaites.

August, 1992

Professor Jozef Zwislocki
The Institute for Sensory Research
Syracuse University
Syracuse, NY   13244

Dear Joe,

Congratulations and best wishes on the occasion of this celebration of your singular accomplishments as a world renowned scientist and a valued member of the faculty at Syracuse University. I regret that I cannot be with you in person during this happy time. However, I add my voice to the chorus of others who sing your praise.

Creating new ways to pay you homage presents some challenges. Your list of honors, recognitions, awards, publications, advances, and various accolades is justifiably classified as remarkable. The prodigious output of your fertile mind and your single-minded dedication to science place you among the world's best scholars.

I can, however, thank you for the honor you have brought this University. Your contributions to the climate of discovery have enriched not only the work of the Institute for Sensory Research but also the whole community of creators, discoverers, and innovators. Your example has stimulated the work of younger scientists and scholars. Your championing of the importance of pure research has excited the imagination of students, leading them to take the difficult path of research scientist. Your presence as our single member of the National Academy of Sciences adds greatly to the quality of Syracuse University.

In a challenging climate for all of higher education, it is heartening to claim someone whose career is as distinguished as yours. We are reminded of our mission to promote learning through teaching, research, scholarship, creative accomplishment, and service. You, Joe, are a fine example of all of these worthy goals.

Sincerely,

Kenneth A. Shaw

Kenneth A. Shaw

Tribute

Ronald T. Verrillo
Institute for Sensory Research, Syracuse University

We are assembled at this conference to honor Dr. Jozef Zwislocki upon his retirement. We honor his many contributions to Syracuse University, to the Institute for Sensory Research (which he founded in 1957 and guided as Director until 1984), and to science. His contributions to our knowledge of the hydromechanical, neurophysiological, and perceptual mechanisms of the auditory system are truly monumental. His contributions to our comprehension of the mammalian auditory system include not only landmark ideas (he is a fountainhead of creativity) but also include many of the experimental findings in psychoacoustics and peripheral auditory physiology that constitute the data base which has provided a springboard for research in laboratories throughout the world. One of his most far-reaching accomplishments was the bridge he pioneered between the once distant sciences of psychoacoustics and auditory physiology. His efforts to link physics, biology, and psychophysics to create a basis for our understanding of the nervous system has had an influence that extends far beyond the science of acoustics.

Jozef Zwislocki was born in Lwow, Poland on March 22, 1922. He became interested in audition during his studies at the Institute of Technology in Zurich, Switzerland, where his doctoral dissertation, a mathematical description and analysis of a plane-wave model of cochlear hydrodynamics, offered the first complete solution to a model of the cochlea. Today, after more than 40 years, that type of model is still used by investigators to explain cochlear function. More recently, his pioneering ideas about the critical role of outer hair cells in coclear micromechanics are viewed with intense interest. For many years his outstanding contributions to our understanding of middle-ear functions have served as the standard in the field.

In the late 1940s, Dr. Zwislocki began his pioneering studies in psychoacoustics with measurements of forward masking. He suggested that two interactive neurophysiological components, the persistence of excitation and adaptation, could account for the phenomenon. From these observations, he developed his comprehensive theory of temporal summation, a theory that has been shown to extend beyond audition to other sense modalities. During his six years at Harvard's Psychoacoustic Laboratory in the 1950s, he made major contributions to the study of central masking and loudness. These studies have continued unabated since he came to Syracuse University in 1957. He developed a sophisticated theory of central masking from demonstrations of a sharp frequency selectivity, similar to that of auditory-nerve fibers. He applied S. S. Stevens' power law and direct scaling procedures to demonstrate the role of the standard in magnitude estimation and to compare monaural and binaural loudness functions. He developed the method of *absolute* magnitude estimation for scaling psychological magnitude and he discovered that intensity enhancement and summation are two fundamentally distinct mechanisms. In my personal judgment, I would consider one of Dr. Zwislocki's most significant and far-reaching accomplishments to be his empirical and theoretical contributions to the theory of measurement. In a landmark paper published in 1991, he developed his notion of "natural measurement," in which he showed that useful measurements can be made without numbers and that people and animals can be successful in measuring aspects of their environments through the use of their senses, without using instruments. In this paper, he asserts that measurement should be defined as matching common attributes of things or events. Furthermore, when the numbers that are used to characterize physical units are introduced, it becomes possible to express the results of internal matching as functions of associated physical variables, so there is no fundamental difference between natural measurement and psychophysical matching experiments. By this theory, the problem of coupling numbers to subjective impressions has been solved in principle.

In the 1970s, faced with the need for electrophysiological data not to be found in the literature, Dr. Zwislocki trained himself in the techniques of electrophysiology and proceeded to launch himself into an essentially new career. Work on the encoding of acoustic signals by single nerve fibers accomplished by him and his group has led to some very illuminating experimental results and has made substantial contributions to the study of peripheral physiology of cochlear microphonics, neural adaptation, the encoding of time-varying signal amplitudes, and hair-cell receptor potentials.

His activities have not been limited to theory and basic experimentation.

He is one of those rare individuals who is able to make the leap from the fundamentals of his science to the world of practical needs. This is reflected in his many contributions (and patents) to diagnostic, protective, and prosthetic devices. The exceptional farsightedness and soundness of his work is attested by the fact that many of the techniques and ideas that he pioneered decades ago are still in use today.

His honors and awards are far too numerous to list here, but among them are the first Békésy Medal of the Acoustical Society of America, the International Centro Ricerche e Studi Amplifon Prize of Italy, the Medal of the Medical Academy in Poland, the Award of Merit of the Association for Research in Otolaryngology, the first Hugh Knowles Prize, and the Chancellor's Citation for Exceptional Academic Achievement at Syracuse University. He is the first and only faculty member in the history of Syracuse University ever to be elected to the National Academy of Sciences, the highest honor that is bestowed by the scientific community in the United States. In 1991, he received a doctorate *honoris cause* from the Adam Mickiewicz University of Poznan in his native and beloved Poland.

In conclusion, Dr. Zwislocki's contributions to the very many different areas of auditory research may have the surface appearance of being rather segregated. To the contrary, his life's achievements succeed to a remarkable extent in demonstrating how psychoacoustic and physiological data can be united with mathematical modeling techniques to develop powerful theories and valid descriptions of underlying neurophysiological mechanisms. His contributions to our university have been equally impressive, having founded the Institute for Sensory Research, the doctoral program in neuroscience, and having fostered the creation of the department of bioengineering. All of these have made it possible for students to receive an education of the highest quality and so make their own contributions to science. Indeed, more than half of the speakers participating in his conference are former or current students from Syracuse University. And, it would be safe to say that all of the speakers have been influenced by Dr. Zwislocki's thinking and example. It is gratifying that so many former students have returned to Syracuse University to participate in this celebration of a truly remarkable man of science, Jozef Zwislocki. We wish him well.

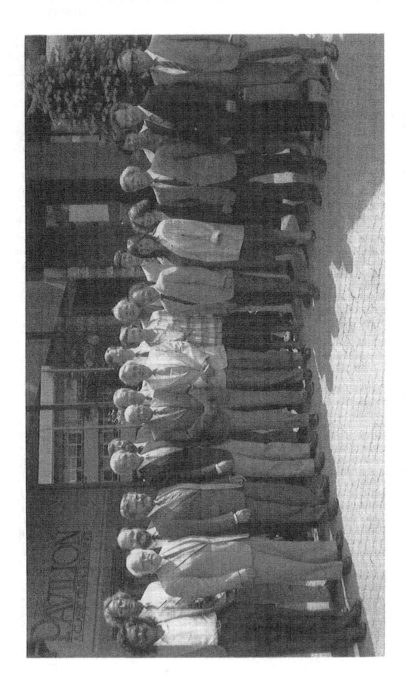

xx

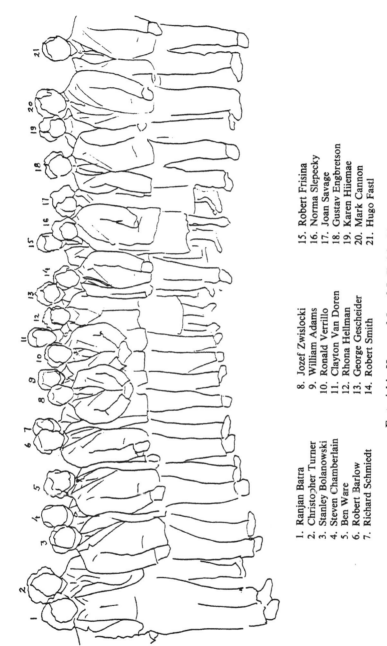

1. Ranjan Batra
2. Christopher Turner
3. Stanley Bolanowski
4. Steven Chamberlain
5. Ben Ware
6. Robert Barlow
7. Richard Schmiedt

8. Jozef Zwislocki
9. William Adams
10. Ronald Verrillo
11. Clayton Van Doren
12. Rhona Hellman
13. George Gescheider
14. Robert Smith

15. Robert Frisina
16. Norma Slepecky
17. Joan Savage
18. Gustav Engbretson
19. Karen Hiiemae
20. Mark Cannon
21. Hugo Fastl

Festspiel in Honor of Jozef J. Zwislocki
August 21, 22, 1992

xxi

List of Contributors

William B. Adams
Department of Pharmacology, Biozentrum, University of Basel, Switzerland
Robert B. Barlow
Institute for Sensory Research, Syracuse University
Ranjan Batra
Department of Anatomy, University of Connecticut Health Center
Stanley J. Bolanowski
Institute for Sensory Research, Syracuse University
Mark W. Cannon
Aerospace Medical Research Laboratories, Wright-Patterson Air Force Base
Steven C. Chamberlain
Institute for Sensory Research, Syracuse University
André Chays
Hopital Nord, Marseille, France
Christine M. Checkosky
Institute for Sensory Research, Syracuse University
Gustav A. Engbretson
Institute for Sensory Research, Syracuse University
Hugo Fastl
Institute of Electroacoustics, Technical University of Munich
Robert D. Frisina
Otolaryngology Division, University of Rochester School of Medicine and Dentistry

George A. Gescheider
Institute for Sensory Research, Syracuse University
Department of Psychology, Hamilton College
Rhona P. Hellman
Department of Psychology, Northeastern University
Karen M. Hiiemae
Department of Bioengineering, Syracuse University
Eric P. Hornstein
Department of Bioengineering, Syracuse University
Ehud Kaplan
Biophysics Laboratory, The Rockefeller University
Kenneth J. Karcich
Otolaryngology Division, University of Rochester School of Medicine
and Dentistry
Lisa L. Menia
Department of Orthopedics, Cleveland Metropolitan General Hospital
Jacques Magnan
Massachusetts Eye and Ear Infirmary
Alain Marchioni
Laboratoire de Mécanique et d'Acoustique, Marseille, France
Joseph Nadol
Hopital Nord, Marseille, France
Joan E. Savage
Institute for Sensory Research, Syracuse University
Bertram Scharf
Department of Psychology, Northeastern University
Laboratoire de Mécanique et d'Acoustique, Marseille, France
Richard A. Schmiedt
ENT Department, Medical University of South Carolina
Norma B. Slepecky
Institute for Sensory Research, Syracuse University
Robert L. Smith
Institute for Sensory Research, Syracuse University
Eduardo C. Solessio
Institute for Sensory Research, Syracuse University
Clayton L. Van Doren
Department of Orthopedics, Cleveland Metropolitan General Hospital
Ronald T. Verrillo
Institute for Sensory Research, Syracuse University

Joseph P. Walton
Otolaryngology Division, University of Rochester School of Medicine and Dentistry
Thomas M. Wengenack
Department of Anatomy and Neurobiology, University of Rochester School of Medicine and Dentistry.

Introduction

On the surface, this book may have appearance of a random collection of unrelated papers assembled to do honor to a distinguished sensory scientist. And, in fact, honor to Jozef Zwislocki can be considered the first unifying theme of the book. The second theme, of course, is that all of the chapters carry a central focus on the sensory systems of hearing, vision, and touch. The scope of the book is broad, not only because it cuts across three sensory systems, but it also encompasses four different experimental methodologies, namely: psychophysics, electrophysiology, cellular anatomy, and neurochemistry.

Chapters by Fastl, Gescheider, Hellman, and Scharf et al. draw upon original experiments and published literature in auditory psychophysics. Fastl (chapter 12) compares two methods of assessing the perception of noise at airports, Gescheider (chapter 13) compares the results of magnitude scaling procedures in hearing and vision, and Hellman (chapter 1) examines loudness functions in persons with hearing loss due to choclear impairment. The chapter by Scharf et al. (chapter 18) deals with the detection of tones in a monaural noise masker and the effect that efferent input to the cochlea has on that detection.

The psychophysical background in hearing is augmented by Batra, Frisina et al., Schmiedt, and Smith with results from auditory electrophysiology. Batra (chapter 9) is concerned with the temporal coding of high-frequency sounds within the inferior colliculus. The mechanisms of neural processing of sound amplitude within the auditory nerve and in the lower brain centers is addressed by Frisina et al. (chapter 10). Schmiedt (chapter 6) has studied the effects of aging on the gerbil cochlea, and Smith (chapter 3) gives us an overview of short-term and rapid adaptation in the auditory periphery. Information from physiological laboratories is dovetailed with the microanatomy and cellular chemistry of auditory hair cells by Savage and Slepecky (chapter 14).

In the world of vision, psychophysical experiments are the principal concern of Cannon (chapter 5), who reports and discusses the effects of spatial frequency, orientation, contrast and surround size on visual suppression. Bolanowski et al. (chapter 8) cover the literature and original experiments on the visual experience under Ganzfeld illumination.

The electrophysiology of the visual system of the horseshoe crab is the purview of Barlow and Kaplan (chapter 4) who explore circadian rhythms and intensity coding in the lateral eye of *Limulus*. Engbretson and Solessio (chapter 15), on the other hand, report on a series of interesting experiments with the parietal eye of the desert lizard and they discuss the functional implications of their results. Chamberlain and Hornstein (chapter 7) have chosen several exotic species to study. They report on seasonal affective disorder and evidence for photostasis in *Limulus, Bathynomus Giganteus* and deep sea shrimps living in the vicinity of hydrothermal vents (black smokers) along the Mid-Atlantic Ridge.

Four investigators targeted their efforts on the sense of touch. Bolanowski et al. (chapter 8) offer a quadruplex model of vibrotaction based on psychophysical and electrophysiological evidence. Hiiemae (chapter 16) has authored a comprehensive review, original experiments and a new model of the process and mechanism for rhythmic behavior in chewing and swallowing. The perception and appreciation of surface textures detected by the skin and its neural code is examined by Van Doren and Menia (chapter 11). Verrillo (chapter 17) considers the effects of aging on the sense of touch based on an extended series of psychophysical experiments conducted by himself and colleagues in his laboratory.

The chapter by Adams (chapter 2) stands apart but is related to all others because his research concerns electrochemical events occurring at the membrane of nerve fibers. He presents data and discusses the nature of the calcium ion as an intracellular second messenger.

It is clear from this assembly of research papers that the study of the human senses is broad indeed, involving human and animal experiments and system modeling, as well as a variety of experimental techniques, and drawing upon multiple modalities to develop intelligent hypotheses or models for how the nervous system works. We respectfully submit that this volume, as its title suggests, represents accurately multimodal perspectives of sensory science.

1 Can Magnitude Scaling Reveal the Growth of Loudness in Cochlear Impairment?

Rhona P. Hellman
Northeastern University and Veterans Administration

INTRODUCTION

Zwislocki's interest and contribution to our understanding of the loudness-intensity relation were sparked by his early studies with Lüscher (Lüscher & Zwislocki, 1948a, 1948b, 1951) and the development of his comprehensive theory of temporal auditory summation which assumes that loudness is directly proportional to neural activity within the auditory system (Zwislocki, 1960, 1969). These pioneering endeavors led him to determine the role of the slope of the loudness function in temporal summation and its extension to central masking, to assess the relation between the acoustic-reflex growth function and loudness, and more generally, to search for the key to an understanding of the form of the sensation-magnitude functions in all sensory systems (Zwislocki, 1965, 1972, 1973, 1974). Underlying much of Zwislocki's loudness work is the assumption that Stevens' power law (1953, 1975), based primarily on direct magnitude-scaling procedures, is determined by the stimulus transformation to a neural loudness code.

One way to ascertain if the outcome of direct magnitude scaling is related to the output of the auditory system is to measure the growth of loudness in cochlear pathology. Cochlear pathology not only produces an elevated threshold, but in the region of impaired hearing it markedly alters the overall shape of the loudness function. This well-documented phenomenon known as *loudness recruitment* is usually measured by loudness matching (e.g., Fowler, 1928, 1936; Hallpike, 1967; Miskolczy-Fodor, 1960; Reger, 1936).

Although an overall description of the loudness-intensity relation can be derived from measured loudness levels, these indirect loudness determinations cannot disclose the actual rate of growth or shape of the loudness functions (Hellman, 1976; Hellman & Zwislocki, 1968), nor can they provide information about the growth of loudness in bilaterally symmetrical impaired hearing (e.g., Marshall, 1981). Thus, despite their significant theoretical and practical ramifications, loudness-growth data spanning the dynamic range of hearing are seldom obtained for the vast majority of the hearing-impaired population. To help solve this thorny but important problem, several recent studies have demonstrated that direct magnitude scaling advocated by Stevens (1959a, 1975) for the measurement of loudness in auditory pathology can be applied to individuals and groups with cochlear-impaired hearing (Hellman, 1988; Hellman & Meiselman, 1990, 1992, 1993). This chapter presents additional evidence confirming the validity of magnitude scaling for measuring loudness in cochlear impairment. In the first section, equal-sensation functions derived from magnitude scaling are shown to be consistent with the results of intramodality matching. The second section shows that the rate of loudness growth is dependent on threshold sensitivity in the region of impaired hearing but not in the region of normal hearing. Finally, the third section shows that Zwislocki's (1965) generalized loudness equation gives a good account of the growth of loudness in cochlear impairment. The results are compared to those predicted by the modified power law in the form $L = K(P^2 - P_o^2)^\theta$ (Ekman, 1956; Luce, 1959; Stevens, 1959b) and to predictions by the alternative form $L = K(P^{2\theta} - P_o^{2\theta})$ subsequently introduced to describe the sensation-magnitude functions in quiet (Zwislocki & Hellman, 1960) and in noise (Lochner & Burger, 1961).

EQUAL-SENSATION FUNCTIONS IN COCHLEAR-IMPAIRED HEARING

Under conditions of minimal experimental constraints and biases Hellman and Zwislocki (1961, 1963, 1964, 1968) showed, in agreement with Stevens (1959a, 1966), that a similar underlying behavior was involved in loudness balances and magnitude scaling, namely matching. The coincidence of equal-sensation matches derived from magnitude scaling with those obtained from direct loudness matching was accomplished by eliminating the confounding effects imposed by either explicit or implicit reference standards and by averaging the individual raw data without any normalization. On the basis of their initial studies, Hellman and Zwislocki postulated that people have the capacity to pair the perceived magnitudes of numbers to sensation magnitudes on an absolute scale. Hence, they reasoned that the outcome of magnitude-scaling experiments can determine both the *slope* and *absolute position* of loudness curves on log–log coordinates. Later experiments corroborated the earlier findings and provided a further demonstration that equal-sensation functions consistent with the results of direct matching procedures can be derived from absolute magnitude scaling (Bolanowski, Zwislocki, & Gescheider, 1991; Collins & Gescheider, 1989; Hellman, 1976; Verrillo, Fraioli, & Smith, 1969; Zwislocki, 1983; Zwislocki & Goodman, 1980). The latter studies were all performed with people who had normal sensory functioning. The present experiments show that the mechanics of absolute scaling also hold for individuals with impaired auditory systems.

Description of Experiments

Equal-sensation functions were generated indirectly from absolute magnitude estimation (AME), absolute magnitude production (AMP), and cross-modality matching (CMM) between loudness and apparent length; they were also generated directly from intramodality matching. Eight listeners with bilateral cochlear impairments of long duration participated. All had clinically normal hearing (≤ 22-dB HL; ANSI, 1969) at one frequency enabling either interfrequency or intrafrequency loudness matches to be performed. Each listener was tested individually in a double-walled sound-proof booth. Listening was monaural through a TDH-49 earphone mounted in an MX-41/AR cushion. Root-mean-square voltages to the earphone were measured daily with a Fluke (8050A) digital voltmeter.

The stimuli were tone bursts that varied in frequency from 500–3,500 Hz and horizontal lines of light displayed one at a time from 35-mm slides. Tone-burst duration was 1 sec, rise-fall time was 10 ms, and the interstimulus interval was 500 ms. The tones were generated by a Krohn-Hite (4141R) oscillator. After appropriate amplification (Crown D-75 amplifier), the levels of the tone were controlled with Hewlett-Packard (350D) attenuators. A Kodak (4600) projector was used to display the lines which were viewed in a dimly lit room through the glass window of the booth.

The experimental protocol for the determination of the sensation-magnitude functions was as follows. First, pure-tone thresholds were measured by the method of limits at two frequencies, one where thresholds were normal, and the second where thresholds were elevated. Next, to increase the stability of the loudness results and to illustrate the concept of an open-ended number scale (Hellman, 1982; Zwislocki, 1983), apparent length was judged by AME for eight previously tested lines with measured projected lengths of 0.52, 1.04, 2.08, 5.2, 10.4, 20.8, 41.6, and 65 cm (Hellman & Meiselman, 1988, 1990). After the judgments of apparent length were completed, loudness was judged by AME in separate sessions at each of the two chosen stimulus frequencies. Loudness judgments were obtained at 7 to 11 sensation levels (SL) spanning the dynamic range of hearing from 4-dB SL to the SL corresponding to the maximal output of the equipment at a sound-pressure level (SPL) of 110 dB. Within a session, AME was followed by AMP (for rationale, see Hellman & Zwislocki, 1963) and by cross-modality matching. A typical stimulus set for AMP consisted of 7 to 11 numbers, and for CMM it consisted of 6 to 7 lines. For AMP the selected stimuli were individually determined from the range of numbers used for AME of loudness; for CMM they were selected from the lines used for AME of apparent length. As in AME of loudness, judgments by AMP and CMM were obtained at each stimulus frequency in a separate session.

The AME procedure was essentially the same for apparent length and loudness. For both tasks, each listener was simply asked to match an appropriate positive number, including decimals and fractions, to the loudness (or length) of the tone (or line), regardless of the number assigned to the previous stimulus. No standard stimulus was prescribed, and no lengthy practice sessions were required. Moreover, all judgments were self-paced; that is, the listeners were permitted to hear a tone (or see a line) more than once before making a response. Order biases arising from the preceding trial are effectively reduced under these conditions (Hellman, 1976). The final averaging was obtained without normalization of the raw data. Geometric means of the second and third judgments provided the estimate of apparent length and of loudness at each stimulus level.

Similarly, the judgments of AMP of loudness and of CMM were obtained without a designated standard. For both AMP of loudness and CMM the levels of the tone were adjusted by the listener until the loudness appeared equal to the perceived magnitude of the assigned number or line. Three adjustments to each stimulus were obtained by a bracketing procedure. The adjustments were made by turning an unmarked black knob attached to a sone potentiometer (60-dB range) external to the booth. To ensure that the listener's settings remained within the middle of the potentiometer's range, the experimenter controlled the input SPL to the potentiometer with a supplementary Hewlett-Packard (350D) attenuator. Just as in AME, the final averages were obtained without normalization of the raw data. Decibel averages of the second and third adjustments provided the average level matched in loudness to each assigned stimulus number or line.

Intramodality matches were obtained in a third listening session with the same apparatus and adjustment procedure used for AMP and CMM. However, rather than match loudness to assigned numbers or lines, six listeners performed intrafrequency matches and two performed interfrequency matches at 6 to 10 levels. The intrafrequency matches were obtained by the traditional alternate binaural loudness balance procedure; the interfrequency matches were performed by the method of alternate monaural loudness balance. In one experimental run the listener adjusted the level of the tone at a frequency in the region of impaired hearing to be as loud as the comparison tone set at a frequency in the region where thresholds were normal. In the second run, the roles of the standard and comparison tones were reversed. During each run, a listener made three separate matches to each standard by varying the sone potentiometer. Decibel averages of the second and third adjustments provided the average equal-loudness match for a given stimulus level.

Figure 1.1 shows the AME functions produced by an individual listener, JC, who had normal hearing at 3.5 kHz in one ear and a 73-dB hearing loss at the same frequency in the contralateral ear. Clearly, the overall shapes of the two functions are very different. Typical of loudness recruitment, the results show that a tone at a given SPL is louder in normal hearing than in impaired hearing (more at moderate than at high SPLs). The data in normal hearing (squares) were fitted by a power function with a slope (re: sound

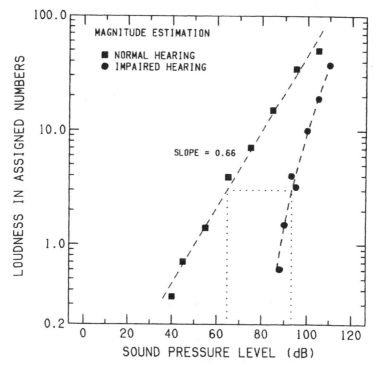

FIG. 1.1. Magnitude estimation of loudness in normal and impaired hearing for listener J.C. at a frequency of 3.5 kHz. The squares are the geometric means in normal hearing; the circles are the corresponding means in impaired hearing. The best-fitting power function to the means in normal hearing has a slope of 0.66. A second-order least-squares fit describes the curvilinear shape of the loudness function in impaired hearing. The dotted lines show the sound-pressure levels that produce equal loudness in normal and impaired hearing.

pressure) of 0.66. As in a previous study (Hellman & Meiselman, 1990), a second-order least-squares fit was used to describe the data (circles) in impaired hearing. Given the assumption inherent in absolute scaling that two sounds assigned the same numerical estimate are perceived to be equally loud, equal-loudness levels were derived from these curves. The dotted lines provide an illustration. In this example, a tone at 65-dB SPL in normal hearing and a tone at 93-dB SPL in impaired hearing are perceived to have a loudness magnitude of 3.0, meaning that the tones at 65-and 93-dB SPL are equally loud. Applying this line of reasoning to all the paired data in normal and impaired hearing, the levels that produced equal loudness were determined over a wide dynamic range.

The same procedure for analyzing the data in Fig. 1.1 was followed to obtain the best-fitting functions to the AMP and CMM data and their derived equal-loudness levels. Figure 1.2 shows the AMP results, and Fig.

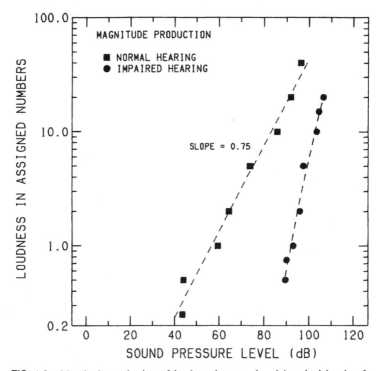

FIG. 1.2. Magnitude production of loudness in normal and impaired hearing for listener J.C. at a frequency of 3.5 kHz. Symbols are the same as in Fig. 1.1. The best-fitting power function to the means in normal hearing has a slope of 0.75. A second-order least-squares fit describes the curvilinear shape of the loudness function in impaired hearing.

1.3 shows those obtained by CMM for listener JC whose AME data are given in Fig. 1.1. A best-fitting power function with a slope of 0.75 provides a good description of the AMP data in normal hearing. The corresponding slope of the power function fitted to the CMM data is 0.66. As in Fig. 1.1, second-order least-squares fits were used to describe the data obtained in impaired hearing. Loudness levels derived according to the procedure employed for listener JC were obtained for the remaining seven listeners. These levels were then compared in the same coordinates to the levels determined directly from intramodality matching.

Figures 1.4 and 1.5 show the SPLs that produce equal loudness for tones located at frequencies in regions of normal and impaired hearing for each of the eight listeners. Results obtained directly from intramodality matching are compared to those obtained indirectly from magnitude scaling. Triangles, squares, and circles indicate equal-loudness levels derived from AME,

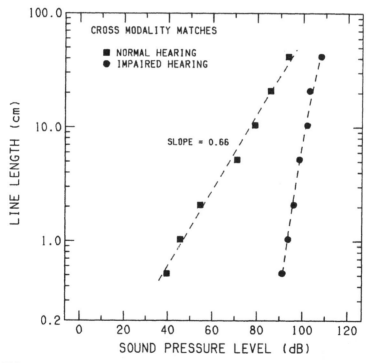

FIG. 1.3. Cross-modality matches between the loudness of a 3.5-kHz tone and apparent length in normal and impaired hearing for listener J.C. Symbols are the same as Fig. 1.1. The best-fitting power function to the means in normal hearing has a slope of 0.66. A second-order least-squares fit describes the shape of the cross-modality matching function in impaired hearing.

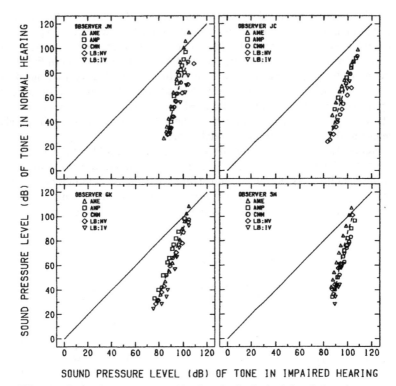

FIG. 1.4. Comparison between equal-loudness levels obtained directly from intramodality matching and those obtained indirectly from magnitude scaling for four individual listeners. Means obtained by the adjustment of the tone in normal hearing are shown by the diamonds; those obtained by the adjustment of the tone in impaired hearing are shown by the inverted triangles. Loudness levels derived from AME, AMP, and CMM are indicated by the triangles, squares, and circles, respectively. The intermittent lines show the second-order least-squares fit to each individual's mean values.

AMP, and CMM, respectively. Equal-loudness levels obtained by adjusting the SPL of the tone set at a frequency in the region of normal hearing are given by the diamonds; those obtained by adjusting the SPL of the tone set at a frequency in the region of impaired hearing are given by the inverted triangles.

Looking first at the complete set of data for listener JC located in the upper right-hand panel of Fig. 1.4, it is evident that the directly and indirectly obtained equal-loudness levels lie within a relatively narrow band. Similarly good agreement among the results of the various procedures is seen for the rest of the listeners in Figs. 1.4 and 1.5. With respect to both

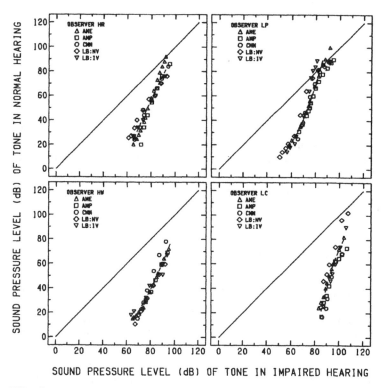

FIG. 1.5. Comparison between equal-loudness levels obtained directly from intramodality matching and those obtained indirectly from magnitude scaling for four individual listeners. (See legend of Fig. 1.4.)

their overall shape and position, the set of data for individual listeners are generally well described by a single function. For a given SPL in normal hearing, the intrasubject variability of the SPLs obtained for equal loudness in impaired hearing ranges, on the average, from 4 to 6 dB across the procedures; the corresponding intersubject variability has a mean value of 4.6 dB. The intermittent lines show the second-order least-squares fits to each individual's mean values. The consistent relation observed between the equal-sensation matches obtained directly from loudness matching and the matches derived indirectly from magnitude scaling could not have been achieved unless individuals were able to refer their judgments to a common internal standard. This fundamental ability, characteristic of "natural measurement" (Zwislocki, 1991), is preserved, despite alterations in the transduction process that severely distort the loudness-intensity relation.

RELATION BETWEEN THE RATE OF LOUDNESS GROWTH
AND THRESHOLDS

Critical to the understanding of loudness magnitude and growth in cochlear impairment is the relation between the rate of growth (slope) and thresholds. In their early studies of loudness scaling Hellman and Zwislocki (1961) showed that the overall shape of the loudness curve in normal hearing depends on the *interaction* between the SL of the reference standard and its numerical designation. Furthermore, they found that the intersubject variability of the loudness estimations is smaller near threshold when SL rather than SPL is the independent variable. The direct relation between the loudness estimations and SL led to the conjecture that loudness recruitment is not present in a population with clinically normal hearing. Evidence to support this hypothesis comes from several recent experiments.

Description of Experiments

In one experimental series (Hellman & Meiselman, 1993), slopes for 32 older listeners (56–72 years) with clinically normal hearing were compared to the slopes for 51 young listeners (16–24 years). Thresholds measured for the older listeners at a midfrequency stimulus tone ranged from 4.5-to 29-dB SPL (-2.5- to 22-dB HL) with a mean of 19-dB SPL; thresholds for the young listeners ranged from 1- to 12-dB SPL with a mean of 7.0 dB. Slopes were obtained from the results of CMM and AME of apparent length using the experimental procedures and stimuli described in the first section. Despite the large intergroup differences in thresholds, the distributions of individual slope values for the two groups turned out to be very similar. Both distributions exhibited a clear peak value near 0.60 with none extending beyond 0.35 and 0.95 (s.d. $=0.13$)). Thus, although threshold-sensitivity was generally poorer and more variable for the older group than for the younger group, the standard slope of 0.60 is a representative value for the loudness function in both groups as long as thresholds lie within normal limits. Determined for the 51 young listeners, the correlation coefficient between the individual slope values and thresholds was -0.16 ($p > 0.05$); for the 32 older listeners a correlation coefficient of 0.32 ($p > 0.05$) was obtained.

The relation between the rate of loudness growth and thresholds was determined in another experiment for 20 listeners ranging in age from 57–72 years (Hellman, 1991; Hellman & Meiselman, 1993). All had normal hearing near 500 Hz (≤ 22-dB HL; ANSI, 1969) and bilateral moderate-to-severe noise-induced sloping high-frequency hearing losses. Like the 32 older listeners who had normal hearing in the midfrequency region, thresholds at 500 Hz ranged from $-$-2.5-to 21.5-dB HL with a mean HL of 13.6 dB.

Loudness was measured at three frequencies, all in the same ear, of each listener. One stimulus frequency was at 500 Hz where hearing was normal, and two were along the sloping section of the threshold contour. Individual slopes were obtained at each frequency from the methods of CMM and AME of apparent length outlined in the first section. In accord with scaling theory (Stevens, 1959a, 1969, 1975) and previous investigations (Hellman & Meiselman, 1988, 1990), slopes derived in this manner are referred to as *predicted values*. The slopes for normal hearing were determined above 30-dB SL where the loudness function in a log–log plot can be approximated by a linear function; for impaired hearing local slopes were determined within the 15- to 30-dB SL range above the elevated threshold. Over this relatively narrow stimulus range, loudness in impaired hearing increases more rapidly with level than in normal hearing (e.g., Hellman & Zwislocki, 1964; Miskolczy-Fodor, 1960; Steinberg & Gardner, 1937; Stevens & Guirao, 1967).

The relation between the slopes predicted from CMM and AME of apparent length and the degree of hearing loss is shown for the 20 individual listeners in Fig. 1.6. The curve is a best-fitting function constructed from two least-squares fits. Its overall shape is consistent with the general shape of the curve obtained for five groups composed of 128 different listeners (Hellman & Meiselman, 1990). A second-order fit, determined from all 60 individual slope values, was used to span the range from 18- to 74-dB HL; a zero-slope least-squares fit line was adjoined to it to represent the points over the range from -2- to 18-dB HL. This linear seqment has an ordinate of 0.61 which is close to the measured group mean of 0.63. In accord with the results obtained for the young and the older listeners cited above, the correlation coefficient between the individual slopes and detection thresholds does not differ significantly from zero ($r = 0.42$; $p > 0.05$) in the region of normal hearing. Therefore, between -2- and 18-dB HL it is appropriate to use a linear function with a zero slope to depict this relation.

Despite the 24-dB threshold range for normal hearing, a nonsignificant correlation coefficient between the individual slope values and detection thresholds is obtained. By comparison, a significant correlation coefficient of 0.69 (p < 0.01) is obtained for the same 20 listeners and a similar threshold range (54–74.5-dB HL) in the frequency region where the thresholds are elevated. These findings imply that the individual slopes are threshold dependent in the region of impaired hearing; whereas no consistent trend is found over a wide range of thresholds in clinically normal hearing. Thus, consistent with earlier theoretical considerations (Hellman & Zwislocki, 1961), the ensemble of results obtained for young and older listeners indicate that the intersubject variability of thresholds at a given

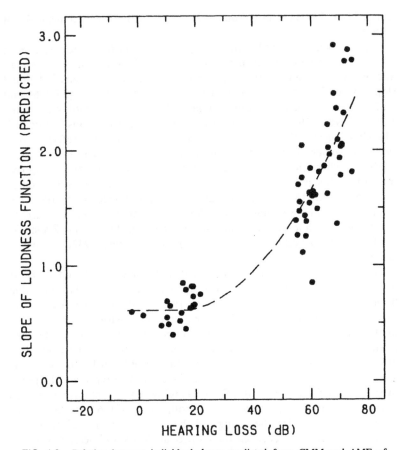

FIG. 1.6. Relation between individual slopes predicted from CMM and AME of
apparent length and the degree of hearing loss for 20 listeners who judged loudness at
three frequencies, one in the region of normal hearing and two in the region of impaired
hearing. The curve was constructed from two best-fitting functions (from Hellman &
Meiselman, 1993).

frequency is not accompanied by loudness recruitment when the thresholds
lie within the range of normal hearing.

MODELING THE LOUDNESS FUNCTION IN COCHLEAR IMPAIRMENT

The positive relation observed between the local slope values and thresholds
for hearing losses exceeding about 30 dB, together with the internal

consistency of the equal-sensation matches, makes it possible to generate loudness functions for groups with similar thresholds from loudness-level functions like those in Figs. 1.4 and 1.5. This was accomplished in a recent study with the help of a monaural loudness function measured in quiet at 1 kHz (Hellman & Meiselman, 1990). Results for three hearing-impaired groups with noise-induced losses of 55, 65, and 75 dB were found to be well described by Zwislocki's (1965) analytical expression for the loudness function in the form:

$$L_s = K[(P_s^2 + P_n^2)^\theta - P_n^{2\theta}] \tag{1}$$

where P_s is the effective sound pressure of the tone, P_n is the effective sound pressure of random noise, and θ, the slope of the loudness function in quiet, has a value of 0.27. Unlike the two more widely employed modifications of Stevens' power law (for review, see Humes & Jesteadt, 1991) given by the equations:

$$L_s = K(P_s^2 - P_o^2)^\theta \tag{2}$$

and its alternative,

$$L_s = K(P_s^{2\theta} - P_o^{2\theta}) \tag{3}$$

the value of θ in Zwislocki's formulation is fixed from experimental determinations of the growth of loudness in quiet and is not free to vary. Only P_n, an additional term not included in the simpler modifications, can be altered. This additional term is of key importance for two reasons: (a) it enables the rate of loudness growth to increase more gradually with level near threshold than either Equations. 2 or 3; and (b) it permits threshold loudness to have a positive magnitude in accord with the operational definition of threshold.

Within the theoretical framework of Zwislocki's (1965) model, $P_n = cP_o$, where c is a multiplicative constant that depends on both the bandwidth of the noise and the CF of the stimulus tone. For the loudness of a tone in quiet, P_n is the equivalent sound pressure of the extrinsic masker surrounding the tone at a given CF. The modifications allowed are consistent with the known response of the auditory system to partially masked sinusoids. Theoretical fits to group results for hearing losses of 55, 65, and 75 dB are displayed in Figs. 1.7, 1.8, and 1.9, respectively. The curves are the calculated functions, and the circles are loudness data obtained from equal-sensation matches. Curve A was generated from Equation 2, curve B was generated from Equation 3, and curve C was generated from Equations 1 and 4. The same value of 0.27 was used for the exponent θ in each example. Also, in all of the computations the sound pressure P_o at the detection threshold for the tone was set at 2.2440 $\times$

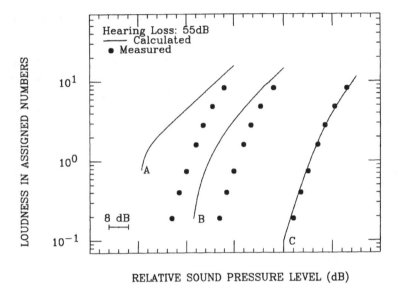

FIG. 1.7.   Measured (circles) and calculated loudness functions (curves) for a group of 24 listeners with a mean noise-induced hearing loss of 55 dB at the stimulus frequency. Curve A was calculated from Equation 2, curve B was calculated from Equation 3, and curve C was calculated from Zwislocki's (1965) generalized expression for the loudness function given in Equations 1 and 4.

10^4 μPa for a 55-dB hearing loss 1.1247 $\times$ 10^5 μPa for a 65-dB hearing loss, and 3.1698 $\times$ 10^5 μPa for a 75-dB hearing loss.

Two additional factors were taken into consideration to obtain the calculated loudness functions according to Zwislocki's model. First, it was assumed that the effect of a noise-induced hearing loss on the shape of the loudness function is similar to the effect of a loss simulated in normal hearing by an extrinsic masking noise 9750-Hz wide. Second, it was assumed that the CF of the stimulus tone was shifted upward from 1000 to 1740 Hz. This assumption required the width of the critical band to be increased from the 160-Hz value used by Zwislocki to 260 Hz. Both assumptions are consistent with experimental evidence (Hellman, 1988; Hellman & Meiselman, 1990). For a noise bandwidth of 9750 Hz and a critical bandwidth of 260 Hz, Equation 1 can be written in the form:

$$L_s = K[(P_s^2 + 93.75P_o^2)^\theta - 3.41P_o^{2\theta}], \tag{4}$$

where the value 93.75 P_o^2 is the equivalent sound pressure of the extrinsic noise. Thus, in Equation 1 $P_n^2 = 93.75 P_o^2$.

Figures 1.7 through 1.9 show that neither of the simpler power-law modifications given by Equations 2 and 3 are able to adequately describe

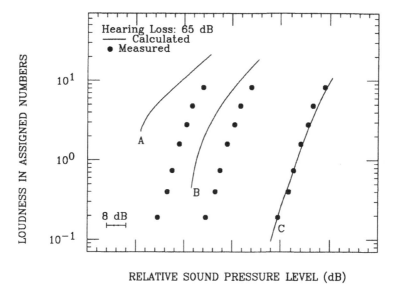

FIG. 1.8. Measured (circles) and calculated loudness functions (curves) for a group of
24 listeners with a mean noise-induced hearing loss of 65 dB at the stimulus frequency.
(See legend of Fig.1.7.)

the growth of loudness in cochlear impairment. These results are consistent
with earlier findings (Gleiss & Zwicker, 1964; Hellman & Zwislocki, 1964).
Zwislocki's proposed modification given by Equation 4 provides a significant improvement. As important, the marked alteration in the shape of the
loudness function in cochlear impairment makes it possible to clearly
distinguish between the subtractive-loudness model (Equation 3) recently
revived by Humes and Jesteadt (1991), and Zwislocki's more general
expression for the loudness function (Equations 1 and 4). Curves B and C
illustrate the differences.

SUMMARY AND CONCLUSIONS

This chapter presents additional evidence to show that loudness relations in
accord with auditory theory can be obtained from magnitude-scaling
procedures. Results in the first section demonstrate that absolute scales of
loudness can be generated for individual listeners with bilateral cochlear-
impaired hearing. The overall agreement found between the equal-sensation
matches determined indirectly from magnitude scaling and the matches
determined directly from intramodality matching means that magnitude

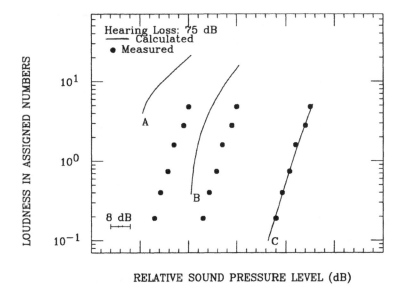

FIG. 1.9.   Measured (circles) and calculated loudness functions (curves) for a group of 19 listeners with a mean noise-induced hearing loss of 75 dB at the stimulus frequency. (See legend of Fig.1.7.)

scaling can reveal both the rate of loudness growth and the magnitude of loudness at the output of the auditory system. Given the precision and accuracy of the individual judgments, especially those from CMM, the functional relation between the rate of loudness growth and threshold sensitivity can be determined for individuals with normal and impaired hearing. This relation, given in the second section, indicates that the rate of loudness growth is threshold dependent in the region of impaired hearing, but not in the region of normal hearing. Moreover, the third section shows that Zwislocki's (1965) generalized loudness equation, which incorporates a number of well-established auditory properties, more accurately describes the overall shape of the loudness function in noise-induced cochlear impairment than either of the power-law modifications $L = K(P^2 - P_o{}^2)^\theta$ and $L = K (P^{2\theta} - P_o{}^{2\theta})$. Although the neurophysiological code for loudness magnitude and growth remains unsolved, psychophysical measurements of loudness continue to provide the clues needed to help unravel this mystery.

ACKNOWLEDGMENTS

I thank Carol H. Meiselman for her able assistance with data collection and analysis. This work was supported by the Rehabilitation Research & Development Service of the Veterans Administration.

REFERENCES

American National Standards Institute (ANSI). (1969). *ANSI S3.6-1969, Specifications for audiometers*. New York: American National Standards Institute.

Bolanowski, S. J., Zwislocki, J. J., & Gescheider G. A. (1991). In S. J. Bolanowski, Jr. & G. A. Gescheider (Eds.), *Ratio scaling of psychological magnitude — In honor of the memory of S. S. Stevens* (pp. 277-293). Hillsdale, NJ: Lawrence Erlbaum Associates.

Collins, A. A., & Gescheider, G. A. (1989). The measurement of loudness in individual children and adults by absolute magnitude estimation and cross-modality matching. *Journal of the Acoustical Society of America, 85*, 2012-2021.

Ekman, G. (1956). *Subjective power functions and the method of fractionation* (Reports from the Department of Psychology, No. 34). Stockholm: University of Stockholm.

Fowler, E. P. (1928). Marked deafened areas in normal ears. *Archives of Otolaryngology, 8*, 151-155.

Fowler, E. P. (1936). A method for the early detection of otosclerosis. *Archives of Otolaryngology, 24*, 731-741.

Gleiss, N., & Zwicker, E. (1964). Loudness function in the presence of a masking noise. *Journal of the Acoustical Society of American, 36*, 393-394.

Hallpike, C. S. (1967). The loudness recruitment phenomenon: A clinical contribution to the neurology of hearing. In A. B. Graham (Ed.), *Sensorineural hearing processes and disorders* (pp. 489-499). Boston: Little Brown.

Hellman, R. P. (1976). Growth of loudness at 1000 and 3000 Hz. *Journal of the Acoustical Society of America, 60*, 672-679.

Hellman, R. P. (1982). Loudness, annoyance, and noisiness produced by single-tone-noise complexes. *Journal of the Acoustical Society of America, 72*, 62-73.

Hellman, R. P. (1988). Loudness functions in noise-induced and noise-simulated hearing losses. In B. Berglund, U. Berglund, J. Karlsson, & T. Lindvall (Eds.), *Proceedings of the 5th International Congress on Noise as a Public Health Problem* (Vol. 2, pp. 105-110). Stockholm: Swedish Council for Building Research.

Hellman, R. P. (1991, November). *Development of cross-modality matching for individual loudness measurement*. Paper presented at the annual American Speech-Language-Hearing Association meeting, Atlanta, GA.

Hellman, R. P., & Meiselman, C. H. (1988). Prediction of individual loudness exponents from cross-modality matching. *Journal of Speech & Hearing Research, 31*, 605-615.

Hellman, R. P., & Meiselman, C. H. (1990). Loudness relations for individuals and groups in normal and impaired hearing. *Journal of the Acoustical Society of America, 88*, 2596-2606.

Hellman, R. P., & Meiselman, C. H. (1992). Role of high-frequency excitation in the growth of loudness. *Midwinter Research Meeting, Association for Research in Otolaryngology, 15*, 267.

Hellman, R. P., & Meiselman, C. H. (1993). Rate of loudness growth for pure tones in normal and impaired hearing. *Journal of the Acoustical Society of America, 93*, 966-975.

Hellman, R. P., & Zwislocki, J. J. (1961). Some factors affecting the estimation of loudness. *Journal of the Acoustical Society of America, 33*, 687-694.

Hellman, R. P., & Zwislocki, J. J. (1963). Monaural loudness function at 1000 cps and interaural summation. *Journal of the Acoustical Society of America, 35*, 856-865.

Hellman, R. P., & Zwislocki, J. J. (1964). Loudness function of a 1000-cps tone in the presence of a masking noise. *Journal of the Acoustical Society of America, 36*, 1618-1624.

Hellman, R. P., & Zwislocki, J. J. (1968). Loudness determination at low sound frequencies. *Journal of the Acoustical Society of America, 43*, 60-64.

Humes, L., & Jesteadt, W. (1991). Models of the effects of threshold on loudness growth and summation. *Journal of the Acoustical Society of America, 90*, 1933-1943.

Lochner, J. P. A., & Burger, J. F. (1961). Form of the loudness function in the presence of masking noise. *Journal of the Acoustical Society of America, 33*, 1705-1707.

Lüscher, E., & Zwislocki, J. (1948a). Eine einfache Methode zur monauralen Bestimmung des Lautstarkeausgleichs [*Archives Ohren-u. Kehlkopfheilk, 155*, 323-334.

Lüscher, E., & Zwislocki, J. (1948b). A simple method for indirect monaural determination of the recruitment phenomenon (Difference limen in intensity in different types of deafness). *Acta Ototlaryngologica, Suppl. 78*, 156-168.

Lüscher, E., & Zwislocki, J. (1951). Comparison of various methods employed in determination of the recruitment phenomenon. *Journal of Laryngology & Otology, 65*, 187-195.

Luce, R. D. (1959). On the possible psychophysical laws. *Psychological Review, 66*, 81-95.

Marshall, L. (1981). Auditory processing in aging listeners. *Journal of Speech & Hearing Disorders, 46*, 226-240.

Miskolczy-Fodor, F. (1960). Relation between loudness and duration of tonal pulses III. Responses in cases of abnormal loudness function. *Journal of the Acoustical Society of America, 32*, 486-492.

Reger, S. N. (1936). Differences in loudness response of normal and hard-of-hearing ears at intensity levels slightly above threshold. *Annals of Otology, 45*, 1029-1039.

Steinberg, J. C., & Gardner, M. B. (1937). The dependence of hearing impairment on sound intensity. *Journal of the Acoustical Society of America, 9*, 11-23.

Stevens, S. S. (1953). On the brightness of lights and the loudness of sounds. *Science, 118*, 576.

Stevens, S. S. (1959a). On the validity of the loudness scale. *Journal of the Acoustical Society of America, 31*, 995-1003.

Stevens, S. S. (1959b). Tactile vibration: Dynamics of sensory intensity. *Journal of Experimental Psychology, 59*, 210-218.

Stevens, S. S. (1966). On the operation known as judgment. *American Scientist, 54*, 385-401.

Stevens, S. S. (1969). On predicting exponents for cross-modality matches. *Perception & Psychophysics, 6*, 251-256.

Stevens, S. S. (1975). *Psychophysics* (G. Stevens, Ed.). New York: Wiley.

Stevens, S. S., & Guirao, M. (1967). Loudness functions under inhibition. *Perception & Psychophysics, 1*, 439-446.

Verrillo, R. T., Fraioli, A. J., & Smith, R. L. (1969). Sensation magnitude of vibrotactile stimuli. *Perception & Psychophysics, 2*, 59-64.

Zwislocki, J. J. (1960). Theory of temporal auditory summation. *Journal of the Acoustical Society of America, 32*, 1046-1060.

Zwislocki, J. J. (1965). Analysis of some auditory characteristics. In R. R. Bush, E. Galanter, & R. D. Luce (Eds.), *Handbook of mathematical psychology* (Vol. 11, pp. 3-97). New York: Wiley.

Zwislocki, J. J. (1969). Temporal summation of loudness: An analysis. *Journal of the Acoustical Society of America,46*, 431-441.

Zwislocki, J. J. (1972). A theory of central masking and its partial validation. *Journal of the Acoustical Society of America, 52*, 644-659.

Zwislocki, J. J. (1973). On intensity characteristics of sensory receptors: A generalized function. *Kybernetik, 12*, 169-183.

Zwislocki, J. J. (1974). A power function for sensory receptors. In H. R. Moskowitz, B. Scharf, & J. C. Stevens (Eds.), *Sensation and measurement — Papers in honor of S. S. Stevens* (pp. 185-197) Dordrecht: Reidel.

Zwislocki, J. J. (1983). Group and individual relations between sensation magnitudes and their numerical estimates. *Perception & Psychophysics, 33*, 460-468.

Zwislocki, J. J. (1991). Natural measurement. In S. J. Bolanowski, Jr. & G. A. Gescheider (Eds.), *Ratio scaling of psychological magnitude — In honor of the memory of S. S. Stevens* (pp. 18-26). Hillsdale, NJ: Lawrence Erlbaum Associates.

Zwislocki, J. J., & Goodman, D. A. (1980). Absolute scaling of sensory magnitudes: A validation. *Perception & Psychophysics, 28*, 28-38.

Zwislocki, J. J., & Hellman, R. P. (1960). On the psychophysical law. *Journal of the Acoustical Society of America, 32*, 924.

2 Control of Rhythmic Firing in *Aplysia* Neuron R15: A Calcium Riddle

William B. Adams
Biozentrum der Uni, Basel University

DEDICATION

It is with great pleasure that I dedicate this chapter to Jozef J. Zwislocki. It was his influence that instilled in me the true nature of scientific research as a "search for truth." In an endeavor in which the pressures of advancement and funding all too often see hasty publications followed by equally hasty retractions, the encouragement to be patient while pursuing the "truth" has guided my research throughout my scientific career.

INTRODUCTION

Neuron R15 from the abdominal ganglion of *Aplysia californica* is one of the best studied cells in neurobiology (Adams & Benson, 1985). A number of reasons have contributed to its popularity as an experimental preparation. The abdominal ganglion can be removed from the animal and kept alive and healthy in simple culture conditions for many days. R15 is large enough to use as a "living test tube" for biochemical experiments, and it is readily accessible for penetration by several electrodes for studying its electrophysiology. These features were crucial for the experiments that provided the first demonstration of a neural response mediated by cyclic-AMP (cAMP) and cAMP-dependent protein phosphorylation (Adams & Levitan, 1982; Drummond, Benson, & Levitan, 1980; Drummond, Bucher, & Levitan, 1980; Lemos, Novak-Hofer, & Levitan, 1982, 1985).

R15 also displays several interesting forms of electrical activity. These

19

include a variety of synaptic responses that last from milliseconds to hours (cf. Adams & Benson, 1985) and an endogenous rhythmic activity known as *bursting* in which action potentials are produced in discrete groups (Arvanitaki & Cardot, 1941). The bursting activity has been well characterized and has a number of features in common with other systems. As a result, R15 has been used as a model for everything from bursting spinal cord neurons to vertebrate heart pacemarkers. Despite this, and despite the investigations of many labs over the years, several features of the bursting mechanisms in R15 remain unclear. This is especially true of the way in which intracellular Ca^{++} controls the currents that produce rhythmic activity, which is the subject of this chapter.

Figure 2.1 illustrates the bursting activity of R15 in normal medium, at room temperature, and in an abdominal ganglion isolated from the animal. The pattern of bursting in an isolated ganglion is very stable and will continue, essentially without change, for many days. Between animals, the details of the bursting pattern differ somewhat in detail. Bursts usually occur at rates between 1 and 10 per minute. They may have as few as 3 or 4 action potentials or as many as 30 or 40, and the action potentials are very important in shaping the burst. In every cell, the burst begins slowly, speeds up, then slows down again. The intervals between action potentials closely describe a parabola, which led Strumwasser (1965) to name this cell the *parabolic burster*. The burst ends with a characteristic depolarizing after-potential, followed by a rapid swoop into the interburst hyperpolarizing phase. During the course of the burst there are a number of changes in the shapes of the action potentials. The positive overshoot of the first action

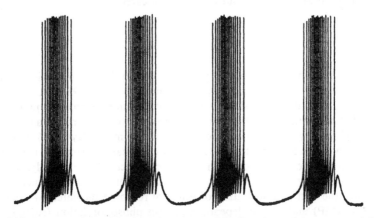

FIG. 2.1. Bursting activity in *Aplysia* neuron R15. Bursting activity was recorded from R15 in an abdominal ganglion isolated from the animal. The ganglion was bathed in medium with salt concentrations similar to those found in seawater with the addition of glucose and Tris buffer. Recordings were made at room temperature.

potential is small and then increases in plateau fashion. The negative undershoot also changes, first decreasing and then increasing again toward the end of the burst. During the burst, successive action potentials become broader.

Before moving to a description of the currents that mediate bursting activity in R15, I will try a thought experiment, based on some hindsight, about how such rhythmic activity might be produced. Generation of a burst of the sort seen in R15 requires three components. I shall illustrate these burst components with a series of cartoons that I hope will not be taken literally.

In many cells, the activity that one finds after penetrating with a microelectrode is illustrated in Fig. 2.2a. The top line represents zero membrane potential, the second line the threshold for generating action potentials, and the bottom line the resting potential of the cell. As mentioned previously, action potentials play an important role in shaping the bursting activity, so that what is needed first is some way to move the membrane potential toward threshold.

Figure 2.2b introduces the first burst component. I've identified it with the initials NSR for reasons that will be explained later. NSR has the job of depolarizing the cell. If the cell is sufficiently depolarized, threshold will be reached, and an action potential will be generated as shown in Fig. 2.2c. NSR exerts a steady-state depolarizing influence, and its action will result in the cell generating a repetitive train of action potentials. Clearly, now that the cell has been started firing action potentials, a way is needed to stop the firing if we want to produce action potentials that are grouped into bursts.

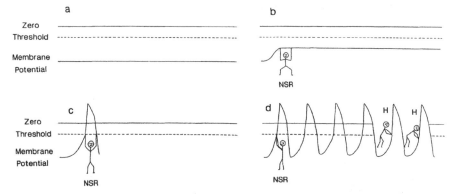

FIG. 2.2. Components for generating a burst. a. A silent cell. The top line represents zero membrane potential, the second line the threshold for generating action potentials, and the bottom line the resting potential of the cell. b. A steady-state depolarizing influence, identified with the initials NSR. c. If the cell is sufficiently depolarized, threshold will be reached, and an action potential will be generated. d. A transient hyperpolarizing burst component, identified by the initial H, that acts to stop the firing.

Stopping the burst is the job of a hyperpolarizing burst component, as identified in Fig. 2.2d by the initial H. The actions of H are elicited by the train of action potentials that NSR has started. At the right of Fig. 2.2d, H can be seen pushing down to repolarize the cell and pushing harder after more action potentials have occurred.

It might seem that these two burst components, NSR and H, would be sufficient to shape the firing pattern of the cell. NSR would get the burst started, and H would stop it. This is not the case, however. With only two burst components, the firing pattern will settle down to a repetitive train, slower than before, but a train nonetheless. This is illustrated in Fig. 2.3a. NSR depolarizes the cell and, following each action potential, H hyperpolarizes for a while and then relaxes. It is possible to generate bursts of action potentials with only two burst components, but only if the hyperpolarizing component is given bizarre kinetics, kinetics that are not in accord with what is observed physiologically.

In order to generate a true burst we need the presence of a transient depolarizing burst component, which is identified in Fig. 2.3b by the initial D. Following each action potential, D gives the membrane potential a "kick" back toward threshold. The effect of the kick doesn't last very long, but it is enough to accelerate the depolarization of the cell and make it fire faster.

Figure 2.3c shows the interactions of the three burst components working together to produce a burst. NSR, shown on the left, provides a steady depolarization of the membrane potential toward threshold and gets the burst started. Following the first action potential, D adds an additional increment of depolarizing influence. With only one action potential, the

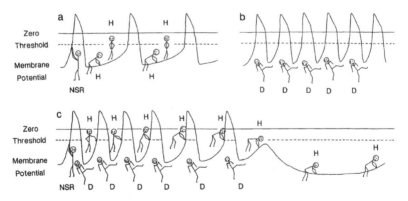

FIG. 2.3. Interaction of burst components. a. Interaction of NSR and H produce slower firing, but are not sufficient to produce bursting. b. A transient depolarizing burst component identified by the initial D. c. Interactions of the three burst components to produce a burst.

hyperpolarizing influence H is still fairly small and has little effect. Following the second action potential, and a second kick by D, the hyperpolarizing influence begins to become more effective, but the rate of action potential production is still increasing. As the burst continues, the hyperpolarizing influence continues to grow, and the firing rate decreases until, at the end of the burst, the last kick by D produces a depolarizing after potential that isn't large enough to reach threshold. The cell enters the interburst hyperpolarizing phase and remains silent until H relaxes sufficiently for the steady depolarization produced by NSR to begin to move the membrane potential back again toward threshold and toward the start of the next burst.

In a real cell, of course, the only way to change the membrane potential is by having electrical current flow across the membrane. The next step, therefore, is to look at the electrophysiology of R15 to see if the three burst components from the cartoons can be identified with particular currents.

When the cell is held in a steady state under voltage clamp, and the current that flows across the membrane is plotted as a function of membrane voltage, the shape of the I–V curve is rather unusual. At large negative voltages, below about $-80\,mV$, the I–V curve is nearly linear. The current in this range of potentials is carried primarily by K^+ (Benson & Levitan, 1983), and it appears as though this part of the curve would intersect the zero-current axis close to the K^+ equilibrium potential (E_K) at $-80\,mV$. As the cell is further depolarized, however, two things begin to happen. First, the K^+ channels that carried the current begin to close, because they are inwardly rectifying or anomalously rectifying channels (Benson & Levitan, 1983). Second, an inward or depolarizing current is activated (Partridge, Thompson, Smith, & Connor, 1979). This current activates more with further depolarization, allowing a larger inward current, and produces a region of negative slope conductance in the I–V curve. More traditionally, this is called a *region of negative slope resistance* or *NSR*. We have named the inward current responsible for producing this region I_{NSR} (Adams & Benson, 1985). It isn't so much the odd shape of the I–V curve that is important as the fact that I_{NSR} provides a continual inward or depolarizing current over the entire range of subthreshold voltages. Thus it accounts for the continual depolarizing influence that we have assigned to the burst component NSR in Figs. 2.2 and 2.3.

The two other burst components, H and D, were spurred into activity by action potentials. So in order to find their physiological counterparts, we need to produce action potentials and examine what happens afterward. There are two ways to do this. The cell can be held under voltage clamp, released to produce an action potential, or a series of action potentials, and then reclamped to measure the currents that have been activated. Data from experiments such as these are shown in the upper two traces of Fig. 2.4.

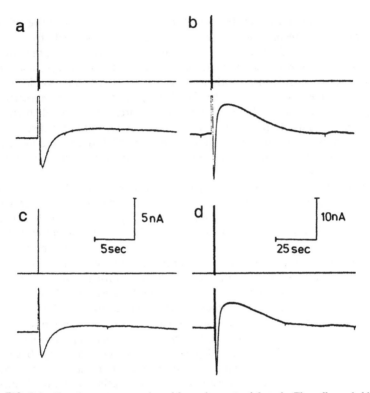

FIG. 2.4. Transient currents activated by action potentials. a,b. The cell was held under voltage clamp, released to produce an action potential (a), or a series of five action potentials (b), and then reclamped to measure the activated currents. c,d. The cell was held continuously under voltage clamp. Action potentials were simulated with 10 ms pulses to +50 mV. c. Single pulse. d. Five pulses at 0.5-sec intervals. In each panel, the upper trace plots membrane voltage and the lower trace membrane current. Note the different calibrations for a,c and b,d. (From Adams, 1985).

Following a single action potential, an inward current can be seen that lasts about a second. Because inward currents depolarize the cell, this current has been named I_D (Adams, 1985). With close examination, a smaller, longer-lasting outward current can also be seen following the action potential. If the cell is allowed to fire several action potentials, as in the trace on the right, the outward current components summate, and a fairly large outward current is seen that lasts for 30 seconds or more. This outward hyperpolarizing current is called I_H (Adams, 1985). I_D and I_H are the physiological counterparts of our cartoon characters D and H.

A second way to activate these currents is to hold the cell under voltage clamp and to simulate action potentials with brief depolarizing pulses. Data from such experiments are shown in the lower traces of Fig. 2.4. We used

10 ms pulses which took the membrane potential to +50 mV. We ignored the currents flowing during the pulses; these often reached amplitudes of microamperes. The currents that were activated by, and followed, the pulses were similar both in their amplitudes and their time courses to those activated by the cell's own action potentials. In practice, it was much easier to deal with these simulated action potentials, especially when the ionic composition of the bathing medium was changed to look at the effects on I_D and I_H.

The steady state current I_{NSR}, together with the kinetics of the two transient currents, I_D and I_H, are sufficient to account for the pattern of rhythmic activity produced by R15. In particular, no special voltage dependences are required. This is illustrated in Fig. 2.5. I_{NSR} was simulated by a linear leak resistance and I_D and I_H by exponentially decaying inward and outward currents with incremental amplitudes and time constants

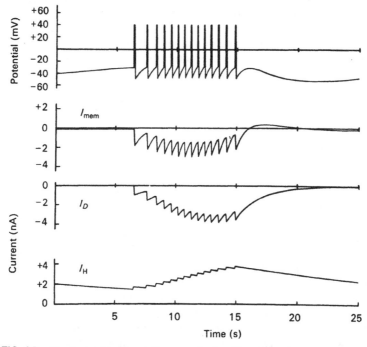

FIG. 2.5. Simple simulated burst. I_{NSR} was simulated by a linear leak resistance. I_D and I_H were simulated by currents that increased incrementally with each action potential and then decayed exponentially. Amplitudes, time constants, and the membrane capacitance were similar to those measured experimentally. Action potentials were produced by a threshold-driven pulse generator which took the membrane potential to +40 mV and then back to −50 mV. I_{mem} plots the sum of I_{NSR}, I_D, and I_H. (From Adams, 1985).

similar to those measured experimentally. Action potentials were produced by a threshold-driven pulse generator. The only other component was the membrane capacitance. The transient depolarizing currents I_D summate over the first several action potentials, leading to the increase in firing rate that is observed in R15. Each hyperpolarizing current increment to I_H is smaller than those for I_D, but the summation time constant for I_H is much longer. As a result, the I_H components summate over the entire burst. After the last action potential, I_D produces a depolarizing after potential, but it isn't large enough to reach threshold. The net current is now outward so that the cell begins to hyperpolarize. The rapid swoop of hyperpolarization is not due to the sudden activation of a hyperpolarizing current, but to the decay of I_D.

Of course, this simple model doesn't show the changes in action potential shape that are seen in R15. We have shown, however, with more complex simulations, that the shape changes arise from the usual activation and inactivation kinetics of the Na^+, K^+, and Ca^{++} currents that produce the action potentials, together with changes in E_K that result from K^+ accumulation in the membrane infoldings (Adams & Benson, 1985).

The next question concerns the nature of these currents, their charge carriers, and their methods of activation. Determining the charge carrier for the steady state current I_{NSR} turned out to be problematic, as several other labs had found (cf. Adams & Benson, 1985). The safest conclusion seems to be that I_{NSR} is carried by both Na^+ and Ca^{++}, although the channels that carry the current, and their exact pharmacology, remain unknown. For the transient currents I_D and I_H, a certain amount of information was available. It was known that the depolarizing phase of action potentials in R15 is produced by roughly equal currents carried by Na^+ and Ca^{++} (Adams & Gage, 1979b, Carpenter & Gunn, 1970) and that repolarization is produced by one or more K^+ currents (Adams & Gage, 1979a, Thompson, 1977). It had also been demonstrated that injection of Ca^{++} into R15 can elicit a Ca^{++}-activated K^+ current $I_K(Ca^{++})$ (Meech & Strumwasser, 1970). Thus, there was reason to believe that the activators for I_D and I_H might be the influx of Ca^{++} into the cell that occurs during the action potential.

The first test, therefore, was to change the concentration of Ca^{++} in the bathing medium and look at the effects on I_D and I_H. For this purpose, a single simulated action potential was used to activate I_D, and a train of five simulated action potentials was used to activate I_H (Fig. 2.6a). The preparation was allowed to stabilize in normal medium, and the Ca^{++} concentration was then reduced from its normal of 11 mM down to 2 mM to reduce its electrochemical gradient. Both I_D and I_H decreased with decreased Ca^{++}.

When measured at a number of Ca^{++} concentrations (Fig. 2.6b), I_D

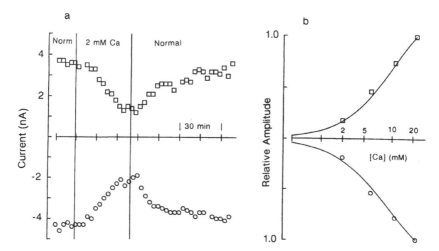

FIG. 2.6. Effects of changes in Ca^{++} concentration on I_D and I_H. a. I_D and I_H were activated by depolarizing pulses as in Fig. 2.4 c,d. Measurements of I_D and I_H were made alternately every 90 secs. During the indicated period the Ca^{++} concentration in the bathing medium was reduced from 11 mM to 2 mM. Osmolarity was held constant by adjusting the Na^+ concentration. b. The amplitudes of I_D and I_H as a function of Ca^{++} concentration. Amplitudes are scaled to 1 in normal medium. Squares indicate I_H, circles I_D. (From Adams & Levitan, 1985).

and I_H were affected in roughly the same way by decreasing Ca^{++} concentration. The effects of inorganic Ca^{++} channel blockers, such as cobalt, cadmium, nickel, lanthanum, and manganese, were also tested and found to block I_D and I_H in a manner similar to reducing the Ca^{++} concentration (Adams & Levitan, 1985).

The next ion investigated was Na^+. Figure 2.7a illustrates one experiment in which the Na^+ concentration in the bathing medium was reduced from its normal of about 500 mM to 100 mM. The inward transient current I_D was decreased, but the outward transient hyperpolarizing current I_H was not affected. Figure 2.7b plots the results pooled from several experiments. I_D decreased roughly in proportion to Na^+ concentration. I_H was unaffected by reductions in Na^+ as long as the concentration remained at least 5% to 10% of normal. Below this level, I_H also decreased; but we think that this is a second-order effect due to a disruption of a Na^+–Ca^{++} exchange, which appears to play an important role in the regulation of intracellular Ca^{++} concentration in R15.

Thus far we have shown that I_D is dependent on both Ca^{++} and Na^+, while I_H depends only on Ca^{++}. Because an $I_K(Ca^{++})$ had been demonstrated in R15, it was thought that it might account for I_H. In fact, it has been part of textbook gospel for many years that I_H is carried by an $I_K(Ca^{++})$. To test this possibility, the K^+ concentration in the bathing

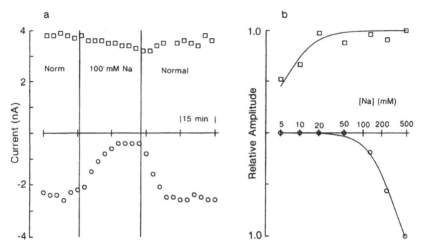

FIG. 2.7. Effects of changes in Na$^+$ concentration on I_D and I_H. Measurements as in Fig. 2.6. Tris was substituted for Na$^+$ to maintain osmolarity. (From Adams & Levitan, 1985).

medium was increased from 10 mM to 40 mM to reduce its electrochemical gradient (Fig. 2.8). There was no effect on the amplitudes of either I_D or I_H. The effects of K$^+$ channel blocking agents, including TEA, cesium, and 4-amino pyridine, were also examined. Even at high concentrations, these agents had no effect on the transient currents (Adams & Levitan, 1985). As an independent test, the voltage dependences of I_D and I_H were examined, looking for a current that reversed at E_K. No such reversal was found. Over a range of membrane potentials between -20 and -120 mV, I_D remained an inward current, and I_H remained an outward current (Adams & Levitan, 1985).

At this point in the investigation, we were a bit concerned that our blocking agents might not be effective. To test this possibility, we made direct measurements of I_H and $I_K(Ca^{++})$, in the same cell, at the same time, and looked at the effects of TEA, a potent blocker of $I_K(Ca^{++})$ in R15. I_H was activated with a train of five simulated action potentials, as before, and $I_K(Ca^{++})$ was activated with intracellular ionophoretic injections of Ca^{++}. The Ca^{++} injections were verified by monitoring the voltage-clamp holding current. Figure 2.9 shows the results. An addition of 10 mM TEA to the bathing medium had no effect on I_H, but totally blocked $I_K(Ca^{++})$ within 5 minutes. In fact, in the presence of TEA, the Ca^{++} injections elicited no outward current of any kind; the only current elicited was a transient inward current. Kramer and Zucker (1985a) have shown a close resemblance between this Ca^{++}-activated inward current and I_D, the transient inward current activated by action potentials.

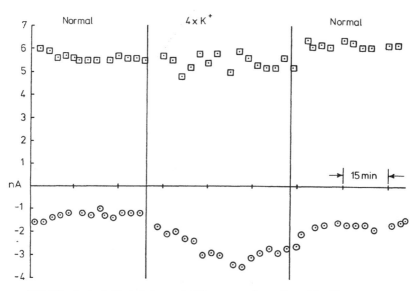

FIG. 2.8.   Lack of effect of changes in K^+ concentration on I_D and I_H. Measurements as in Figs. 2.6 and 2.7. Taken from Adams & Levitan (1985).

Taken together, the results suggest that I_D, the transient inward current, is carried by Na^+, or perhaps Na^+ and Ca^{++}, and is activated by increases in intracellular Ca^{++}. I_H, the transient outward current, depends only on Ca^{++}. However, because the Ca^{++} current flows into the cell, I_H must represent a decrease in a steady-state inward Ca^{++} current that is, a Ca^{++} dependent inactivation of the Ca^{++} current (Eckert & Tillotson, 1981). A similar mechanism has been proposed for an activity-dependent hyperpolarizing current found in bursting neurons from the upper-left quadrant of the abdominal ganglion of *Aplysia* (Kramer & Zucker, 1985b). These conclusions are summarized in Table 2.1 I_{NSR} is a steady-state inward Na^+ and Ca^{++} current. I_D can be activated by a Ca^{++} influx or Ca^{++} injections and is carried by Na^+ and possibly Ca^{++} as well. I_D may well be carried by some of the same channels that carry I_{NSR}. I_H is activated by a Ca^{++} influx, but not by Ca^{++} injections, and arises from a decrease in a steady-state Ca^{++} current. In fact, because the steady-state current necessarily forms a part of I_{NSR}, I_H can be thought of as a decrease in the Ca^{++} component of I_{NSR}. $I_K(Ca^{++})$, the Ca^{++}-activated K^+ current, is activated by Ca^{++} injections, but not by an influx of Ca^{++} across the membrane.

Although it may not be obvious immediately, there is a problem with these results, and that problem forms the "calcium riddle" that is part of the title of this chapter. I illustrate this problem with another series of cartoons.

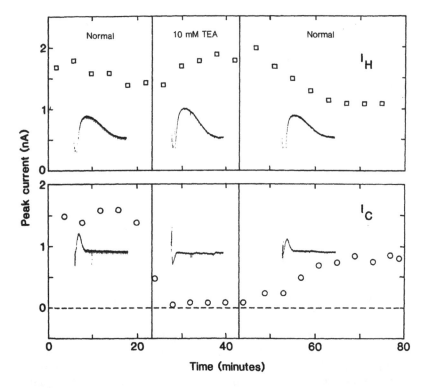

FIG. 2.9. Effects of TEA on I_H and $I_K(Ca^{++})$. I_H was activated as in Figs. 2.6–2.8. $I_K(Ca^{++})$ was activated with 1-sec 200 nA intracellular ionophoretic injections of Ca^{++}. During the indicated period 10 mM TEA was added hyperosmotically to the bathing medium. Squares indicate I_H, circles $I_K(Ca^{++})$. (From Adams & Levitan, 1985).

Figure 2.10a illustrates the means, natural and artificial, by which Ca^{++} can get into a cell. One method of entry, of course, is through Ca^{++} channels, specifically those voltage-dependent channels that are open during the action potential. The second method of Ca^{++} entry, which can be produced experimentally, is a Ca^{++} injection through a micro-pipette.

The data previously presented show that Ca^{++} that comes into the cell during the action potential activates the transient inward current I_D, as shown in Fig. 2.10b. An influx of Ca^{++} also activates the transient outward current I_H, as shown in Fig.2.10c. In this illustration, it is noted more specifically that I_H represents a reduction in the Ca^{++} component of I_{NSR}. Injection of Ca^{++}, as illustrated in Fig.2.10d, is also capable of activating I_D and, in addition, of activating $I_K(Ca^{++})$.

The problems arise with the lines that are still missing in Fig.2.10b. If

TABLE 2.1
Summary

Current	Activator
I_{NSR} I_{Na} + I_{Ca}	Steady-state
I_D ↑ I_{Na} (↑ I_{NSR}?)	Ca^{++} influx, Ca^{++} injection
I_H ↓ $I_{Ca,NSR}$	Ca^{++} influx
$I_K(Ca^{++})$ ↑ I_K	Ca^{++} injection

Note. I_{NSR} = steady-state inward Na^+ and Ca^{++} current. I_D = transient increase in Na^+ current activated by Ca^{++} influx or Ca^{++} injections. I_H = transient decrease in the Ca^{++}: component of I_{NSR} activated by Ca^{++} influx, but not by Ca^{++} injections. $I_K(Ca^{++})$ = increase in K^+ current activated by Ca^{++} injections, but not by influx of Ca^{++} across the membrane.

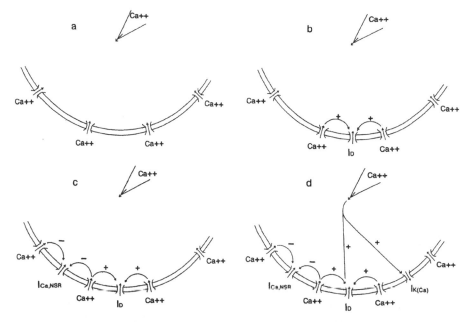

FIG. 2.10. Activation of currents by Ca^{++} influx and Ca^{++} injection. a. Entry of Ca^{++} into a cell through voltage-dependent Ca^{++} channels and by injection through a micropipette. b. Activation of I_D by Ca^{++} influx. c. Activation of I_H by Ca^{++} influx, shown specifically as a reduction in the Ca^{++} component of I_{NSR}. d. Activation of I_D and $I_K(Ca^{++})$ by Ca^{++} injection.

$I_K(Ca^{++})$ is activated by a Ca^{++} injection, why isn't it activated by Ca^{++} that comes in during the action potential (Fig. 2.11a)? Also, as illustrated in Fig. 2.11b, why isn't I_H affected by a Ca^{++} injection?

Although there is little direct evidence, there are some experimental findings that might provide suggestions about the mechanisms that lead to the discrepancies. Several years ago, Tillotson and Gorman (1980) made use

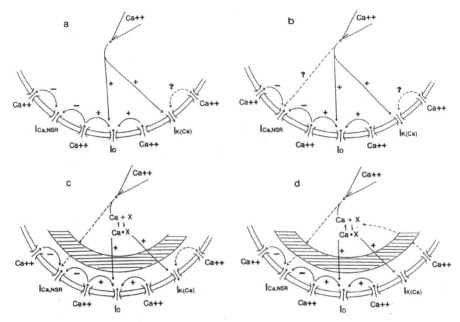

FIG. 2.11. The missing links: Nonactivation of current by Ca^{++} influx and Ca^{++} injection. a. Ca^{++} influx does not activate $I_K(Ca^{++})$. b. Ca^{++} injection does not activate I_H. c. A layer of high Ca^{++} buffering capacity may prevent injected Ca^{++} from reaching the membrane sites necessary to activate I_H. d. A high Ca^{++}-buffering capacity may also prevent Ca^{++} that enters through Ca^{++} channels from reaching the sites necessary to activate molecule X, which then activates $I_K(Ca^{++})$.

of Ca^{++}-sensitive dyes to look at the Ca^{++}-buffering capacity of R15. An important finding of theirs was that the Ca^{++}-buffering capacity is not uniform throughout the cytoplasm of R15, but is low near the center of the cell and high closer to the cell membrane. It may well be that this layer of high buffering capacity close to the membrane prevents injected Ca^{++} from reaching the membrane sites necessary to activate I_H (Fig.2.11c).

Calcium buffering may also play a role in explaining why $I_K(Ca^{++})$ is activated by a Ca^{++} injection but not by a Ca^{++} influx. It is clear that there is considerable variation in the characteristics of Ca^{++} activated K^+ channels (Kaczmarek & Levitan, 1987). Although many such channels appear to be activated directly by binding Ca^{++}, activation of the channels in R15 may not be so simple. In particular, they may require the binding of a Ca^{++} complex, for example, Ca^{++}-calmodulin, or of a molecule that requires Ca^{++}-dependent phosphorylation for its activity. This is illustrated schematically as molecule "X" in Fig. 2.11d. If this molecule were plentiful in the center of the cell, but in short supply near the membrane, then injected Ca^{++} could exert its action, and the resulting complex could diffuse through the

Ca^{++}-buffering region to reach the K^+ channels. In contrast, Ca^{++} entering through Ca^{++} channels would not be able to pass through the buffering region to activate the molecule.

One thing that has become clear over the years is the ubiquitous nature of Ca^{++} as an intracellular second messenger. It has been assigned roles ranging from channel modulation to synaptic release to control of nucleic acid transcription. What is less clear in many cases are the mechanisms that mediate the second messenger activities of Ca^{++} and that direct them to their correct end effectors. Of course, we would like to know how Ca^{++} exerts its effects in R15. But more signigficantly, understanding the actions of Ca^{++} in R15 will likely enhance our general understanding of the roles of this most important ion.

REFERENCES

Adams, D. J., & Gage, P. W. (1979a). Ionic currents in response to membrane depolarization in an *Aplysia* neurone. *Journal of Physiology, 289*, 115–141.

Adams, D. J., & Gage, P. W. (1979b). Characteristics of sodium and calcium conductance changes produced by membrane depolarization in an *Aplysia* neurone. *Journal of Physiology, 289*, 143–161.

Adams, W. B. (1985). Slow depolarizing and hyperpolarizing currents which mediate bursting in *Aplysia* neurone R15. *Journal of Physiology, 360*, 51–68.

Adams, W. B., & Benson, J. A. (1985). The generation and modulation of endogenous rhythmicity in the *Aplysia* bursting pacemaker neurone R15. *Progress in Biophysics and Molecular Biology, 46*, 1–49.

Adams, W. B., & Levitan, I. B., (1982). Intracellular injection of protein kinase inhibitor blocks the serotonin-induced increase in K^+ conductance in *Aplysia* neuron R15. *Proceedings of the National Academy of Sciences, 76*, 3877–3880.

Adams, W. B., & Levitan, I. B. (1985). Voltage and ion dependences of the slow currents which mediate bursting in *Aplysia* neurone R15. *Journal of Physiology, 360*, 69–93.

Arvanitaki, A., & Cardot, H. (1941). Les charactéristics de l'activité rythmique ganglionnaire "spontanée" chez l'Aplysie. *Comptes Rendu Seance Societe Biologie, 1351, 1201–1211.*

Benson, J. A., & Levitan, I. B. (1983). Serotonin increases an anomalously rectifying K^+ current in the Aplysia neuron R15. *Procedures of the National Academy of Sciences, 80*, 3522–3525.

Carpenter, D., & Gunn, R., (1970). The dependence of pacemaker discharge of Aplysia neurons upon Na^+ and Ca^{++}. *Journal of Cellular Physiology, 7521, 121–128.*

Drummond, A. H., Benson, J. A., and Levitan, I. B. (1980). Serotonin-induced hyperpolarization of an identified *Aplysia* neuron is mediated by cyclic AMP. *Proceedings of the National Academy of Sciences, 77*, 5013–5017.

Drummond, A. H., Bucher, F., & Levitan, I. B. (1980). Distribution of serotonin and dopamine receptors in Aplysia tissues: Analysis by [3H]LSD binding and adenylate cyclase stimulation. *Brain Research, 184*, 163–177.

Eckert, R., & Tillotson D. L. (1981). Calcium-mediated inactivation of the calcium conductance in caesium-loaded giant neurones of Aplysia californica. *Journal of Physiology, 314*, 265–280.

Kaczmarek, L. K., & Levitan, I. B. (Eds.). (1987). *Neuromodulation*. New York and Oxford: Oxford University Press.

Kramer, R. H., & Zucker, R. S. (1985a). Calcium-dependent inward current in Aplysia bursting pace-maker neurones. *Journal of Physiology, 362,* 107–130.

Kramer, R. H., & Zucker, R. S. (1985b). Calcium-induced inactivation of calcium current causes the interburst hyperpolarization of Aplysia bursting pace-maker neurones.*Journal of Physiology, 362,* 131–160.

Lemos, J. R., Novak-Hofer, I., & Levitan, I. B. (1982). Serotonin alters the phosphorylation of specific proteins inside a single living nerve cell. *Nature, 298,* 64–65.

Lemos, J. R., Novak-Hofer, I., & Levitan, I. B. (1985). Phosphoproteins associated with the regulation of a specific potassium channel in the identified Aplysia neuron R15. *Journal of Biological Chemistry, 260,* 3207–3214.

Meech, R. W., & Strumwasser, F., (1970). Intracellular calcium injection activates potassium conductance in Aplysia nerve cells. *Federation Procedures, 29,* 834.

Partridge, L. D., Thompson, S. H., Smith, S. J., & Connor, J. A. (1979). Current-voltage relationships of repetitively firing neurons. *Brain Research, 164,* 69–79.

Strumwasser, F. (1965). The demonstration and manipulation of a circadian rhythm in a single neuron. In J. Aschoff (Ed.), *Circadian clocks* (pp. 442–462). Amsterdam: North-Holland Publishing Co.

Thompson, S. H. (1977). Three pharmacologically distinct potassium channels in molluscan neurons. *Journal of Physiology, 265,* 464–488.

Tillotson, D., & Gorman, A. L. F. (1980). Non-uniform Ca^{2+} buffer distribution in a nerve cell body. *Nature, 286,* 816–817.

3 Adaptation and Dynamic Responses in the Auditory Periphery

Robert L. Smith
Syracuse University

INTRODUCTION

When Dr. Josef Zwislocki was my dissertation advisor, he asked me if I could perform a few experiments to clarify the nature of adaptation in the auditory nerve. At the time it was known that adaptation was a characteristic property of auditory-nerve fibers (e.g., Kiang, Watanabe, Thomas, & Clark, 1965). Specifically, in response to a tone of constant sound intensity, auditory-nerve firing rate was maximum at stimulus onset and then adapted or decayed to a constant value. However, not much else was known. This chapter reviews the course of the studies that have resulted as I tried to respond to Dr. Zwislocki's charge, and presents some recent findings and remaining questions. In addition, some attempts to develop simple measures of dynamic response that involve the compound action potential are described.

Before entering into specifics, it is appropriate to ask, "why study auditory adaptation?" One answer, from a purely scientific perspective, is "because it's there." In addition, adaptation has important bioengineering implications. This is because adaptation appears to reflect a dynamic process that plays an important role in the processing of changes or fluctuations in sound intensity. Changes in intensity, in turn, provide meaningful auditory information, be they present in speech, music, or other sounds.

Adaptation to changes in intensity has been implicated in a variety of psychophysical tasks, although the detailed role remains the subject of disagreement (e.g., Viemeister, 1988). For example, Carlyon and Moore (1986) provide evidence that the transient response at tone onset is important for the detection of a tone burst in the presence of an ongoing background sound. Florentine (1986) hypothesizes that the onset response conveys more information about an auditory stimulus than is available after adaptation. Adaptation may also play an important role in speech communication, for example, by producing a temporal contrast that accentuates changes in the stimulus frequency spectrum (e.g., Delgutte, 1980; Delgutte & Kiang, 1984). In addition, the increased dynamic operating range at onset, described later in the chapter, allows spectral analysis to occur over a wider range of intensities at the onset of a speech-like stimulus rather than after adaptation has occurred and many units are saturated (e.g., Miller & Sachs, 1983; Sachs, Young, & Miller, 1983). Onset responses also appear to provide information about some stop consonants even in the presence of relatively high background noise levels (Geisler & Gamble, 1989). Consequently, inclusion of adaptation in a speech recognition system reportedly improves performance (Cohen, 1989). Finally, adaptation would appear to play a role in the psychophysically determined overshoot phenomena in which masking is greatest at the onset of a masker and then decays with time (e.g., Bacon & Moore, 1986; Bacon & Viemeister 1985; see also the review by Bacon & Smith, 1991). The overshoot would appear to consist of two components, one of which is frequency independent, and the other dependent on the frequency difference between background and masker (Kimberley, Nelson, & Bacon, 1989). A number of reports (see the review by Bacon & Smith, 1991) suggest that overshoot depends on onset responses or adaptation occurring in frequency regions removed from the region of signal energy, suggesting central involvement at least in monitoring peripheral adaptation.

SUMMARY OF EARLY RESULTS

Let me begin by summarizing some of our earliest results which were obtained in direct collaboration with Dr. Zwislocki and set the stage for subsequent studies. Our first experiments were performed on cochlear nucleus units which showed "primary-like" adaptation (Smith & Zwislocki, 1971). We varied the time delay from the onset of a background tone to the onset of a superimposed probe tone. We found, to a first order of approximation, that the change in firing rate produced by the probe tone, or increment, was independent of time delay. In other words, if the probe was applied at background onset, it would add a certain firing rate to the onset response. If the probe was applied after adaptation, it would produce the same change in firing rate, but added to the steady-state response. We concluded that "The finding that the incremental response does not depend on time delay from the pedestal onset may have considerable significance with respect to receptor processes," that "Whatever process produces the decay, it does not affect the incremental response," and that "no currently available neural models account for these relationships" (p. 1525). Since then we have been investigating the generality of these conclusions and attempted to generate an appropriate neural model. We also speculated that "From the psychophysical point of view, the constant incremental response . . . in conjunction with the decreasing pedestal response, may provide an explanation for the results of some detection experiments in which the detectability of a signal was found to improve with time delay for a pedestal or masker onset" (p.1525). This is the so-called *psychophysical overshoot phenomena*. At the time we suggested that we could account for about 5 dB of overshoot in this manner. In terms of the most recent psychophysical results, this may represent the so-called "frequency independent" component of overshoot. This early study and the questions that it raised set the stage for a rather extensive line of studies that are reviewed next.

SHORT-TERM AND RAPID ADAPTATION

Our first series of experiments involved short-term adaptation, a component of the dynamic response characterized by a decay with a time constant on the order of 60 ms. The incremental experiments described previously led to the hypothesis that short-term adaptation was basically additive or linear in nature. Furthermore, several lines of evidence led to the conclusion that a static saturating nonlinearity preceded additive short-term adaptation in the chain of peripheral auditory signal processing. For example, it was observed that to a first order of approximation the onset rate-intensity function had the same shape as the steady-state function (Smith, 1979; Smith & Zwislocki, 1975) and in general that the time constant of short-term adaptation was independent of sound intensity. In addition, when the intensity of a conditioning tone was increased, the decrement in response to the test tone increased in proportion to the driven response to the conditioning tone (Harris & Dallos, 1979; Smith, 1977). Hence, the same nonlinearity appeared to control the effects of stimulus intensity in all of the above situations and was apparently followed by an adapting process that was additive and proportional to the response to the adapting tone, that is, the output of the peripheral nonlinearity (Smith, 1979). A functional model was produced to account for the results and consisted of two stages in cascade: a saturating static nonlinearity followed by a linear adapting stage that obeyed superposition (Smith, 1979; Smith & Zwislocki, 1975).

The initial studies of adaptation were purposely insensitive to a second, faster, dynamic component known as *rapid adaptation* that occurs during the first few milliseconds of an adapting response. The short-term studies used time intervals of 10 ms or more to measure response firing rates and effectively smoothed out the more rapid process. However, when Brachman, Frisina, Westerman, and I began investigating events occurring during the first few milliseconds of the dynamic response, and began applying sinusoidal amplitude modulation to induce controllable intensity fluctuations, some new and distinguishing features of rapid adaptation became evident (Brachman 1980; Smith & Brachman, 1980a, 1980b, 1980c; Smith, Brachman, & Frisina, 1985; Westerman, 1985; Westerman & Smith, 1984). In particular, it was observed that the operating range at onset, that is, measured during the first few milliseconds of response, was generally greater than the steady-state operating range.

In addition, responses to sinusoidal amplitude modulation were controlled by the onset or dynamic operating range as opposed to the steady-state operating range. Rapid adaptation appears to have an exponential time course with a time constant of 1 to 10 ms, that is, an order of magnitude smaller than short-term adaptation. Furthermore, time constant is a misnomer, because this parameter varies with intensity and decreases with increases in intensity. This decrease is accompanied by an increase in amplitude of the rapid component. As sound intensity increases, the amplitude of rapid adaptation increases more rapidly than the amplitude of short-term adaptation, resulting in the increased operating range at onset. The increased operating range at onset occurred in spite of refractory limitations in the firing rate. Westerman and I found that the onset operating range was still greater when refractory effects were compensated for (Smith, 1988; Westerman, 1985; Westerman & Smith, 1987). These results were all consistent with the hypothesis that the large operating range at onset was the result of a dynamic process that was not fully subject to the static operating range that limited short-term and steady-state responses.

SOME UNRESOLVED ISSUES

Because of the brief nature of rapid adaptation, some of its features and properties still remain unresolved. One question concerns the potential role of neural refractoriness in producing adaptation-like dynamic phenomena. Specifically, when the auditory nerve is initially firing at a high rate at response onset, is the occurrence of spikes sufficient to produce rapid adaptation? A number of lines of evidence can be raised against this possibility, but perhaps the most convincing measurement is shown in Fig. 3.1 (Smith & Westerman, 1988; Westerman, 1985). The probability of first firing, that is, the conditional probability of the time of the occurrence of the next spike, is plotted as a function of time since the previous spike for two conditions: onset and steady state. The onset function was determined

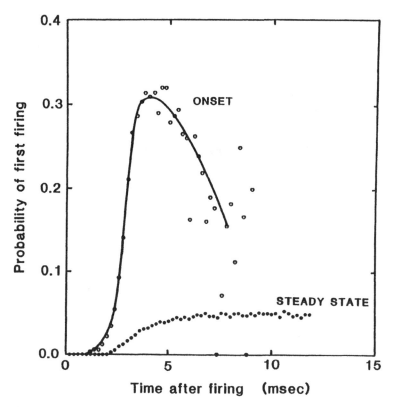

FIG. 3.1. The conditional probability of a spike plotted as a function of time since the previous spike. The onset function was determined for the first spike after the onset spike in response to a CF tone at 43 dB above threshold. The steady-state function is the standard "hazard function" obtained during the last 200 msec of a 300-msec-long tone burst. Unit CF = 4.39 kHz.

for the first spike after the onset spike in response to an intense tone. The steady-state function is the standard "hazard function" obtained during steady-state firing (e.g., Gaumond, Molnar, & Kim, 1982). In both cases the conditional probability is reduced immediately following a spike and then recovers, presumably because of neural refractoriness. Hence, dynamic responses are bound to be influenced by refractoriness as suggested earlier. In addition, the conditional probability at onset reaches a maximum and then, if no spike occurs, begins to decrease. This decrease was seen at tone onset, but not in the steady state, suggesting that there is also an underlying decay in excitation or generator potential that underlies rapid adaptation at response onset.

Data also suggest that at high intensities, for stimuli with short rise times, the two-component description of adaptation breaks down. In the presence of very high firing rates near onset, plateaus and/or nonmonotonicities can occur in PST histograms, apparently as a result of higher-order discharge-history effects (Lütkenhöner & Smith, 1986a, 1986b, 1992). Recent data on auditory-nerve responses to electrical stimulation also suggest that the occurrence of spikes can lead to subsequent reductions in neural threshold (Dynes & Delgutte, 1992; Javel, 1990). Hence, synaptic transmission and the generator process alone may not be adequate to account for all aspects of dynamic responses.

Another question that can be asked is whether rapid adaptation reflects the frequency splatter produced at stimulus onset. Turning on and off a tone generates transient energy at frequencies surrounding the tone frequency, and this energy could conceivably produce a neural response. Indeed, when units are stimulated far from their characteristic frequencies, they sometimes respond only at tone onset and offset, apparently in response to transient energy falling near their characteristic frequency (e.g., Rhode & Smith, 1985). The more rapid the stimulus onset, the greater is the frequency splatter. However, these effects do not appear to influence rapid or short-term adaptation in response to CF stimuli (Smith & Westerman, 1988; Westerman, 1985). As can be seen in Figs. 3.2 and 3.3, a tone's rise time has no appreciable effect on either the time constant (Fig. 3.2) or magnitude (Fig. 3.3) of rapid adaptation.

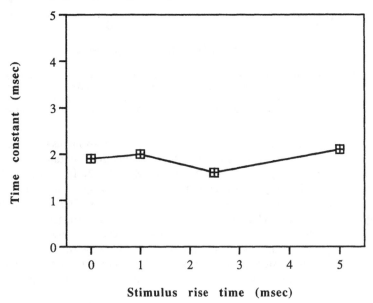

FIG. 3.2.   The time constant of rapid adaptation plotted as a function of stimulus rise time. Mean values for 6 fibers and tone bursts 40 dB above stimulus threshold.

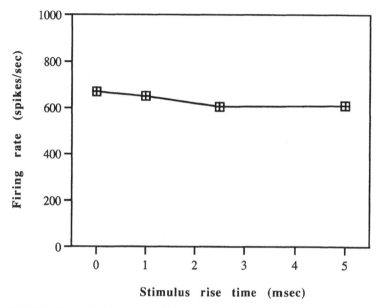

FIG. 3.3.   The amplitude of the rapid adaptation component plotted as a function of stimulus rise time. Mean values as in Fig.3.2.

These kinds of data support the concept that rapid adaptation is a result of the generator process producing spikes. Adaptation is presumably a reflection of synaptic transmission because hair-cell receptor potentials do not adapt (e.g., Goodman, Smith, & Chamberlain, 1982). Consequently, adaptation should directly reflect the amount of excitation produced, not specifically the frequency of stimulation. Some evidence supporting this view is shown by the single unit responses in Figs. 3.4 through 3.6. In this experiment, adapting tones of various frequencies and intensities were applied, and the responses to the adapting tone and a poststimulatory test tone were obtained. The test tone was at units CF, 15 ms long, and occurred about 10 ms after the end of the adapting tone. In each of the graphs, the average response to the adapting tone is given along the ordinate and is a measure of the excitation produced by the stimulus. The symbols represent different stimulus frequencies. Figure 3.4 shows the maximum onset response to the adapting tone. It can be seen that the onset response increases motonically with the average response, and the function is relatively independent of the frequency producing the average response. Similarly, it can be seen in Fig. 3.5 that the onset response to the test tone, a measure of the rapidly adapting response, decreases with average response to the adapting tone, and again the functions are independent of adapting frequency. Finally, the average response to the test tone, which is dominated by the short-term component, also decreases with adapting response

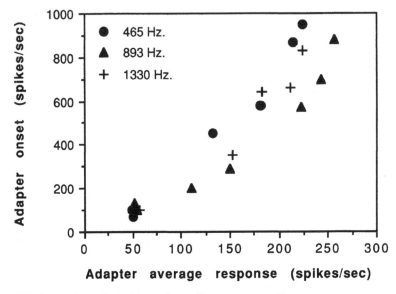

FIG. 3.4.   Effects of sound frequency on the onset response. The onset response to an adapting tone is plotted as a function of the average response to the adapting tone for three adapting tone frequencies. The onset response was the maximum response measured over a 1-ms interval. Unit CF = 893 Hz.

in a manner independent of the adapting frequency as can be seen in Fig. 3.6. These data are in partial conflict with some earlier reports of Westerman and Smith (1984, 1985), which illustrated that the time constant of rapid adaptation could depend on tone frequency, and the reasons for the difference remain to be determined. It is conceivable, however, that frequency splatter may have influenced the non-CF responses in the earlier studies by generating transient energy in the CF region and confounding the estimation of the rapid adaptation time constant. Responses to the poststimulatory test tone should be minimally effected by such splatter.

Other questions that remain unanswered concern the nature of recovery from adaptation and possible differential properties of the rapid and short-term components (Smith & Westerman, 1988; Westerman, 1985). An example is shown Fig. 3.7, in which two recovery curves are plotted for a poststimulatory test tone that was preceded by a 300-ms-long adapting or masking tone. The ordinate is the time after the end of the masker, that is, the silent interval before the test tone. The onset response to the test tone, a reflection of the rapidly adapting component, recovered with a time constant of about 49 ms. The short-term component was characterized by the firing rate in a 20-ms interval beginning 10 ms after test onset. For this unit it recovered with a larger time constant of 63 ms. Based on 12 single

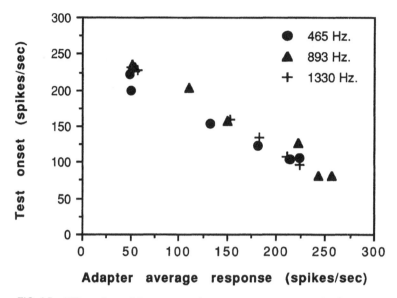

FIG. 3.5.   Effects of sound frequency on the onset response to a poststimulatory test tone. The adapting tone as in Fig. 3.4. The test tone was at CF and had a fixed intensity, and its onset response was the maximum response measured over a 1-ms interval.

units, the mean time constants for recovery of these two components were 48 ms for the rapid component and 169 ms for the recovery of the short-term component. For the same units, the average time constant for the perstimulatory short-term adaptation was 58 ms (Westerman, 1985). Hence, it would appear that comprehensive models of these effects will have to account for the variety of time constants that exist and include dichotomies between perstimulatory and poststimulatory time constants and between rapid and short-term properties. Stimuli were about 40 dB above threshold for these measurements, and effects of adapting and probe intensity remain to be determined. An additional complication is the fact that a unit's spontaneous activity classification appears to play a key role in the recovery from adaptation (Relkin & Doucet, 1991). Results such as these illustrate the need for further studies of of the adaptation process before a comprehensive model can be developed.

ADAPTATION AND THE COMPOUND ACTION POTENTIAL

A complete understanding of auditory-nerve response dynamics will undoubtedly require additional studies of large numbers of single units.

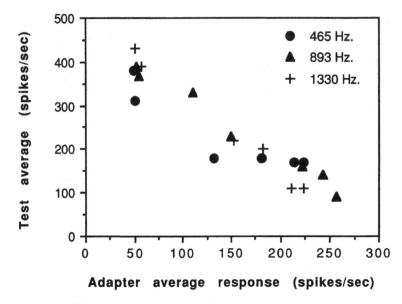

FIG. 3.6.   Effects of sound frequency on the average response to a poststimulatory test tone. The adapting and test tone as in Fig. 3.4 and 3.5. The response to the test tone was averaged over its 15-ms-long duration.

However, another approach which should help to provide insights into single-unit properties and to guide future experiments is to utilize the compound action potential (CAP) measured at the round window as an indirect monitor of single-unit responses. The CAP depends on the temporal and spatial contributions of spikes in individual fibers, making it notoriously difficult to interpret. Nevertheless, it also reflects summated or average population responses, and sometimes provides a surprisingly good match to psychophysical phenomena such as loudness (Zwislocki, 1974) and the growth of forward masking (Relkin & Smith, 1991). CAP measurement is relatively noninvasive and can be obtained in both anesthetized mammals and in humans, so that the CAP can provide a guide in making physiological comparisons across species. For reasons such as these, I attempted to determine the extent to which adaptation and dynamic response properties comparable to those in single units can be quantitatively obtained from CAP measurements. Some of the results have been quite encouraging, although anomalies and questions remain.

The CAP reflects biphasic contributions of single-unit action potentials (e.g., Teas, Eldridge, & Davis, 1962) which tend to cancel one another unless the single-unit spikes are sufficiently synchronized. Hence, a CAP only appears at the onset of a tone burst and does not directly reflect

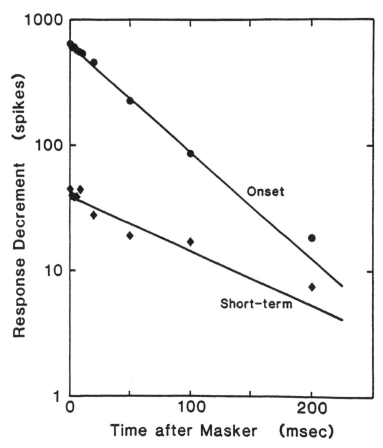

FIG. 3.7. Recovery of onset and short-term response components. Paradigm as described in the text.

adaptation during an ongoing tone, because the spikes across units are uncorrelated in time. One way to bypass this problem is to observe adaptation in response to a train of tone bursts, as outlined schematically in Fig. 3.8. When such a train is applied, CAPs in response to successive tone bursts decrease gradually in size as a result of adaptation to the preceding pulses (e.g., Peake, Goldstein, & Kiang, 1962). This paradigm was used to answer two simple questions: How does adaptation depend on tone frequency, and how does it depend on tone intensity (Smith, Chatterjee, & Relkin 1990)?

Tone bursts were generally 5 ms in duration, with 2-ms rise-fall times and 5-msec off times between tones. Figures 3.9 and 3.10 contain some normalized data showing the general shape of the decay functions for the

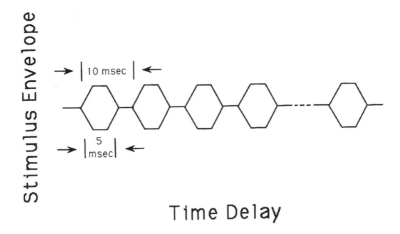

FIG. 3.8.   Schematic diagram of a train of tone bursts used to produce adaptation of the compound action potential.

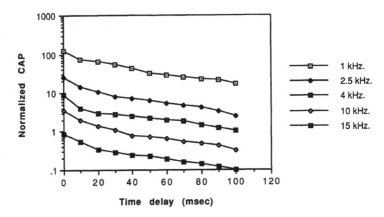

FIG. 3.9.   Plot of compound action potential versus time delay for successive tone bursts as in Fig. 3.8, with tone-burst frequency as a parameter. Data normalized as described in the text. Intensity at 4 dB above visual threshold for the CAP.

magnitude of the N1 component of the CAP. Figure 3.9 was obtained with sound frequency as a parameter. The curves are shifted by arbitrary amounts along the logarithmic ordinate in order to separate the various frequencies which run from 1 to 15 kHz in going from the top to the bottom. Each curve was normalized by first subtracting the quasi steady-state value which was reached at about 150 ms. Notice that the curves are approximately parallel for the semilogarithmic coordinates used. Further,

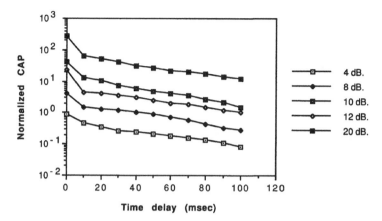

FIG. 3.10.   Plot of compound action potential versus time delay for successive tone bursts as in Fig. 3.8, with tone-burst intensity as a parameter. Data normalized as described in the text. Intensity at specified dB above visual threshold for the CAP. Tone-burst frequency = 2.5 kHz.

with the exception of the first one or two points, the functions can be approximated by a straight line, indicating an exponential decay.

In order to compare the several time courses, the data were fit with a single exponential plus a constant term. The first point, which suggests an additional onset or rapid decay that is beyond the resolution of this technique, was omitted from the procedure. The average value of the best-fit time constants was about 60 ms and was independent of sound frequency. An analogous independence of sound intensity is shown in Fig. 3.10, in which normalized curves at a number of intensities are shown. Again, the curves were parallel with time constants of about 60 ms. Hence, the CAP data are consistent with the conclusion from single-fiber experiments that the time course of short-term adaptation is independent of the intensity and of the frequency of stimulation. It should also be noted that the close agreement with the single-unit time constant of short-term adaptation may be somewhat fortuitous, because the effects of stimulus duration and off times were not investigated.

From the discussed series it would appear that the properties of short-term adaptation seen in the CAP are a fairly close reflection of the corresponding single-unit characteristics. However, this paradigm does not provide information about rapid adaptation. Consequently, an additional paradigm was utilized which is outlined in Fig. 3.11. In this case the adapting duration, T, is varied, and the CAP in response to the poststimulatory test tone is measured. As previously pointed out by Abbas and Gorga (1981), based on the single-unit results (Harris & Dallos, 1979; Smith, 1977;

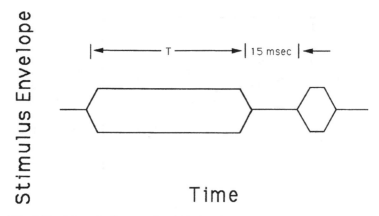

FIG. 3.11.   Schematic diagram of variable-duration masker used to produce adaptation in the compound action potential.

Smith, Brachman, & Goodman, 1983), it is expected that the decrement in test response would be an indirect measure of the adaptation to the first tone. However, the CAP data of Abbas and Gorga (1981) were fit with a single exponential. In contrast, in this experiment it was possible to obtain increased resolution near onset, and consequently resolve the rapidly adapting component, by obtaining more points for short durations.

A typical series of results is plotted in Fig. 3.12 (Smith et al., 1990), showing the CAP as a function of masker duration for various frequencies. Note that for a given curve the masker and probe were always at the same frequency and intensity, so that the CAP at the onset of the adapting tone served as a control for the probe response. In order to characterize the results, the data were fit with the sum of two exponentials and a constant. One time constant averaged about 6 ms across the conditions studied and is presumably related to rapid adaptation which has a time constant of between 1 and 10 msec in single auditory-nerve fibers. The other time constant averaged about 94 ms, somewhat longer than expected from single-unit short-term adaptation or from the first CAP experiment. The reason for this difference is not immediately apparent, but may be partly methodological due to the long durations used in this series.

Figure 3.13 shows the time constants for the various frequencies in the previous data. It can be seen that both time constants are relatively independent of frequency. For the longer time constant, that is, short-term adaptation, this is consistent with the single-unit data. However, in contrast to this constancy of the CAP rapid time constant, the single-unit results suggested that the rapid time constant varies with frequency and was higher at low frequencies (Westerman & Smith, 1984). The reason for this discrepancy is not known. It was observed, however, that the shapes of the

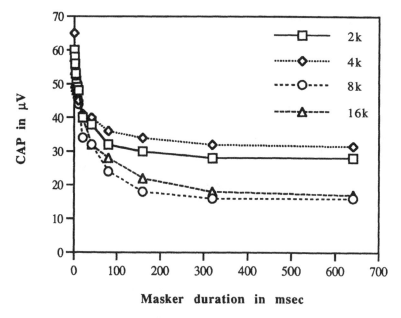

FIG. 3.12. Poststimulatory CAP response as a function of masker duration for the paradigm of Fig. 3.11, with sound frequency as a parameter.

normalized CAP functions did vary with frequency. This variation could be accounted for by changes in the relative sizes of the coefficients of the two components. There is apparently more rapid adaptation at high frequencies. It is not known whether or not this is true of the single-unit data.

These two series of adaptation experiments suggest that at least to a first order of approximation both rapid and short-term adaptation can be observed in the CAP experiments, albeit some unresolved differences remain in comparison to the single-unit data.

CONCLUSIONS

These results should serve to demonstrate that a substantial line of research was initiated when Zwislocki suggested that I solve the "adaptation problem" in the auditory nerve. The problem has not been fully resolved, but interesting results have been obtained along the way. The CAP also appears to provide additional insights in peripheral adaptation. Recent experiments involved investigating counterparts of psychophysical overshoot in the CAP (Chatterjee & Smith, in press; Chatterjee et al., 1990), with

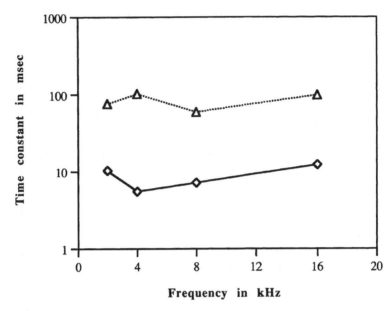

FIG. 3.13. Time constants for rapid (solid line) and short-term (dashed line) components that fit the data of Fig. 3.12.

results that suggest some possible bases for the overshoot that also relate back to Zwislocki's initial insights. In addition, sinusoidal amplitude modulation had been used to generate compound responses with an adapting component at the modulation frequency. This may provide the best technique yet for noninvasive determination of peripheral adaptation (Smith & Passaglia, 1992; Smith et al., 1993). Hence, the seed that Zwislocki planted in this area remains alive and healthy, still yielding fruit.

ACKNOWLEDGMENTS

This work was supported by NSF grant BNS 8920418, and NIH grants DC 00074 and DC 00380. Thanks to Chris Stathatos for his assistance with the preparation of figures and manuscript.

REFERENCES

Abbas, P. J., & Gorga, M. P. (1981). AP responses in forward-masking paradigms and their relationship to responses of auditory-nerve fibers. *Journal of the Acoustical Society of America, 69,* 492–499.
Bacon, S. P., & Moore, B. C. J. (1986). Temporal effects in simultaneous pure-tone masking:

Effects of signal frequency, masker/signal frequency ratio, and masker level. *Hearing Research, 23,* 257-266.

Bacon, S. P., & Smith, M. A. (1991). Spectral, intensive, and temporal factors influencing overshoot. *Quarterly Journal of Experimental Psychology, 43A,* 373-399.

Bacon, S. P., & Viemeister, N. F. (1985). The temporal course of simultaneous tone-on-tone masking. *Journal of the Acoustical Society of America, 78,* 1231-1235.

Brachman, M. L. (1980). *Dynamic response characteristics of single auditory-nerve fibers.* Unpublished doctoral dissertation and special report ISR-S-19, Institute for Sensory Research, Syracuse University, Syracuse, NY.

Carlyon, R. P., & Moore, B. C. J. (1986). Continuous versus gated pedestals and the "severe departure" from Weber's law. *Journal of the Acoustical Society of America, 79,* 453-460.

Chatterjee, M., & Smith, R. L. (in press). *Physiological overshoot and the compound action potential. Hearing Research.*

Chatterjee, M., Smith, R. L., & Relkin, E. M. (1990). Some temporal effects on the sensitivity of the CAP to changes in sound intensity and frequency. *Journal of the Acoustical Society of America, 1, 87* (Suppl. 1), S101.

Cohen, J. R. (1989). Application of an auditory model to speech recognition. *Journal of Acoustical Society of America, 85,* 2623-2629.

Delgutte, B. (1980). Representation of speech-like sounds in the discharge patterns of auditory-nerve fibers. *Journal of the Acoustical Society of America, 68,* 843-857.

Delgutte, B., & Kiang, N. Y.-S. (1984). Speech coding in the auditory nerve IV. Sounds with consonant-like dynamic characteristics. *Journal of the Acoustical Society of America, 75,* 897-907.

Dynes, S. B. C., & Delgutte, B. (1992). Phase-locking of auditory nerve discharges to sinusoidal electrical stimulation of the cochlea. *Hearing Research, 58,* 79-90.

Florentine, M. (1986). Level discrimination of tones as a function of duration. *Journal of the Acoustical Society of America, 79,* 792-798.

Gaumond, R. P., Molnar, C. E., & Kim, D. O. (1982). Stimulus and recovery dependence of cat cochlear nerve fiber spike discharge probability. *Journal of Neurophysiology, 48,* 856-873.

Geisler, C. D., & Gambler, T. (1989). Responses of "high-spontaneous" auditory-nerve fibers to consonant-vowel syllables in noise. *Journal of the Acoustical Society of America, 85,* 1639-1652.

Goodman, D. A., Smith, R. L., & Chamberlain, S. C. (1982). Intracellular and extracellular responses in the organ of Corti of the gerbil. *Hearing Research, 7,* 161-169.

Harris, D. M., & Dallos, P. (1979). Forward masking of auditory nerve fiber responses. *Journal of Neurophysiology, 42,* 1083-1107.

Javel, E. (1990). Acoustic and electrical encoding of temporal information. In J. Miller & F. Spelman (Eds.). *Cochlear implants: Models of the electrically stimulated ear* (pp. 247-295). New York: Springer-Verlag.

Kiang, N. Y.-S., Watanabe, T., Thomas, E. C., & Clark, L. F. (1965). *Response patterns of single fibers in the cat's auditory nerve* (MIT Research Monograph 35). Cambridge, MA: MIT Press.

Kimberley, B. P., Nelson, D. A., & Bacon, S. P. (1989). Temporal overshoot in simultaneous masked psychophysical tuning curves from normal and hearing-impaired listeners. *Journal of the Acoustical Society of America, 85,* 1660-1665.

Lütkenhöner, B., & Smith, R. L. (1986a). Rapid adaptation of auditory-nerve fibers: Fine structure at high stimulus intensities. *Hearing Research, 23,* 223-232.

Lütkenhöner, B., & Smith, R. L. (1986b). The role of discharge-history effects in rapid adaptation of auditory-nerve fibers. *Journal of the Acoustical Society of America, 79,* S33.

Lütkenhöner, B., & Smith, R. L. (1992). A theoretical basis for conditional probability analyses of neural discharge activity. *Biological Cybernetics, 67,* 1-10.

Miller, M. I., & Sachs, M. B. (1983). Representation of stop consonants in the discharge patterns of auditory-nerve fibers. *Journal of the Acoustical Society of America, 74,* 502–517.

Peake, W. T., Goldstein, M. J., Jr., & Kiang, N. Y.-S. (1962). Responses of the auditory nerve to repetitive acoustic stimuli. *Journal of the Acoustical Society of America, 34,* 562–570.

Relkin, E. M., & Doucet, J. R. (1991). Recovery from prior stimulation. I. Relationship to spontaneous firing rates of primary auditory neurons. *Hearing Research, 55,* 215–224.

Relkin, E. M., & Smith, R. L. (1991). Forward masking of the compound action potential: Thresholds for detection of the N_1 peak. *Hearing Research, 53,* 131–140.

Rhode, W. S., & Smith, P. H. (1985). Characteristics of tone-pip response patterns in relationship to spontaneous rate in cat auditory nerve fibers. *Hearing Research, 18,* 159–168.

Sachs, M. B., Young, E. D., & Miller, M. I. (1983). Speech encoding in the auditory nerve: Implications for cochlear implants. *Annals of the New York Academy of Sciences, 405,* 95–113.

Smith, R. L. (1977). Short-term adaptation in single auditory-nerve fibers — some poststimulatory effects. *Journal of Neurophysiology, 40,* 1098–1112.

Smith, R. L. (1979). Adaptation, saturation and physiological masking in single auditory-nerve fibers. *Journal of the Acoustical Society of America, 65,* 166–178.

Smith, R. L. (1988). Encoding of sound intensity by auditory neurons. In G. Edelman, W. Gall, & W. Cowan (Eds.), *Auditory function: Neurobiological basis for hearing* (pp. 243–273) New York: John Wiley & Sons.

Smith, R. L., & Brachman, M. L. (1980a). Dynamic response of single auditory-nerve fibers — some effects of intensity and time. In G. van den Brink & F. A. Bilsen (Eds.), *International symposium on psychophysical, physiological and behavioral studies in hearing* (pp. 312–319). The Netherlands: Delft University Press.

Smith, R. L., & Brachman, M. L. (1980b). Operating range and maximum response of single auditory-nerve fibers. *Brain Research, 184,* 499–505.

Smith, R. L., & Brachman, M. L. (1980c). Response modulation of auditory-nerve fibers by AM stimuli: Effects of average intensity. *Hearing Research, 2,* 123–133.

Smith, R. L., Brachman, M. L., & Goodman, D. A. (1983). Adaptation in the auditory periphery. *Annals of the New York Academy of Sciences, 405,* 79–94.

Smith, R. L., Chatterjee, M., & Relkin, E. M. (1990, February). Auditory-nerve adaptation and the compound action potential. *Abstracts of 13th Midwinter Meeting of the Association for Research in Otolaryngology, 191.*

Smith, R. L., & Passaglia, C. L. (1992, February). Auditory-nerve neurophonic in response to amplitude modulation? *Abstracts of the 15th Midwinter Meeting of the Association for Research in Otolaryngology,* p. 101.

Smith, R. L., Passaglia, C., Relkin, E. M., Prieve, B., Nguyen, M., & Murname, O. (1993, February). Modulation-following responses from the auditory periphery: Some results from gerbils and humans. *Abstracts of 16th Midwinter Meeting of the Association for Research in Otolaryngology,* p. 93.

Smith, R. L., & Westerman, L. A. (1988). Comparison of rapid and short-term adaptation in the auditory nerve. *Journal of the Acoustical Society of America, 84,* S55.

Smith, R. L., & Zwislocki, J. J. (1971). Responses of some neurons of the cochlear nucleus to tone-intensity increments. *Journal of the Acoustical Society of America, 50,* 1520–1525.

Smith, R. L., & Zwislocki, J. J. (1975). Short-term adaptation and incremental responses of single auditory-nerve fibers. *Biological Cybernetics, 17,* 169–182.

Smith, R. L., Brachman, L., & Frisina, R. D. (1985). Sensitivity of auditory nerve fibers in changes in intensity: A dichotomy between increments and decrements. *Journal of the Acoustical Society of America, 78,* 1310–1316.

Teas, D. C., Eldredge, D. H., & Davis, H. (1962). Cochlear responses to acoustic transients:

An interpretation of whole-nerve action potentials. *Journal of the Acoustical Society of America, 34,* 1438–1459.

Viemeister, N. F. (1988). Intensity coding and the dynamic range problem. *Hearing Research, 34,* 267–274.

Westerman, L. A. (1985). *Adaptation and recovery of auditory nerve responses.* Unpublished doctoral dissertation and special rep. ISR-S-24, Institute for Sensory Research, Syracuse University, Syracuse, NY.

Westerman, L. A., & Smith, R. L. (1984). Rapid and short-term adaptation in auditory nerve responses. *Hearing Research, 15,* 249–260.

Westerman, L. A., & Smith, R. L. (1985). Rapid adaptation depends on the characteristic frequency of auditory nerve fibers. *Hearing Research, 17,* 197–198.

Westerman, L. A., & Smith, R. L. (1987). Conservation of adapting components in auditory-nerve responses. *Journal of the Acoustical Society of America, 81,* 680–691.

Zwislocki, J. J. (1974). A power function for sensory receptors. In H. Moskowitz, B. Scharf, & J Stevens (Eds.), *Sensation and measurement* (pp. 185–197). Dordrecht, The Netherlands: D. Reidel.

4 Intensity Coding and Circadian Rhythms in the *Limulus* Lateral Eye

Robert B. Barlow
Syracuse University

Ehud Kaplan
Rockfeller University

THE *LIMULUS* LATERAL EYE: A BRIEF HISTORY

The lateral eye of the horseshoe crab, *Limulus polyphemus*, occupies a special place in vision research. Its long, distinguished history began in 1926 at the Marine Biological Laboratory in Woods Hole, MA. H. Keffer Hartline, then a student at John Hopkins Medical School, had developed a keen interest in the neural events leading from photochemical reactions in the eye to an animal's behavior. However, when studying frogs, cats, and humans he became weary of the complexity of light-evolved electrical responses — electroretinograms (ERGs) — he was able to record from their eyes (Hartline, 1925). He traveled to Woods Hole in search of a simpler visual system and was immediately impressed with the prominent lateral eyes of *Limulus*. They contained hundreds of receptor units, ommatidia, so large he could see them without using a magnifying glass.

Hartline reasoned that if he could see individual retinal receptors, perhaps he could record from them. At about the same time, Adrian's Laboratory in Cambridge, England was revolutionizing neurophysiology by recording and analyzing the electrical activity of single nerve cells. Hartline moved quickly after learning of the rapid advances taking place in Cambridge. He constructed a vacuum tube amplifier, acquired an oscillating reed oscillograph, and returned to Woods Hole in 1931 with Clarence Graham hoping to achieve with the *Limulus* optic nerve what Adrian and Bronk (1928) did with the rabbit phrenic nerve: record from single nerve fibers.

Hartline and Graham excised a lateral eye of a juvenile animal, dissected the optic-nerve trunk, and were frustrated to find that they could not isolate

55

the responses of a single fiber from the mass discharge of large numbers of fibers. They repeated the experiment many times without success. Only a few days before their departure from Woods Hole they decided to test the eye of the last animal in the saltwater tank, which happened to be an adult. Their success was immediate. They found that the rate of discharge of optic-nerve impulses from a single ommatidium increased with light intensity over a range of intensities of at least 1 to 10,000 (Hartline & Graham, 1932).

The single fiber experiments yielded information on almost every aspect of vision and led to the formulation of basic mechanisms of retinal function applicable to many species (Hartline, 1972; Ratliff, 1974). Hartline and his colleagues found that a wide range of visual phenomena, such as light and dark adaptation, flicker fusion, contrast enhancement, and spectral sensitivity, originated in the retina of this primitive animal. In this chapter we discuss the intensity coding properties of the *Limulus* eye and how our knowledge has evolved from the original work of Hartline.

THE LABORATORY OF SENSORY COMMUNICATION

In 1967 one of us (R.B.) joined the budding Laboratory of Sensory Communication (LSC) at Syracuse University after completing graduate studies in the laboratory of Hartline and Ratliff at Rockefeller University. Housed in a refurbished two-story wooden structure, LSC was indeed an austere setting for a modern research facility. It was, however, the realization of its founder, Jozef J. Zwislocki, who we honor with this collection of papers by colleagues and former associates and students. Zwislocki firmly believed that comparative and multidisciplinary approaches provided the best chance of understanding how the nervous system processes sensory information.

His goal was to investigate the major sensory systems—audition, taction, and vision—with the tools of psychophysics, physiology, and anatomy, together with a heavy dose of systems analysis. The evolution of LSC to the highly successful Institute for Sensory Research confirms the wisdom of Zwislocki's approach.

The Laboratory of Sensory Communication had strong research programs in audition and taction before 1967. The arrival that year of one of us (R.B.) initiated research in the field of vision. Leaving the cloistered halls of Rockefeller University to occupy two small rooms in the basement of a wooden house was quite a shock. A groove cut in the cement floor of the basement carried runoff from leaking walls during the rainy season. Nevertheless, through strong support of both Syracuse University and Joe Zwislocki, a first-rate facility for vision research was established by 1969. The other of us (E.K.) arrived that year to pursue a doctorate in Sensory

Science. Our first research project in the Vision Laboratory was to repeat Hartline's classic experiment of recording from single optic-nerve fibers of the *Limulus* eye, but without removing the eye from the animal.

INTACT VERSUS EXCISED LIMULUS EYES: OUR FIRST SURPRISE

Knowledge of the functioning of the *Limulus* lateral eye in the late 1960s was based entirely on studies in which the eye had been excised from the animal (Wolbarsht & Yeandle, 1967). Although the technique of excising the eye is relatively easy and well suited for many types of experiments, an important drawback is that excision causes a gradual decline in the eye's sensitivity to light. This is particularly troublesome in studies of inhibitory interactions in the retina (Hartline & Ratliff, 1972), because reduced responses to light may be misinterpreted as effects of lateral inhibition. Excised eyes remained relatively stable for only about 4 to 5 hours. Experiments requiring longer recording times (~ 10 hours), such as those to measure the spread of inhibition in the retina (Barlow, 1969), were difficult to carry out with excised eyes.

To achieve greater stability we set out to record activity from single optic-nerve fibers without exercising the eye or impairing its blood supply. We were thankful that *Limulus* cooperated by running each lateral optic-nerve trunk directly under the shell as it leaves the eye before diving deep into the body and entering the brain. However, we were not at all thankful that *Limulus* located each optic-nerve trunk inside a blood vessel. We cut a hole in the carapace, exposed and opened the blood vessel, and dissected single fibers from the nerve trunk attempting to repeat Hartline's elegant technique, but with the eye still in the animal. We were continually frustrated by a seemingly unending supply of blood that gushed forth from the blood vessel. We overcame the problem by fashioning a small chamber which fit snugly in the hole in the carapace and had a small hole to accommodate the cut end of the optic nerve. With the chamber, we finally succeeded in recording the activity of a single optic-nerve fiber.

The light-evoked responses were a great surprise They differed significantly from those of the excised eye. No matter how much we attenuated the incident light intensity with available neutral density filters, the light-evoked responses persisted. We were convinced our fiber-optics illumination system had a light leak around the filter box allowing light to enter the light pipe without attenuation. To check on possible light leaks, one of us (E.K.) crawled inside the Faraday cage, and the other (R.B.) sealed the cage as if his colleague were an experimental preparation. After 30 minutes of dark adaption inside the cage, E.K. looked into the exit port of the illumination system expecting to see a light leak with the shutter closed. But it was pitch black—no light was detected. Fearing asphyxiation because no air could be piped into the cramped cage from outside, we held a running conversation about how to account for the strange responses of the intact eye in the event no light leaks were detected.

Figure 4.1a (filled circles) shows an experiment we performed after acquiring a set of light-attenuating filters with greater densities than those we had for experiments with excised eyes. We focused our attention on responses to light intensities (log I -5 to -10) below those detectable by excised eyes. For comparison Fig. 4.1a also plots an intensity-response function we recorded a year earlier from an excised eye. The growth of response with light intensity and the ranges of intensities over which the excised eye responded agree well with the data of Hartline and others (Hartline & McDonald, 1947; Ratliff, 1974). To assure ourselves that intact and excised eyes shared some common properties, we tested responses of the intact eye to several higher intensities (log I $= -2.5$ and 0.0) and found that they matched those of the excised eye.

We were astonished by the 10-log unit operating range of single receptors in the *Limulus* eyes. To our knowledge no other sensory receptor has been found with an equally large range. Vertebrate photoreceptors have ~4 log-unit range (Baylor & Fuortes, 1970), and auditory receptors of the noctuid moth have ~5 log-unit range (Adams, 1971).

We were also astonished to find that no matter how much we attenuated the incident light intensity, a single ommatidium remained active: It fired nerve impulses in darkness. (Note that the response to Log I $= -9.5$ is only slightly lower than that to Log I $= -9.0$) Although not shown in Fig 4.1a, the single optic-nerve fiber fired ~1.1 impulses/s when the shutter was closed. Hartline (personal communication, 1970) was highly skeptical of this result. He cautioned us that spontaneous activity was a clear sign of an eye in poor physiological condition. His criticism weighed heavily on us as we discuss here.

TWO RECEPTOR MECHANISMS: ZWISLOCKI'S CONTRIBUTION

We drew a dashed line through the incomplete set of data in Fig. 4.1a and rushed off to show Joe Zwislocki what we found. He had a keen interest in the intensity-responses properties of sensory receptors, and we were anxious to show him a set of data that spanned a greater range of intensities than any others we had seen. Zwislocki was also intrigued by our finding and was particularly struck by the interesting divergence of responses from our handdrawn line in the range of Log I $= -7$ to -5. He took a pencil and drew a double-sigmoid curve (solid line in Fig. 4.1b) and suggested that the eye may use more than one receptor mechanism to code light intensity.

We returned to the laboratory, repeated the experiment on another animal, and found that Joe was right: The intensity-response function had a clear plateau at intermediate light intensities (Fig. 4.2). The second experiment also exhibited wide-range intensity coding and spontaneous activity in the dark. We found also that the transient response at the onset of the light stimulus increased monotonically over a relatively narrow range and saturated at high intensities (Barlow & Kaplan, 1971). In the next series of experiments we investigated the differences between intact and excised eyes.

We tested directly the possibility that the difference between intact eyes and excised eyes resulted from cutting off the blood supply. After measuring an intensity-response characteristic for an ommatidium of a fully dark-adapted eye, we cut the animal's heart in half without disturbing the optical isolation of the unit or its state of adaptation. Within minutes the rate of spontaneous activity of the recorded ommatidium began to decrease and after about 1 hour, it stopped entirely. We measured the intensity-response function periodically, and after six hours it stabilized with the range and shape of the excised eye characteristic shown in Fig. 4.1a.

Hartline was intrigued by the new results, but remained skeptical of the spontaneous activity we recorded in complete darkness. He strongly recommended we go to the Marine Biological Laboratory, where he had initiated his studies, and repeat our experiments on freshly collected animals before submitting our results for publication. It was Spring 1971, and we had just finished writing a paper on this work for *Science*. However, we welcomed his suggestion, because one of us (R.B.) spent two summers at MBL during his graduate years and relished the opportunity to expose his graduate student (E.K.) to such an exciting environment. Time was short, and we had just two weeks to complete our work at MBL. Needless to say, it was an interesting challenge to assemble the necessary equipment and set up a working laboratory in that time span. We could not transport to MBL the large, shielded Faraday cage that only a short time ago had been home to one of us. Unfortunately, all of the Faraday cages at MBL were in use. Luckily we found in the dumpster a large cardboard box for shipping a children's toy (Johnny Lightning). We covered the box with aluminum foil for an electrical shield and filled all light leaks. The Johnny Lightning Faraday cage enjoyed a long life. We used if for the next 3 or 4 summers at MBL.

Our Woods Hole data matched perfectly those recorded in Syracuse. Spontaneous activity was the same rate (0.5 to 1.0 impulses/s) as we recorded in Syracuse. Hartline was satisfied. We submitted our paper in July, and *Science* published it in December (Barlow & Kaplan, 1971).

At that time Zwislocki was developing a generalized mathematical expression to describe the intensity-response (I-R) characteristics of sensory

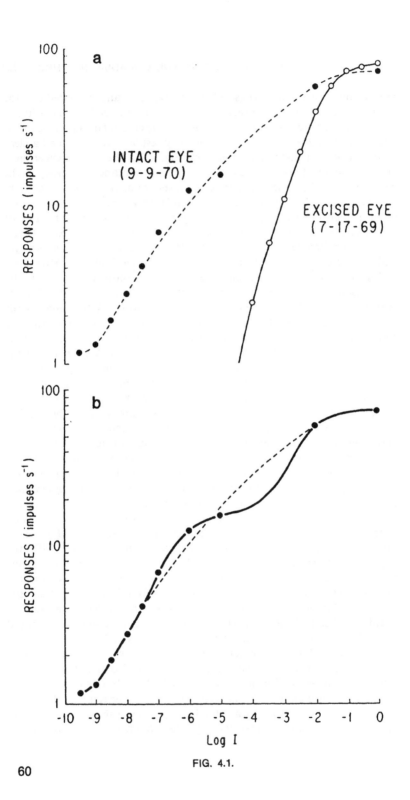

FIG. 4.1.

receptors (Zwislocki, 1973). He hypothesized that sensory transducers linearly integrate energy and perform a power-function transformation on the result. Any internal noise is linearly added to extrinsic signal energy. At low stimulus levels responses are directly proportional to stimulus energy. An exponential function models response saturation at high stimulus levels. Figure 4.2 shows that Zwislocki's theory for two independent receptor mechanisms (curve) fit well the physiological data we recorded from an intact eye.

Our next goal was to determine whether two receptor mechanisms did in fact encode light intensity in the intact eye as Zwislocki had suggested. The 10-log unit range of light intensity of *Limulus* ommatidia was about equal to the range of the human visual system measured psychophysically (see Barlow & Verrillo, 1976). Intensity coding in the human as in many other vertebrates is served by two receptors – rods and cones. *Limulus* ommatidia possess only a single photoreceptor – a retinular cell. If two receptor mechanisms exist, they must be within a single cell.

TWO RECEPTOR MECHANISM: PHYSIOLOGICAL EVIDENCE

To test the hypothesis that two receptor mechanisms encode light intensity in the intact *Limulus* eye, we studied the properties of incremental sensitivity, spectral sensitivity, light and dark adaptation, and the temporal properties of the impulse discharge of single ommatidia (Kaplan & Barlow, 1975). We briefly recount the results of these studies in this section.

The increment threshold function for steady-state responses contains two characteristic $\Delta I/I$ functions which meet at a "knee" corresponding to the plateau region in the I-R function in Fig. 4.2. This is not unexpected, because the entire $\Delta I/I$ function can be constructed directly from the I-R function simply by choosing a criterion for the increment response and reading the value of the increment threshold (ΔI) for each background level (I).

Light and dark adaptation also provided evidence for two receptor mechanisms. Light adaptation to an intermediate intensity (Log I = – 4) reduced the range of the I-R function from 10 to 5 log units with no substantial change in the shape of the function at high intensities. The

---

FIG. 4.1. (Opposite page) Intensity-response data for ommatidia in intact and excised lateral eyes of *Limulus*. a. Filled circles show first responses recorded by Kaplan and Barlow from an intact eye. Plotted are the mean steady-state responses measured in the last 5 sec of a 10 sec flash. All data are plotted as a log of the impulse discharge on the ordinate versus log of the relative light intensity on the abscissa. At log I = 0 approximately 10^{12} photons/s were incident on the ommatidium at the cornea between 400 and 700 nm. The dashed line was drawn by eye. (b) Unfilled circles show a typical I-R function for an excised eye. Excising the eye reduces sensitivity as much as 5 log units.

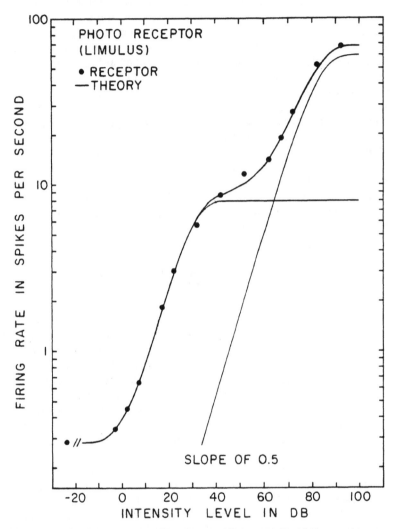

FIG. 4.2. Filled circles give the intensity-response function of an ommatidium in an unexcised *Limulus* eye (Kaplan & Barlow, unpublished data). The curves are theoretical. The thin lines were calculated from Zwislocki's model for receptors with two different sensitivities; the heavy line gives the linear sum of the two components. The left most data point represents spontaneous activity measured in complete darkness. (Adapted from "On Intensity Characteristics of Sensory Receptors: A Generalized Function," by J. J. Zwislocki, 1973, *Kybernetik*, *12*, p. 179. Copyright 1973 by Springer-Verlag. Reprinted by permission.)

light-adapted I-R function of the intact eye matched well that of the excised eye, suggesting that both light adaptation and excision desensitize one receptor mechanism more than the other. Dark adaptation mirrored the light adaptation results. Namely, the sensitivity of an ommatidum to bright-test flashes recovers almost immediately, whereas those to dim-test flashes recovers slowly, suggesting that a less-sensitive mechanism dark adapts rapidly, and a more-sensitive mechanism adapts slowly. Spectral sensitivity was unchanged by the state of adaptation of the eye, indicating that if two mechanisms generate the steady-state response, both utilize the same visual pigment hypothesized by Graham and Hartline (1935) and extracted by Hubbard and Wald (1960).

The temporal properties of the discharge of a single ommatiduim also point to two receptor mechanisms. At low-light intensities the discharge is irregular consisting mainly of bursts of nerve impulses. At higher intensities the bursts of nerve impulses disappear, and the discharge becomes regular as is generally recorded from excised eyes. In sum, two receptor mechanisms appear to function in the eye *in situ*: one at low light intensities (threshold ~ 1 absorbed photon), and the other at high intensities (threshold $\sim 10^5$ absorbed photon). Together they enable an ommatidium to operate over an intensity range of 10 log units. Table 4.1 taken from Kaplan and Barlow (1975) summarizes their properties.

The dual nature of the *Limulus* eye response appears to originate in the primary photoreceptor—the retinular cell. Figure 4.3 shows typical intracellular recordings from a retinular and second-order eccentric cell which receives its input from retinular cells and generates the optic-nerve discharge. The retinular cell exhibits two types of potential fluctuation: small potential fluctuations (SPFs) normally less then 20 mV in amplitude, and large potential fluctuations (LPFs) of up to 80 mV in amplitude (Barlow & Kaplan, 1977). The SPFs are the well-known quantum bumps that occur in darkness and can be evoked by single photons (Adolph, 1964; Yeandle,

TABLE 4.1
Properties of the Two Hypothesized Receptor Mechanisms

	A	B
Threshold (absorbed photons)	~ 1	10^5
Operating range	5 log units	5 log units
Shape of intensity function	Similar for both	
Spontaneous activity	Yes	No
Firing pattern	Irregular (bursting)	Regular
Dark adaptation	slow	Rapid
Increment threshold (slope of linear segment)	1.0 for both	
Spectral sensitivity	Same for both	
Survival after eye excision	Short	Long

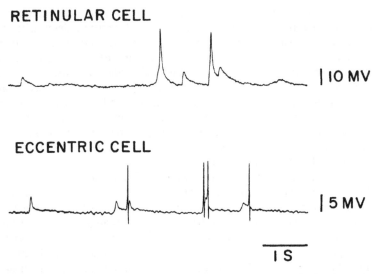

FIG. 4.3.   Intracellular recordings from dark-adapted cells *in situ* in the dark. The retinular cell spontaneously generated two types of potential fluctuations: quantum bumps (SPFs) and regenerative-like potentials (LPFs). Small depolarizing potentials in the eccentric cell often triggered one or more impulses in the optic-nerve fiber. These data were recorded in darkness. Light can trigger SPFs which in turn trigger LPFs and optic-nerve impulses. Amplitude of nerve impulses was attenuated 50% by the bandpass characteristic of the recorder. All other potentials in both cells are faithfully reproduced. Data were recorded from different eyes. (From Barlow & Kaplan, 1977. Reprinted with permission from the *Journal of General Physiology*.)

1958). The LPFs are regenerative events triggered by SPFs that enable single photons absorbed by retinular cells to fire off nerve impulses in the eccentric cell. LPFs dominate the receptor potential at low light levels, but are suppressed at high light levels where SPFs sum together to produce the receptor potential (Dodge, Knight, & Toyoda, 1968). LPFs and SPFs together provide wide-range intensity coding in single photoreceptor cells. Excising the adult lateral eye or cutting off its blood supply generally abolishes LPFs, although under optimal conditions, Dowling (1968) was able to record them from the excised eyes of juvenile *Limulus*. The two types of potentials—LPFs and SPFs—appear to underlie most of the dual-response characteristics we detected in the optic-nerve discharge of the intact lateral eye.

CIRCADIAN MODULATION OF THE RETINA: A SECOND SURPRISE

When we cut the optic nerve to pull it into the recording chamber attached to the carpace, we often wondered what type of information the eye lost from the brain. At about the time we were uncovering the differences between intact and excised eyes, Fahrenbach was publishing evidence for efferent fibers in the optic-nerve trunk (Fahrenbach, 1971) and efferent terminals on both retinular and eccentric cells (Fahrenbach, 1969, 1973). We wanted to first clarify the intact-excised eye dichotomy before tackling more complex issues, such as the role of the efferent input from the brain. However, in Summer 1973 while at the Marine Biological Laboratory we received a call from Mildred Behrens, Masonic Research Laboratory, Utica, NY, who was studying the effects of light and dark on the structure of the *Limulus* ommatidium. She asked if we would catch animals in the wild and fix their eyes at various times of the day and night under natural lighting. Hartline had recommended we repeat our Syracuse experiments with freshly collected animals at MBL, and now Behrens wanted to be certain her experiments in Utica could be replicated with animals caught in the wild.

We were more than willing to help Behrens and hoped she would also help us. Specifically, we asked her to check the structure of eyes excised and fixed at various times of day and night from animals maintained in constant darkness. We were well aware of the reports of endogenous circadian rhythms in the structure of compound invertebrate eyes (Welsh, 1938), their possible influence on retinal responses (Jahn & Crescitelli, 1940), and the involvement of both neural and humoral processes in the rhythmic changes of screening pigment and visual responses in the crayfish eye (Aréchiga & Wiersma, 1969). She agreed with our request, but could not think of a rapid fixation method that would avoid structural changes after excision similar to the physiological changes we had detected (Fig. 4.1a). William Miller from Yale Medical School, well-known for his earlier anatomical studies of the *Limulus* eye (Miller, 1958), suggested we excise the eyes and fix them by dropping them in boiling water. Using a propane camp stove, we excised and fixed eyes both day and night on Cape Cod beaches under natural lighting and in darkness in our MBL laboratory.

Behrens phoned us the following year (1974) in disbelief: The structure of eyes under both diurnal lighting and complete darkness changed with the time of day. Retinal structure appeared to possess a circadian rhythm, and light appeared to enhance the rhythm (Behrens, 1974). Because such structural rhythms were never detected in experiments that cut the optic nerve, we immediately suspected they were mediated by the efferent optic-nerve fibers found by Fahrenbach. We also suspected that the structural rhythms would induce daily oscillations in retinal response.

THE INSTITUTE FOR SENSORY RESEARCH: VISION PHYSIOLOGY COURSE

The next chapter in research on the *Limulus* lateral eye had to be put on hold until we finished moving the Laboratory of Sensory Communication from its humble two-story house to a magnificent facility at Skytop on South

Campus at Syracuse University. Zwislocki had succeeded in convincing the University that expansion was essential and well deserved. We changed the name of our research facility to the Institute for Sensory Research (ISR), and we renamed our educational program to Neuroscience. The year before our move one of us (E.K.) completed his doctorate and was invited by Hartline to carry out postdoctoral research at Rockefeller University. Hartline had an open invitation for the "first born" of R.B. William Adams (Chapter 2, this volume) was R.B.'s first student, but he continued research in auditory physiology after graduation. The second student, E.K., accepted Hartline's invitation and has been on the faculty of Rockefeller ever since.

The Vision Physiology course of the Neuroscience doctoral program was taught for the first time in the new quarters of ISR in 1975. New expanded facilities afforded excellent opportunities for more ambitious laboratory exercises in all courses. Past students in the course had learned to record ERGs using excised *Limulus* eyes. Now it was possible to use various preparations including the unexcised eye. Of course, I did not tell them of what we had suspected from Behren's data. I (R.B.) thought it would be great fun for students to discover circadian rhythms in the *Limulus* eye, if in fact they excised. Shortly after beginning the ERG experiment, two students — Stanley Bolanowski and Michael Brachman — came to me depressed. They complained they were unable to keep the visual sensitivity of the animal stable — it seemed to fluctuate day and night, even though the animal remained in complete darkness (Figure 4.4a). I was delighted to hear the news and asked whether they thought cutting the optic nerve would abolish the day–night changes and produce stable responses. Quickly a pool was formed, and students and faculty placed $1 bets on the outcome of optic-nerve section. It is not hard to imagine how I was betting.

Figure 4.4a shows that the ERG exhibited a circadian rhythm, and that cutting the optic nerve did indeed block the rhythm. It was immediately clear that efferent fibers in the optic nerve mediated circadian rhythms in retinal sensitivity. The laboratory was a beehive of activity as Bolanowski, Brachman, and I explored what was certain to be the next major chapter in research on the *Limulus* eye. The following summer Bolanowski and I went to MBL to study what effects the efferent input had on the afferent output of the retina. Figure 4.4b shows what we expected: The clock's input to the retina increased the optic-nerve response at night. We were surprised to find that the day–night changes in retinal sensitivity could be as much as 1,000,000 (Barlow, 1988).

MULTIPLE CIRCADIAN MECHANISMS MODULATE INTENSITY CODING

How does a circadian clock increase lateral-eye sensitivity 10^6 times at night? What are the cellular mechanisms? We turned our attention to these

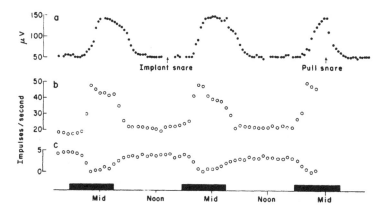

FIG. 4.4.   a. Circadian rhythm in the amplitude of the electroretinogram (ERG) of the lateral eye. Points give the peak amplitudes of the ERG in response to 50-ms test flashes of constant light intensity presented every 30 min while the animal remained in darkness. Cutting the optic nerve ("pull snare") on the third day of the experiment abolished the free-running rhythm in the ERG responses. b. Circadian rhythm in the optic-nerve response of a single dark-adapted ommatidium. Each point gives the mean firing rate of the ommatidium during the last 3 sec of 6 sec flashes presented every hour while the animal remained in darkness. The test flash delivered 10^5 quanta/s to the ommatidium at the cornea from 400 to 650 nm (corresponds to log I = −7 in Fig. 4.1.) c. Circadian rhythm in the spontaneous activity of a single dark-adapted ommatidium. Each point gives the mean rate of discharge of nerve impulses in a 25 sec interval in the dark. The data in (b) and (c) were recorded from the same optic-nerve fiber. d. Dark bars give the periods of general efferent optic-nerve activity recorded with a suction electrode from the proximal stump of the cut optic nerve. The animals remained in the dark throughout each 3-day experiment. (From "Efferent Optic Nerve Fibers Mediate Circadian Rhythms in the Limulus Eye," by R. B. Barlow, Jr., S. J. Bolanowski, and M. L. Brachman, 1977, *Science, 197*, p. 87. Copyright 1977 by AAAS. Reprinted by permission.)

questions with research carried out both at ISR and MBL. To summarize briefly, we discovered that circadian rhythms in photon catch, gain, and noise dramatically change intensity coding of the *Limulus* eye day and night.

Steven Chamberlain discovered that major circadian changes in retinal structure increase the photon-catching ability of the eye (Chamberlain & Barlow, 1984). He also discovered that the clock has a critical role in controlling the daily turnover of rhodopsin-containing membranes in the photoreceptor cells (Chamberlain & Barlow, 1979, 1984). Takehito Saito (Tsukuba University, Japan), George Renninger (Guelph University, Ontario), and Keith Purpura (Rockefeller University, New York) joined us in an intensive series of experiments to understand the clock's action at the cellular level by recording intracellularly from single photoreceptor cells. Without question, recording membrane potentials from single photoreceptor cells in the eyes of unanesthetized animals for several days were the most ambitious and difficult experiments ever attempted in our laboratory.

However, the results were worth the effort. We found that at night the clock's input lowered photoreceptor noise (Kaplan & Barlow, 1980), changed quantum bump shape (Kaplan, Barlow, Renninger, & Purpura, 1990), and increased photoreceptor gain (Barlow, Kaplan, Renninger, & Saito, 1987). Building on the earlier work of Barbara-Ann Battelle (1980), Leonard Kass (University of Maine) showed that the neuromodulator — octopamine — mimicked the clock's action on retinal sensitivity (Kass & Barlow, 1984) and structure (unpublished observation).

With Janice Pelletier (University of Maine) and Renninger, Kass also demonstrated the action of octopamine on noise and gain at the cellular level (Kass, Pelletier, Renninger, & Barlow, 1988). Ranjan Batra (University of Connecticut) discovered the clock's action on lateral inhibition (Batra & Barlow, 1982) and on the temporal transfer characteristics of the eye (Batra & Barlow, 1990). Kass and Berent (1988) showed that the clock could influence the dark adaptation of the eye. Table 4.2 lists the multiple circadian rhythms detected thus far in the *Limulus* eye.

The first in the list — efferent input — mediates all the others. All exhibit endogenous rhythms that combine with mechanisms of dark adaptation to increase retinal sensitivity as much as 1,000,000 times at night (last in the list). Behavioral studies in the field show conclusively that *Limulus* use there eyes to find mates (Barlow, Ireland, & Kass, 1982), and that they can see nearly as well at night as during the day (Powers, Barlow, & Kass, 1991).

Circadian neuromodulators, octopamine, and a putative neuropeptide act together with a blood-borne substance to form a push–pull mechanism controlling retinal structure and function (Barlow, Chamberlain, & Lehman, 1989). Herman Lehman (University of Arizona) and Bruce Calman (University of Florida) had key roles in establishing the existence of a critical factor in the blood (Chamberlain et al., 1987).

Circadian rhythms in photon catch, gain, and noise have the greatest influence, of those factors in Table 4.2, on the modulation of intensity coding. Figure 4.5 shows how these three factors combine to shift the intensity-response function of a single dark-adapted ommatidium from day to night. The "Day" function is graded over about 9 log units and has a shape characteristic of the intact eye with the optic nerve cut, which is expected because the circadian clock does not transmit efferent activity to the eye during the day (Barlow, Bolanowski, & Brachman, 1977). The onset of efferent activity causes a rapid increase in "gain" (upward arrow) and a rapid decrease in "noise" (downward arrow) producing an intermediate function (dashed line). Efferent input appears to reduce retinal noise by stabilizing the visual pigment — rhodopsin — via protonation of the Schiff-base linkage of retinal to opsin (Barlow, Birge, Kaplan, & Tallent, 1992). The increase in gain in the optic-nerve response at intermediate intensities represents an increase in membrane depolarization per absorbed photon.

TABLE 4.2
Circadian Rhythms in the *Limulus* Lateral Eye

Retinal property	Day	Night	Reference
Physiology			
Efferent input	Absent	Present	Barlow et al. (1977); Barlow (1983)
Gain	Low	High	Barlow et al. (1987); Renninger et al. (1984)
Noise	High	Low	Barlow et al. (1987, 1977); Kaplan and Barlow (1980)
Quantum bumps	Short	Long	Kaplan et al. (1990)
Frequency response	Fast	Slow	Batra (1983); Renninger (1983)
Dark adaptation	Fast	Slow	Kass and Berent (1988)
Lateral inhibition	Strong	Weak	Renninger and Barlow (1979); Batra and Barlow (1982)
Anatomy			
Cell position	Proximal	Distal	Chamberlain and Barlow (1977)
Pigment granules	Clustered	Dispersed	Barlow and Chamberlain (1980)
Aperture	Constructed	Dilated	Chamberlain and Barlow (1977)
Acceptance angle	6°	13°	Barlow et al. (1980)
Photomechanical movements	Trigger	Prime	Chamberlain and Barlow (1987)
Photon catch	Low	High	Barlow et al. (1980)
Metabolism			
Photoreceptor membrane turnover	Trigger	Prime	Chamberlain and Barlow (1979, 1984)
Intense light effects	Protected	Labile	(unpublished results)
Behavior			
Visual sensitivity	Low	High	Powers and Barlow (1985); Powers et al. (1991)

Studies of *Limulus* ventral photoreceptors (Pepose & Lisman, 1978) suggest that the efferent input may increase gain by reducing the efficacy of voltage-dependent K+ channels that repolarize the membrane potential during light exposure. In effect, the clock's input appears to increase response by suppressing a membrane mechanism of light adaptation. Prolonged input by the clock slowly changes retinal structure, which in turn increases the number of photons caught by each ommatidium and shifts the I-R function to the left by 1–1.3 log units. The clock's input produces about a 50-fold increase in the signal-to-noise characteristics of dark-adapted ommatidia.

Intensity coding changes significantly from day to night. Response is nearly a monotonic increasing function with light intensity at night. The clock's input nearly abolishes the intermediate plateau which we considered earlier in this chapter to be evidence of dual mechanisms for encoding light intensity (see Fig. 4.2). The dual receptor potentials — SPFs and LPFs — are

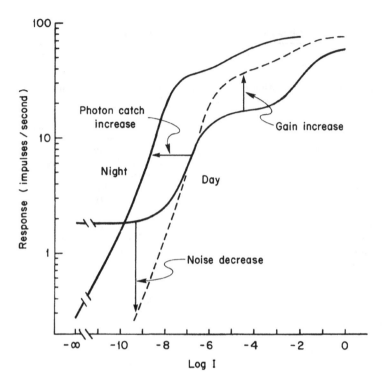

FIG. 4.5. Scheme of how circadian rhythms in noise, gain, and photon catch change the intensity coding properties of the *Limulus* eye. The onset of efferent activity at night causes a rapid increase in gain and decrease in noise producing an intermediate function (dashed line). Continued efferent input slowly increases photon catch which moves the I-R function to the left to produce the nighttime state. (From "Circadian Rhythms in Invertebrate Vision," by R. B. Barlow, Jr., S. C. Chamberlain, and H. K. Lehman, 1989, *Facets of Vision*, edited by D. C. Stavenga and R. C. Hardie, p. 268. Copyright 1989 by Springer-Verlag. Reprinted by permission.)

the building blocks of the photoreceptor response both day and night (Barlow et al., 1987). The plateau in the daytime I-R function appears to be shaped more by voltage-dependent conductances than by intensity-dependent shifts from LPFs to SPFs. As the clock suppresses voltage-dependent conductances at night, increasing light intensity induces a smooth transition from LPS to SPFs.

Research on the *Limulus* lateral eye has contributed significantly to our understanding of how sensory organs encode information and how properties of sensory organs may be modulated to optimize their performance under changing environmental conditions such as the day–night cycle of ambient illumination. We and our colleagues at the Laboratory of Sensory Communication, Institute for Sensory Research, and the Marine Biological

Laboratory extended the original studies of Hartline and his colleagues to the unexcised eye of *Limulus* and were richly rewarded for our efforts. It is indeed appropriate in this tribute to Jozef Zwislocki to acknowledge his many contributions to our studies. He created the research facilities, both LSC and ISR, supported the establishment of the Vision Laboratory, and offered many insightful suggestions as our research evolved. Although he has not appeared as a coauthor on any of our research reports, his footprints are certainly there.

ACKNOWLEDGMENTS

The authors gratefully acknowledge support from Grant BNS-9012069, National Science Foundation, and Grant EY-00667, National Institute of Health, Department of Health and Human Services.

REFERENCES

Adams, W. B. (1971). Intensity characteristics of the noctuid acoustic receptor. *Journal of General Physiology, 58*, 562–579.

Adolph, A. R. (1964). Spontaneous slow potential fluctuation in the *Limulus* photoreceptor. *Journal of General Physiology, 48*, 297–322.

Adrian, E. D., & Bronk, D. W. (1928). The discharge of impulses in motor nerve fibers. *Journal of Physiology, 66*, 81–101.

Aréchiga, H., & Wiersma, C. A. G. (1969). Circadian rhythm of responsiveness in crayfish visual units. *Journal of Neurobiology, 1*, 71–85.

Barlow, R. B., Jr. (1969). Inhibitory fields in the Limulus lateral eye. *Journal of General Physiology, 54*, 383–396.

Barlow, R. B., Jr. (1983). Circadian rhythms in the *Limulus* visual system. *Journal of Neuroscience, 3*, 856–870.

Barlow, R. B., Jr. (1988). A paradoxical result: Inhibition increases optic nerve activity. *Society Neuroscience Abstracts, 14*, 603.

Barlow, R. B., Jr. Birge, R. R., Kaplan, E., & Tallent, J. (1992). *On the molecular origin of photoreceptor noise.* Manuscript submitted for review.

Barlow, R. B., Jr., Bolanowski, S. J., & Brachman, M. L. (1977). Efferent optic nerve fibers mediate circadian rhythms in the *Limulus* eye. *Science, 197*, 86–89.

Barlow, R. B., Jr. & Chamberlain S. C. (1980). Light and a circadian clock modulate structure and function in *Limulus* photoreceptors. In T. P. Williams & B. N. Baker (Eds.), *The effects of constant light on visual processes* (pp. 247–269). New York: Plenum.

Barlow, R. B., Jr., Chamberlain S. C., Levinson J. Z. (1980). *Limulus* brain modulates the structure and function of the lateral eye. *Science, 210*, 1037–1039.

Barlow, R. B., Jr., Chamberlain, S. C., & Lehman, H. K. (1989). Circadian rhythms in invertebrate vision. In D. C. Stavenga & R. C. Hardie (Eds.), *Facets of vision* (pp. 257–280). Berlin-Heidelberg: Springer-Verlag.

Barlow, R. B., Jr., Ireland, L. C., & Kass, L.(1982). Vision has a role in *Limulus* mating behavior. *Nature, 296*, 65–66.

Barlow, R. B., Jr., & Kaplan, E. (1971). *Limulus* lateral eye. Properties of receptor units in the excised eye. *Science, 174*, 1027–1029.

Barlow, R. B., Jr., & Kaplan, E. (1977). Properties of visual cells in the lateral eye of *Limulus* in situ: Intracellular recording. *Journal of General Physiology*, *69*, 203–220.

Barlow, R. B., Jr., Kaplan, E., Renninger, G. H., & Saito, T. (1987). Circadian rhythms in Limulus photoreceptors. I. Intracellular recordings. *Journal of General Physiology*, *89*, 353–378.

Barlow, R. B., Jr., & Verrillo, R. T. (1976). Brightness sensation in a ganzfeld. *Vision Research*, *16*, 1291–1297.

Batra, R. (1983). *Efferent control of visual processing in the lateral eye of the horseshoe crab*. Unpublished doctoral dissertation, Institute for Sensory Research, Syracuse University, Syracuse, NY.

Batra, R., & Barlow, R. B., Jr. (1982). Efferent control of pattern vision in *Limulus*. *Society for Neuroscience Abstracts*, *8*, 49.

Batra, R., & Barlow, R. B., Jr. (1990). Circadian rhythms in the temporal response of the Limulus lateral eye. *Journal of General Physiology*, *95*, 229–224.

Battelle, B. -A. (1980). Neurotransmitter candidates in the visual system of *Limulus* polyphemus: Synthesis and distribution of octopamine. *Vision Research*, *20*, 911–922.

Baylor, D. A., & Fuortes, M. G. F. (1970). Electrical responses of single cones in the retinal of the turtle. *Journal of Physiology*, *20*, 77–92.

Behrens, M. E. (1974). Photomechanical changes in the ommatidia of the *Limulus* lateral eye during light and dark adaptation. *Journal of Comparative Physiology*, *89*, 45–57.

Chamberlain, S. C., Barlow, R. B., Jr., (1977). Morphological correlates of efferent circadian activity and light adaptation in the *Limulus* lateral eye. *Biological Bull. 153*: 418–419 (Abstr).

Chamberlain, S. C., & Barlow, R. B., Jr. (1979). Light and efferent activity control rhabdom turnover in *Limulus* photoreceptors. *Science*, *206*, 361–363.

Chamberlain, S. C., & Barlow, R. B., Jr. (1984). Transient membrane shedding in *Limulus* photoreceptors: Control mechanisms under natural lighting. *Journal of Neuroscience*, *42*, 792–2810.

Chamberlain, S. C., Barlow, R. B., Jr., (1987). Control of structural rhythms in the lateral eye of *Limulus*. Interactions of diurnal lighting and circadian efferent activity. *Journal of Neuroscience*, *7*, 2135–2144.

Chamberlain, S. C., Lehman, H. K., Schuyler, R. R., Vadasz, A., Calman, B. G., & Barlow, R. B., Jr. (1987). Efferent activity and circulating hormones: Dual roles in controlling the structure and mechanical movements of the *Limulus* lateral eye. *Investigative Ophthalmology, and Visual Science* (Supp., 28, 186).

Dodge, F. A., Jr., Knight, B. W., & Toyoda, J. (1968). Voltage noise in *Limulus* visual cells. *Science*, *160*, 88–90.

Dowling, J. E. (1968). Discrete potentials in the dark-adapted eye of the crab *Limulus*. *Nature*, *217*, 28–31.

Fahrenbach, W. H. (1969). The morphology of the eyes of *Limulus*. II. Ommatidia of the compound eye. *Zeitschrift Zellforschung Mikroskopisch Anatomie*, *93*, 451–483.

Fahrenbach, W. H. (1971). The morphology of the Limulus visual system IV. The lateral optic nerve. *Zeitschrift Zellforschung*, *114*, 532–545.

Fahrenbach, W. H. (1973). The morphology of the *Limulus* visual system. V. Protocerebral neurosecretion and ocular innervation. *Zeitschrift Zellforschung*, *144*, 153–166.

Graham, C., & Hartline, H. K. (1935). The response of single visual sense cells to lights of different wave lengths. *Journal of General Physiology*, *18*, 917–931.

Hartline, H. K. (1925). The electrical response to illumination of the eye in intact animals, including the human subject, and in decerebrate preparations. *American Journal of Physiology*, *73*, 600–612.

Hartline, H. K. (1972). Visual receptors and retinal interaction. In *Nobel Lectures: Physiology of Medicine 1963–1970* (pp. 269–288). New York: Elsevier.

Hartline, H. K., & Graham, C. (1932). Nerve impulses from single receptors in the eye. *Journal of Cellular and Comparative Physiology, 1*, 227–295.

Hartline, H. K., & McDonald, P. R. (1947). Light and dark adaptation of single photoreceptor elements in the eye of *Limulus. Journal of Cellular and Comparative Physiology, 30*, 225–253.

Hartline, H. K., & Ratliff, F. (1972). Inhibitory interaction in the retina of the *Limulus*. In M. G. F. Fourtes (Ed.), *Physiology of photoreceptor organs, Handbook of sensory physiology*. (Vol. VII/2, pp. 381–447). Berlin: Springer-Verlag.

Hubbard, R., & Wald, G. (1960). Visual pigment of the horseshoe crab, *Limulus polyphemus, Nature, 186*, 212–215.

Jahn, T. L., & Crescitelli, F. (1940). Diurnal changes in the electrical response of the compound eye. *Biological Bulletin, 78*, 42–52.

Kaplan, E., & Barlow, R. B., Jr. (1975). Properties of visual cells in the lateral eye of *Limulus* in situ. *Journal of General Physiology, 66*, 303–32.

Kaplan, E., & Barlow, R. B., Jr. (1980). Circadian clock in *Limulus* brain increases response and decreases noise of retinal photoreceptors. *Nature, 286*, 393–395.

Kaplan, E., Barlow, R. B. Jr., Renninger, G., & Purpura, K. (1990). Circadian rhythms in *Limulus* photoreceptors II. Quantum bumps. *Journal of General Physiology, 96*, 665–685.

Kass, L., & Barlow, R. B., Jr. (1984). Efferent neurotransmission of circadian rhythms in *Limulus* lateral eye. I. Octopamine-induced increases in retinal sensitivity. *Journal of Neuroscience, 4*, 904–917.

Kass, L., & Berent, M. D. (1988). Circadian rhythms in adaptation to light of *Limulus* photoreception. *Comparative Biochemistry and Physiology, C91*, 229–239.

Kass, L., Pelletier, J. L., Renninger, G. H., & Barlow, R. B., Jr. (1988). Efferent neurotransmission of circadian rhythms in *Limulus* lateral eye. *Journal of Comparative Physiology A, 164*, 95–105.

Miller, W. H. (1958). Fine structure of some invertebrate photoreceptors. *Anuals of the New York Academy of Sciences, 74*, 204–209.

Pepose, J. S., & Lisman, J. E. (1978). Voltage-sensitive potassium channels in Limulus ventral photoreceptors. *Journal of General Physiology, 71*, 101–120.

Powers, M. K., Barlow, R. B., Jr. (1985). Behavioral correlates of circadian rhythms in the *Limulus* visual system. *Biological Bulletin, 169*, 578–591.

Powers, M. K., Barlow, R. B., Jr. & Kass, L. (1991). Visual performance of horseshoe crabs day and night. *Visual Neuroscience, 7*, 179–189.

Renninger, G. H. (1983). Circadian changes in the frequency response of visual cells in the *Limulus* compound eye. *Society for Neuroscience Abstracts, 9*, 217.

Renninger, G. H., & Barlow, R. B., Jr. (1979). Lateral inhibition, excitation, and the circadian rhythm of the *Limulus* compound eye. *Society for Neuroscience Abstracts, 5*, 804.

Renninger, G. H., Kaplan, E., & Barlow, R. B., Jr., (1984). A circadian clock increases the gain of photoreceptor cells of the *Limulus* lateral eye. *Biological Bulletin, 167*, 532 (Abstr).

Ratliff, F. (1974). *Studies on excitation and inhibition in the retina: A collection of papers from the laboratories of H. K. Hartline*. New York: Rockefeller University Press.

Welsh, J. H. (1983). Diurnal rhythms. *Quarterly Review of Biology, 13*, 123–139.

Wolbarsht, M. L., & Yeandle, S. S. (1967). Visual processes in the Limulus eye. *Annual Review of Physiology, 29*, 513–532.

Yeandle, S. (1958). Electrophysiology of the visual system-discussion. *American Journal of Ophthalmology, 46*, 82–85.

Zwislocki, J. J. (1973). On intensity characteristics of sensory receptors: A generalized function. *Kybernetik, 12*, 169–183.

5 The Influence of Long-Range Spatial Interactions on Human Contrast Perception

Mark W. Cannon
Armstrong Laboratory AL/CFHP
Wright-Patterson Air Force Base

INTRODUCTION

An understanding of contrast perception is crucial to the development of models that can account for the human observer's ability to identify objects in the presence of complex backgrounds. Research over several decades has demonstrated that many facets of human contrast detection and perception can be explained by assuming that contrast information in the visual system is mediated by the responses of filter mechanisms tuned to a variety of spatial positions, spatial frequencies, and orientations (Blakemore & Campbell, 1969). This research has resulted in the publication of several computational models for contrast detection and contrast perception (Bergen, Wilson, & Cowan, 1979; Cannon & Fullenkamp, 1991a; Wilson & Bergen, 1979). One of the characteristics of these models is the assumed independence of the filter mechanisms across the spatial dimension. There are well-known spatial summation effects near threshold, where the threshold contrast of a sine-wave grating patch decreases as the number of cycles in the patch is increased, but these effects have been attributed to probability summation among independent noisy filter mechanisms (Quick, 1974). The spatial independence theory was reinforced by experiments showing that perceived contrasts for suprathreshold gabor-function stimuli (a sine-wave grating multiplied by a gaussian envelope) were apparently independent of the number of sine-wave cycles visible in the envelope (Cannon & Fullenkamp, 1988). The spatial-independence theory implied that any interference with the detection or perception of targets in a scene due to the presence of adjacent objects or texture regions must be attributed

75

to a processing stage more central than the processing that mediates the sensation of contrast. However, recent experiments from several laboratories have demonstrated changes in the apparent contrast of a centrally viewed stimulus due to the presence of adjacent patterns in the visual field. The data also indicate that the distance over which this lateral interaction is active is larger than the "receptive field" size proposed for most spatial filter mechanisms. These results indicate that models of early visual processing will require substantial revision.

Experiments by Chubb, Sperling, and Solomon (1989) showed that the apparent contrast of a patch of texture presented at the center of a rectangular texture-filled surround was suppressed when the texture in the surround had higher physical contrast than the texture in the center. Suppression was also strong when the central and surround textures were narrow-band filtered with identical spatial filters. However, suppression was reduced if the center and surround were filtered by bandpass filters tuned to different spatial frequency ranges. This implied that suppression was mediated by interconnections among mechanisms tuned to similar spatial frequencies.

Cannon and Fullenkamp (1991b) investigated this phenomenon using sine-wave gratings presented in a circular central patch embedded in the center of various grating-filled annular surrounds. The experiments were designed so that suppression could be studied as a function of the spatial frequency, orientation, contrast, and size of the surround grating. This chapter discusses some of these experiments, adds the results of more recent experiments, and indicates general properties of the lateral interaction network that can be inferred from both sets of experiments.

METHODS

Typical stimuli used for studying spatial contrast effects are shown in Fig. 5.1. The experiments were conducted to determine how the apparent contrast of the small sine-wave-filled central patch was affected by the presence of a sine-wave-filled annular surround. Three surround-to-center contrast ratios are shown in the figure. The panel labeled "high surround" contains a surround sine wave equal to twice the physical contrast of the central sine-wave patch. The "low-surround panel" contains a sine wave equal to $\frac{1}{2}$ the physical contrast of the central sine-wave patch. In the "equal"-surround panel the central and surround sine waves obviously have the same contrast.

The sine-wave gratings were digitized and displayed on a video monitor using an analog contrast controller, built in house. All gratings were in sine phase with the center of the display, so they have an average luminance equal to the average luminance of the background (about $100cd/m^2$). The

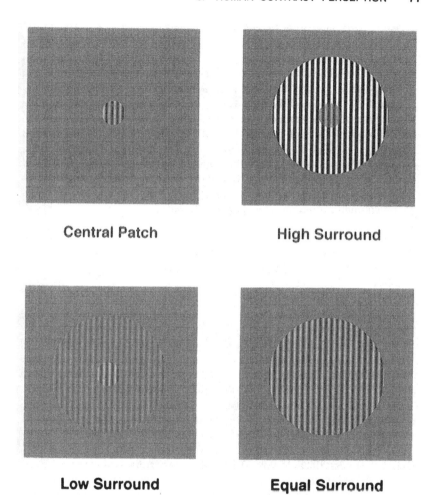

Central Patch   **High Surround**

Low Surround   **Equal Surround**

FIG. 5.1.   Typical stimuli used to measure spatial interactions.

boundary between the central patch and the surround was marked by very small dots placed on the monitor screen at the top and bottom of the central patch region. These fixation aids showed the observers where to attend in the case where the surround and central patch had equal contrasts. A method of constant stimulus-matching paradigm was used. The contrast of the embedded patch and surround was fixed in each experimental session. The contrast of the isolated central patch was presented at one of eight contrasts spanning a range chosen in a preliminary experiment to bracket an exact match. Embedded and isolated patches were each presented for 1 sec in one of two consecutive 2-sec viewing intervals marked by auditory tones. Presentations were counterbalanced so that embedded and isolated patches appeared in the first interval an equal number of times. Observers indicated, by pressing a two-position switch, which interval contained the central patch of greater contrast. Each isolated central-patch contrast was presented 10 times, and the data were plotted as a histogram showing the number of times the isolated patch had higher apparent contrast than the embedded patch for each contrast level of the isolated patch. The histogram amplitudes, divided by 10, approximated a psychometric function which expressed the probability that the isolated patch had higher apparent contrast than the embedded one versus the contrast of the isolated patch. The contrast of perceptual equality was the isolated patch contrast at which the psychometric function crossed the 50% point.

RESULTS FOR FIXED SURROUND AND CENTER CONTRASTS

The Effect of Surround Size

The experiments discussed in this section were performed with three observers and measured apparent contrast of the central grating patch as a function of surround width in cycles when the surround-to-center contrast ratio was fixed at 2.0, with the central patch contrast at 0.25 and the surround contrast at 0.5. Both center and surround contained gratings of the same spatial frequency. Results of three observers and three spatial frequencies are illustrated in Fig. 5.2. The vertical axis in these plots is the central-patch apparent contrast divided by the central-patch physical contrast. This ratio was chosen, because a match of the isolated central patch with itself was almost always veridical, that is, the matching contrast was always very close to 0.25. All subsequent figures conform to this same normalization procedure for the vertical axis. The horizontal axis is the width of the surround annulus in cycles, measured along a radius from the edge of the central patch to the outer edge of the annulus. The horizontal line at a ratio of 1 indicates a veridical match with the isolated patch. Any points below this line indicate that the apparent contrast of the embedded patch has been suppressed by the presence of the surround. Apparent contrast for all three observers declines with surround width, and the curves for different spatial frequencies lie almost on top of each other when surround width is expressed in cycles. The data imply that contributions to suppression come from surround regions as far away as 10 cycles from the center of the embedded patch (the embedded patch has a radius of 2 cycles), although most of the suppression occurs within the first 4 cycles. Note that if the surround width had been expressed in degrees, the 2-cycle-per-degree (c/deg) curves would have decreased much

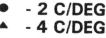
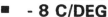

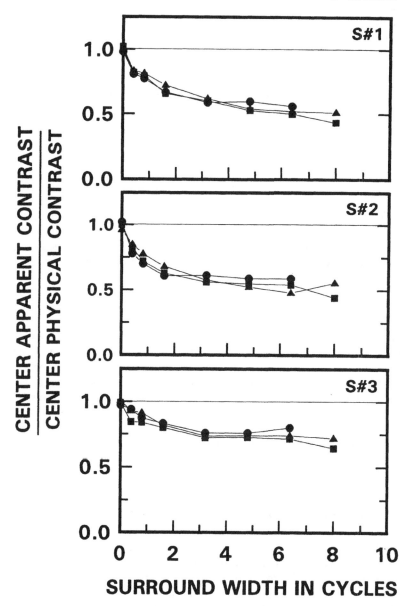

FIG. 5.2. Suppression of central-patch apparent contrast by fixed-contrast surrounds of increasing width at three different spatial frequencies. Both center and surround contained gratings of the same spatial frequency.

more slowly with surround width than the 8-c/deg curves. Thus, the spatial weighting function associated with suppression of the 8-c/deg stimulus is of smaller spatial extent in degrees than the spatial weighting function associated with suppression of the 2-c/deg stimulus, but has about the same halfwidth in cycles. The data imply that the halfwidth of the weighting function describing the inhibitory effect of a peripheral mechanism on a target mechanism attending to the central patch, when both are tuned to the same spatial frequency, is proportional to the period of the spatial frequency to which the mechanisms are tuned.

The Effect of Surround Orientation

The same three observers matched the isolated patch to an embedded patch as the orientation of the surround grating was changed from 0° to 90°. The data are shown in Fig. 5.3. The spatial frequency was 8 c/deg, the surround size was maintained at 8 cycles, and the surround to center contrast ratio was 2.0. Note that the apparent contrast of the central patch increases steeply as the surround orientation changes by 15° and increases much more slowly thereafter. The suppression effect never completely disappears, even when the surround orientation reaches 90°.

The Effect of Spatial Frequency

The three observers matched an isolated central patch to an embedded central patch as the spatial frequency of the surround was changed from one octave below the spatial frequency of the central patch to one octave above. Central patch spatial frequencies were 2, 4, and 8 c/deg. In each case the central patch had a diameter of 4 cycles, and the surround width was 6.4 cycles. The data are illustrated in Fig. 5.4. Suppression at 8 c/deg is strongest when surround and center are at the same spatial frequency and declines as the surround spatial frequency is set above or below this value. At a center spatial frequency of 2 c/deg, however, the suppression is essentially constant at all surround spatial frequencies.

CONCLUSIONS FROM FIXED-CONTRAST EXPERIMENTS

The data from these experiments imply a complex-interconnection scheme among contrast-sensitive tuned mechanisms responding to the central sine-wave grating and those responding to the surround sine-wave grating. Apparently, mechanisms responding to the sine-wave grating in the central patch receive inhibitory inputs from spatially distant mechanisms tuned to different spatial frequencies and orientations. The strength of this interac-

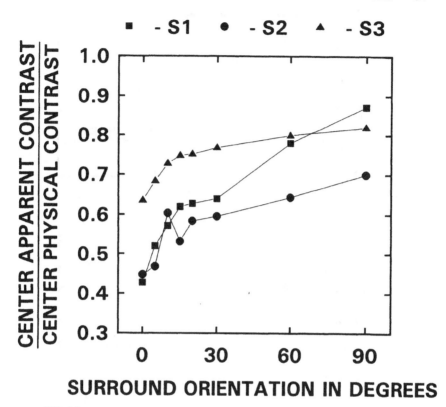

FIG. 5.3. Suppression of central-patch apparent contrast by fixed-contrast surrounds containing gratings of different orientations. Central-patch grating orientation remained vertical.

tion versus the distance between interacting mechanisms can be described in terms of a spatial weighting function. The spatial weighting functions responsible for the inhibition may have several components. (a) The weighting function falls off with distance, because most of the inhibitory effects in Fig. 5.2 occur within about 6 cycles of the center of the embedded grating patch. (b) Mechanisms tuned to 8 c/deg appear to have a weighting-function component that falls off rapidly with a spatial-frequency difference between mechanisms responding to center and surround and another component that increases slowly with the absolute spatial frequency of mechanisms responding to the surround (Fig.5.4). (c)Mechanisms mediating contrast perception for the 2-c/deg central patch are suppressed equally by all surround spatial frequencies studied. This implies that they receive inhibitory inputs of the same strength from distant mechanisms tuned to spatial frequencies from 1 to 4 c/deg. The tuned component of

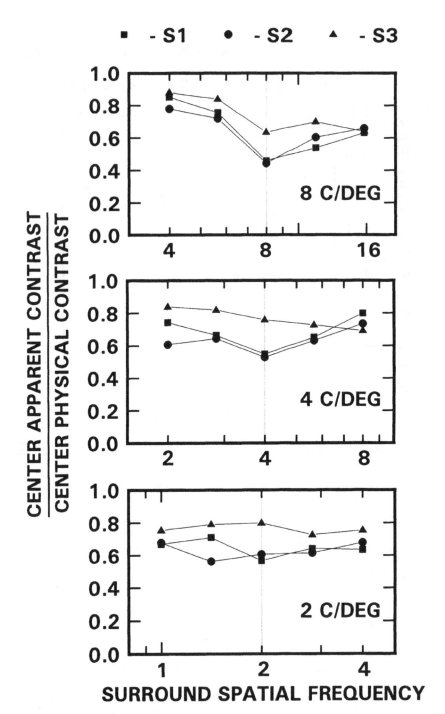

FIG. 5.4. Suppression of central-patch apparent contrast by fixed-contrast surrounds containing gratings of different spatial frequencies. Spatial-frequency tuning is evident at 8 c/deg, but not at 2 c/deg.

inhibition, apparent at 8 c/deg, disappears at 2 c/deg. (d) Mechanisms tuned to 8 c/deg receive inhibitory inputs from spatially distant mechanisms with different orientations. This spatial weighting function also appears to have two components, one of which falls rapidly with an orientation difference between the mechanisms, and the other which declines very slowly with an orientation difference. Thus, the data imply the existence of an extensive inhibitory network linking tuned mechanisms across space. The apparent complexity of this network increased further when we studied the effect of contrast with an expanded observer pool. Some of these observers showed both suppression and enhancement of the central patch, depending on the contrast conditions.

RESULTS OF CHANGES IN SURROUND AND CENTER CONTRAST

Data From Observers Who Showed Only Inhibition

In these experiments, the apparent contrast of the central patch was studied with both center and surround spatial frequencies fixed at 8 c/deg. Three surround-to-center contrast ratios were used (2.0, 1.0, and 0.5), and each of these ratios was studied for four central-patch contrasts (0.03125, 0.0625, 0.125, and 0.25). Data for two observers who showed only suppression of the embedded central patch are shown in Fig. 5.5. The three vertically positioned panels on each side of the figure contain data from the three surround-to-center contrast ratios. These ratios are indicated by the symbol in the upper right-hand corner of the left column of panels. The ratios of 2.0, 1.0, and 0.5 are indicated by 2X, 1X, and 0.5X, respectively. The four curves in each panel represent the four central-patch contrast levels studied for each surround-to-center contrast ratios. The data are plotted in the usual way, as center-apparent contrast/center-physical contrast versus surround width in cycles. Data points below the horizontal line at 1 represent suppression of the central patch by the surround. Data points above the line represent enhancement of the central patch by the surround. These subjects show only suppression. An interesting feature of their data is that all four curves in each panel lie close together and have basically the same shape. Central-patch contrast, for these subjects, has essentially no effect on the inhibition. The strength of suppression varies only with surround-to-center ratio. Higher surround-to-center ratios produce stronger suppression.

Data From Observers Who Showed Both Suppression and Enhancement

The data in Fig. 5.6 are typical of 6 observers who showed enhancement as well as suppression of central-patch apparent contrast. The three lower

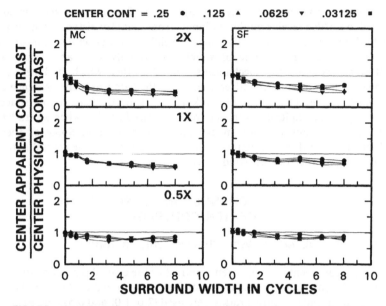

FIG. 5.5. Central-patch apparent contrast as a function of surround size for two observers who show only suppression. Suppression effects are largely independent of central-patch contrast. The graphs show data for four different central-patch contrasts and the three surround-to-center contrasts ratios illustrated in Fig. 5.1.

curves in the 2X panels show suppression effects similar to those seen in Fig. 5.5. The curves corresponding to a central-patch physical contrast of 0.03125, however, show enhancement for small surround sizes and almost no change in central-patch contrast for larger surround sizes. Three observers also showed enhancement for the 1X condition, but the position of the enhancement peak along the surround-size axis was not as consistent as the peak in the 2X condition. Responses for the 0.5X condition were almost all suppressive. In all cases in which enhancement occurred, it was confined to the lowest central-patch contrast condition.

Data From Observers Who Showed Enhancement Under Most Experimental Conditions

The data illustrated in Fig. 5.7 are, with the exception of one panel, completely different from the data produced by any other observers. This exception is the 2X panel for observer DR. These data are similar to the data shown in the 2X panels of Fig. 5.6, except for the fact that DR shows enhancement for small surround sizes at all but the highest central-patch

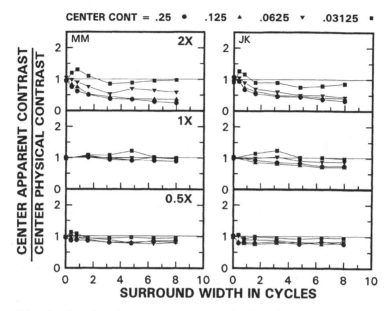

FIG. 5.6. Central-patch apparent contrast as a function of surround size for two observers who show both enhancement and suppression. Enhancement only occurs at the lowest central-patch contrast. The experimental conditions are the same as in Fig. 5.5.

contrast. The other experimental conditions show strong enhancement of the central-patch apparent contrast that increases in strength as the contrast of the central patch decreases.

The 2X data of observer DR showed suppression of central-patch contrast as surround width increased. Because DR had shown only enhancement for lower surround-to-center contrast ratios, it appeared likely that the 2X data were showing some sort of transition from enhancement to suppression. Thus, both DR and KD were tested with a range of surround-to-center ratios that extended from 0.125 to 16.0 with a surround width of 6.4 cycles. Due to the available linear contrast range of our monitor (0 to 0.55), the highest contrast ratios were tested with a low-contrast central patch. The center contrasts used in the experiment were 0.03125, 0.0625, 0.125, and 0.25. Each of these central-patch contrast was tested with surround contrasts of 0.03125, 0.0625, 0.125, 0.25, and 0.5. The results of these experiments are shown in Fig. 5.8. As expected, observer DR showed enhancement at surround-to-center ratios less than or equal to 1. However, DR's central-patch apparent contrast showed only suppression for surround-to-center ratios greater than 1.0. Observer KD also showed suppression, but only for surround-to-center ratios higher than 2.0. Thus, both observers,

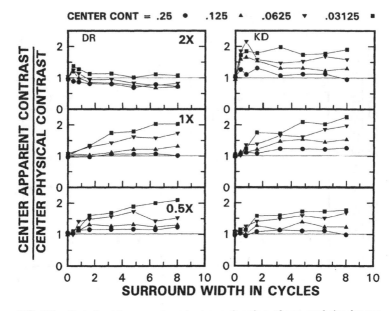

FIG. 5.7. Central-patch apparent contrast as a function of surround size for two observers who show mainly enhancement. Enhancement increases as central-patch contrast decreases. The experimental conditions are the same as in Fig. 5.5.

who showed strong enhancement for the experimental conditions in Fig.5.7, experienced a transition to suppressive behavior as the surround-to-center contrast ratio increased.

CONCLUSIONS FROM VARIABLE-CONTRAST DATA

The data obtained by varying center and surround contrast indicate a much more complex set of interconnections among tuned mechanisms than those deduced from the fixed-contrast data illustrated in Figs. 5.2, 5.3, and 5.4.

Consider the data in Fig. 5.5. These observers show no trace of enhancement; so it can be assumed that their responses reflect, primarily, the operation of the system that mediates suppressive interactions. Because the four curves in each panel lie more or less on top of each other, it appears that the *suppressive* interactions are dependent primarily on the surround-to-center contrast ratio and not dependent on the contrast of the central patch or the average contrast of the entire center-plus-surround stimulus.

Now consider the data in Fig. 5.7. Assume that KD's data represent, primarily, the action of the system that mediates the enhancement interac-

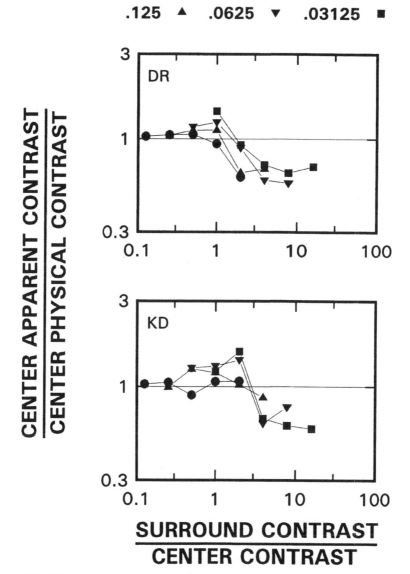

FIG. 5.8. Central-patch apparent contrast as a function of surround-to-center contrast ratio for two observers who showed mainly enhancement in Fig. 5.7. Both observers show suppression as the surround-to-center ratio increases beyond 2.0.

tions. Because the curves are distinctly ordered with central-patch contrast, it appears that *enhancement* interactions depend strongly on the absolute contrast of the central patch or the average contrast of the center plus surround. Enhancement strength increases as contrast decreases. The enhancement system also shows a dependence on surround size as evidenced by the positive slopes for the lower contrast curves in the 1X and 0.5X panels of Fig. 5.7.

Finally, consider the data of Fig. 5.6. Enhancement for those observers, represented by the data in Fig. 5.6, occurred most strongly and consistently for small surround sizes at a surround-to-center ratio of 2. The fact that this effect occurs most consistently when the surround contrast is higher than the center contrast implies that mechanisms responding to the positive contrast change across the edge separating center and surround may be contributing to the enhancement effect. Responses of edge-sensitive mechanisms would remain constant as the surround width increased, and this constant response could explain the separation of the lowest contrast curves in the 2X panels of Fig. 5.6 from the rest of the curves. The reduction in the apparent contrast beyond the peak could be the action of the inhibitory system acting to reduce the edge effect. The fact that KD's data in the 2X panel of Fig. 7 show an initial steep rise for small surround sizes could also be explained by an edge effect. This sharp rise is absent when there is no edge, under the 1X condition, or when the edge is negative, under the 0.5X condition. The data in both Figs. 5.6 and 5.7 imply that this possible edge effect is also contrast dependent. The effect increases as central-patch contrast decreases.

The apparent-contrast data of KD, for the 1X and 0.5X conditions, and of DR, for the 0.5X condition, in Fig. 5.7 show little enhancement for the 0.4- and 0.8-cycle surrounds. However, both observers show a fairly steep rise in enhancement at a surround width of 1.6 cycles, implying that the maximal enhancement for a mechanism responding to the central patch may come from the response of a mechanism responding to a portion of the surround some distance from the central patch. Thus, the nonedge component of the excitatory weighting function may be in the form of an annular surround.

The apparent contrast of the central patch may be analyzed in terms of enhancement due to a contrast-dependent excitatory network that receives inputs from mechanisms responding to both the annular-surround grating and the inner edge of the annular-surround grating, and suppression due to an inhibitory network that responds to the annular-surround grating and is dependent only on the surround-to-center contrast ratio. In this context observers KD and DR show stronger enhancement responses to both the edge and annular surround than the six observers characterized by the data in Fig. 5.6. Both DR and KD appear to show edge effects for all four central-patch contrasts in the 2X panels, while the Fig. 5.6 observers show an effect only for the lowest central-patch contrast. The two observers in Fig. 5.5 must have extremely weak edge and enhancement mechanisms that are completely masked by suppression effects.

GENERAL CONCLUSIONS

These are not the first experiments to observe both enhancement and suppression of the apparent contrast of a grating patch due to the presence of gratings in the surrounding visual field. Ejima and Takahashi (1985) studied the apparent contrast of a rectangular grating patch which was bordered to the right and left or above and below by other rectangular grating patches. When the surround grating was of higher contrast than the central grating, they observed that the apparent contrast of the central grating was suppressed. When the contrast of the surround grating was less than the contrast of the central grating, the apparent contrast of the central grating was enhanced. They only presented data from two observers—the authors—but their results are similar to the results from observers DR and KD shown in Figs. 5.7 and 5.8. The Ejima and Takahashi enhancement values were not as large as those shown by KD and DR, but the Ejima and Takahashi experiment was performed at a lower spatial frequency (3 vs. 8 c/deg), and the geometry of the stimuli were different. Ejima and Takahashi also claimed that the enhancement effect was contrast dependent, while the suppression effect was not. This agrees with the data in Figs. 5.5 and 5.7 discussed previously. The data presented here demonstrate some of the features of what appears to be a complex lateral-interconnection network among tuned contrast-sensitive mechanisms.

There is also neurophysiological evidence for suppression and enhancement of tuned contrast-sensitive cells in the striate cortex of monkeys and cats. DeValois, Thorell, and Albrecht (1985), using sine-wave grating stimuli, found evidence for both inhibitory and facilitatory regions surrounding the classic receptive fields. The optimal receptive-field width for the cells they studied was about 2 cycles. Many cells showed a monotonic decrease in firing rate as the width of the sine-wave grating was extended from 2 to 6 or 7 cycles. Other cells showed a reduction in firing rate followed by an increase for the same range of stimulus size.

Further experiments and quantitative modeling are required to understand the operation of the lateral-interaction system more fully. Both suppression and enhancement effects are quite large with sine-wave grating stimuli, but it is not yet possible to assess what role this system plays in spatial pattern processing for complex real-world scenes.

REFERENCES

Bergen, J. R., Wilson, H. R., & Cowan, J. D. (1979). Further evidence for four mechanisms mediating vision at threshold: Sensitivities to complex gratings and aperiodic stimuli. *Journal of the Optical Society of America, 69*, 1580–1587.

Blakemore, C., & Campbell, F. W. (1969). On the existence of neurones in the human visual system selectively sensitive to the orientation and size of retinal images. *Journal of Physiology, 203*, 237–260.

Cannon, M. W., & Fullenkamp, S. C. (1988). Perceived contrast and stimulus size: Experiment and simulation. *Vision Research, 28*, 695–709.

Cannon, M. W., & Fullenkamp, S. C. (1991a). A transducer model for contrast perception. *Vision Research, 31*, 983–998.

Cannon, M. W., & Fullenkamp, S. C. (1991b). Spatial interactions in apparent contrast: Inhibitory effects among grating patterns of different spatial frequencies, spatial positions and orientations. *Vision Research, 31*, 1985–1998.

Chubb, C., Sperling, G., & Solomon, J. A. (1989). Texture interactions determine perceived contrast. *Proceedings of the National Academy of Sciences, 86*, 9631–9635.

DeValois, R. L., Thorell, L. G., & Albrecht, D. G. (1985). Periodicity of striate-cortex-cell receptive fields. *Journal of the Optical Society of America A, 2*, 1115–1123.

Ejima, Y., & Takahashi, S. (1985). Apparent contrast of a sinusoidal grating in the simultaneous presence of peripheral gratings. *Vision Research, 25*, 1223–1232.

Quick, R. F. (1974). A vector magnitude model of contrast detection. *Kybernetik, 16*, 65–67.

Wilson, H. R., & Bergen, J. R. (1979). A four mechanism model for threshold spatial vision. *Vision Research, 19*, 19–23

6 Cochlear Potentials in Quiet-Aged Gerbils: Does the Aging Cochlea Need a Jump Start?

Richard A. Schmiedt
Medical University of South Carolina

INTRODUCTION

The sense of hearing tends to decline with age, a well-known but poorly understood process that is termed *presbyacusis*. We have been exploring the Mongolian gerbil as a model of presbyacusis using brainstem-evoked responses (BSER), compound action potentials of the auditory nerve (CAP), cochlear microphonics (CM) recorded at the round window (RW), single-fiber recordings in the auditory nerve, and measures of the endocochlear potentials (EP) within scala media (Hellstrom & Schmiedt, 1990, 1991; Mills, Schmiedt, & Kulish, 1990; Schmiedt, Mills, & Adams, 1990; Schulte & Schmiedt, 1992; Tarnowski, Schmiedt, Hellstrom, Lee, & Adams, 1991).

Measures of EP have become an important adjunct to our neural studies for several reasons. First, from anatomical and histological work it is apparent that the stria vascularis in these old gerbils is most often abnormal or even absent at specific locations along the cochlear duct (Schulte & Adams, 1989; Schmiedt & Schulte, 1992; Schulte & Schmiedt, 1992). Second, the hair-cell loss in quiet-aged gerbils is often minimal, characterized by a scattered loss of outer hair cells (OHC) and almost no loss of inner hair cells (IHC) (Tarnowski et al., 1991). Third, the work of Sewell (1984), demonstrating a linear relation between the EP (in mV) and the CAP threshold (in dB SPL) in young cats treated acutely with furosemide, suggests that the degeneration of the stria may play a role in the loss of neural thresholds in these aged gerbils.

In this chapter, dedicated to my mentor, Dr. Josef Zwislocki, some relations between cochlear and neural potentials are examined, and a simple model is developed to explain some of the results that at first seem to be contradictory.

METHODS

The methods used in these studies have all been described before. The CAP data were gathered using techniques as outlined in Hellstrom and Schmiedt (1990), and Schmiedt et al. (1990). The EP values were obtained as described in Schmiedt and Zwislocki (1977). All three groups of gerbils (young controls less than 8 months, 30 months, and 36 months) were born and raised in acoustically treated quarters where ambient sound levels are less than 49 dBA 99% of the time, and median levels are between 35 and 40 dBA (Mills et al., 1990).

Very briefly, CAP and CM are measured with a silver-ball electrode on the bony niche surrounding the round window of the gerbil cochlea (Chamberlain, 1977). Tone pips with 0.75 ms rise/fall times are used to elicit the CAP response; the pips have an overall duration of 1.8 ms and are shaped with an approximately Gaussian envelope.

EP is measured with a single micropipette in scala media. The micropipettes are filled with 0.5 M KCI, and their tips are left unbroken, resulting in impedances of around 10 Mohms. Voltages are always referred to a pellet of chlorided silver surrounded by cotton soaked in saline and embedded in the neck muscles.

The micropipettes are introduced into scala media via 50–100 m diameter holes drilled in the bony lateral wall. The locations of the holes correspond to cochlear best frequencies of 16 kHz (T1), 2 kHz (T2), and 0.5 kHz (T3) (Schmiedt & Zwislocki, 1977). Electrodes are then introduced into the RW, T3, T2, and T1, usually in that order. Junction potentials are recorded before the micropipette is inserted into each hole, and again after the pipette is removed (to control for the possibility of tip breakage).

RESULTS AND DISCUSSION

CAP Thresholds and EP

Average CAP thresholds are shown in the upper panel of Fig. 6.1 for each of the three groups. The mean thresholds of the 30-month group are essentially shifted in parallel to those of the controls. The mean thresholds of the 36-month group are further elevated, with an increased shift at frequencies greater than 4 kHz. The mean EP data from the same three groups of animals are plotted in the lower panel. (Valid EP measures were not always obtained at all four locations for each of the ears; thus, the

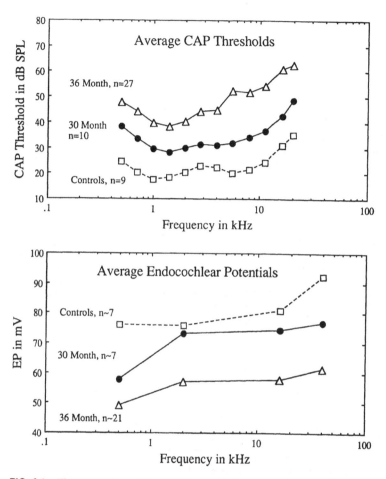

FIG. 6.1. The mean values of the CAP thresholds (upper panel) and the EP (lower panel) plotted as a function of frequency for the three groups of gerbils. The points correspond to the mean data in Tabs. 6.1 and 6.2. There is essentially a parallel shift of CAP thresholds in the 30-month group, and an additional shift, greater at high frequencies, in the 36-month group. The EP decline in the 30-month group is greatest in the base and apex with little shift seen in the midcochlea. At 36 months, however, there is a significant decline of EP throughout the cochlea. A 2 factor ANOVA using the 12 frequencies as repeated measures indicates that the three groups are significantly different at the 95% level for both the CAP and EP data.

number of ears is smaller for the three groups in the lower graph than in the upper one.) It is clear that the EP values measured at the base and apex of the cochlea show the largest declines with age, whereas the midcochlear values are closest to normal.

Tables 6.1 and 6.2 outline the actual mean and standard errors for the

TABLE 6.1
Cap Anova Results [X ± SEM]

kHz	CTRL (N=9)	30M (N=10)	36M (N=27)
0.5	24.7±0.8	38.2±3.8[a]	47.8±17.0[a]
0.7	20.4±0.8	33.6±3.7	44.3± 3.4[a]
1.0	17.6±0.8	29.6±3.4	39.6± 3.5[a]
1.4	18.4±0.4	28.3±2.6	38.4± 3.8[a]
2.0	20.4±0.4	29.9±2.4	40.3± 3.9[a]
2.8	22.9±0.8	31.4±1.8	44.2± 3.9[a,b]
4.0	22.4±0.7	31.1±1.3	44.7± 3.8[a,b]
5.6	20.0±1.3	31.9±1.9	52.3± 3.6[a,b]
8.0	21.6±1.2	34.2±2.0	51.7± 3.4[a,b]
11.3	24.2±1.2	36.5±2.4	54.3± 3.3[a,b]
16.0	30.9±1.6	42.6±2.9	61.2± 3.4[a,b]
20.0	35.3±4.6	48.7±2.2	62.7± 3.8[a,b]

[a]significance at 95% from control group [b]significance at 95% from 30-month group

Mean values of the CAP thresholds in dB SPL obtained at 12 frequencies for the three groups of gerbils. Also shown is the standard error of the mean (SEM) at each frequency measure. The population (n) is the same for all frequencies. Significance was tested at the 95% level using a single-factor ANOVA test. All of the CAP thresholds of the 36-month group are significantly different from those of the controls; those above 2 kHz are significantly different from those of the 30-month group.

TABLE 6.2
EP Anova Results [X ± SEM (N)]

	kHz	CTRL	30M	36M
T3	0.5	76.1±4.7(7)	57.7±7.6 (7)	49.1±4.1[a] (22)
T2	2.0	75.8±4.9(8)	73.1±4.7 (9)	57.0±4.5[a,b](22)
T1	16.0	80.8±3.3(9)	74.2±4.3 (9)	57.8±5.2[a,b](21)
RW	40.0	92.3±2.0(7)	76.7±2.7[a](10)	61.3±3.6[a,b](26)

[a]significance at 95% from control group [b]significance at 95% from 30-month group

Mean values and SEMs of the EPs measured at four cochlear locations in the three groups of gerbils. Because of problems in obtaining a reliable EP value at each location in some animals, the population (n) differs for each measure. Otherwise, the animals represented in this table are from the same population as represented in Tab. 6.1. All of the EP values of the 36-month group are significantly different from those of the controls; the three more basal locations are also different from those of the 30-month group.

CAP and EP data presented in Fig. 6.1. A one-factor analysis of variance (ANOVA) treating each frequency separately shows that all the 36-month data are significantly different from the control data, and some of the 36-month data are significantly different from the 30-month data. A two-factor ANOVA using the frequencies as repeated measures reveals that each of the three groups is significantly different from the others for both the AP and EP data.

According to the acute cat experiments of Sewell (1984), the shifts in CAP thresholds should be linearly related to the shifts in EP. To assess whether this relationship is valid in any of the three groups, the shifts of the EP and those of the associated CAP thresholds were plotted against one another. The shifts were derived by normalizing to the respective mean values obtained from the control group. Thus, the EP shifts at three cochlear locations (T1, T2, and T3) are plotted against the CAP shifts at the associated frequencies (16, 2, and 0.5 kHz, respectively). Round window values were not used, because the frequency associated with this position is around 40 kHz, and no acoustic data are available. Each point in the scatter plots represents a paired measure of CAP and EP data from one animal. Linear regression lines were calculated, and their correlation coefficient (r), slope, and intercept are shown within each graph. Note that a slope of zero forces the correlation coefficient to be zero as well. Examples of regression lines near-zero slopes and correspondingly low r values are found in the top two panels of Fig. 6.2.

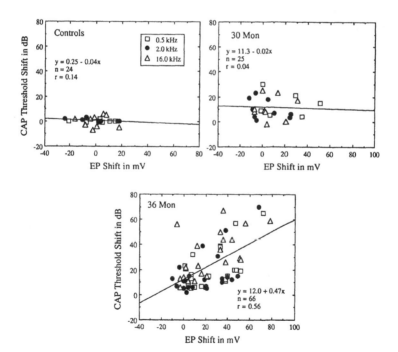

FIG. 6.2.   Scatterplots of CAP threshold shifts and EP shifts for young controls, 30- and 36-month-old gerbils. Each point represents a CAP and EP measurement from one animal. The 0.5, 2, and 16 kHz CAP data are paired with EP data obtained from cochlear turns 3, 2, and 1, respectively. Note that only the oldest group of animals shows a correlation of CAP threshold shifts with EP shifts.

The upper-left panel of Fig. 6.2 illustrates the regression line calculated for the control group. There is little variation in the CAP shift (± 5 dB) with substantial variation in the EP shift (± 20 mV). EP values ranged from 100 to 60 mV in our young control animals; all measures were highly stable and repeatable. We believe the scatter seen in the control EPs is truly a result of interanimal variability and not an artifact of measurement.

The shifts of the 30- and 36-month groups are similarly plotted in the top-right and bottom panels of Fig. 6.2, respectively. The correlation coefficients are low, and the slopes are negative or near zero in the 30-month group at all locations. However, the correlations rise to moderately high values ($r = 0.56$) in the data obtained from the 36-month group. The r value of the 36-month group indicates that around 31% of the variability in the CAP data can be explained with the EP shift.

From Fig. 6.2 it is clear that there can be a relatively large variation in the EP magnitude that is not reflected in the CAP thresholds, even among young controls. Perhaps in gerbils the acute dependence of the CAP threshold is not as tightly coupled to the EP as Sewell (1984) has shown for cats? Figure 6.3 demonstrates that this is not the case: gerbils and cats behave similarly with the application of systemic furosemide. Indeed, there

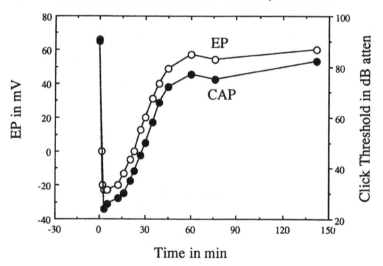

FIG. 6.3. EP and CAP thresholds to clicks for a control gerbil after a bolus of furosemide was administered through the external jugular vein. The total dose of furosemide was 125 mg/kg injected over 1 minute. Note the excellent correlation of the EP and CAP threshold. The correlation follows closely that of Sewell (1984) in cats and is approximately 1 dB/mV.

is a 1 millivolt/dB relation between EP decrease and CAP threshold shift to a click—a relation that also is seen in cats.

The operative word in the above paragraph is *acute*. From our experience with quiet-aged gerbils it seems clear that the transduction mechanism in the cochlea can adapt to chronic decreases in EP. In other words, the CAP thresholds can remain sensitive with little interanimal variation in spite of 40 mV differences in EP. Thus, even though the furosemide studies are informative as to what is going on acutely, their results cannot be applied to the chronic condition.

CAP and CM Input/Output Functions

One of the most apparent changes with age in the cochlear physiology of gerbils is the decrease in the magnitude of the CAP response. Both the slope and maximum amplitude of the input/output (I/O) function are reduced, often dramatically, as shown in Fig. 6.4. Threshold shifts are often far less

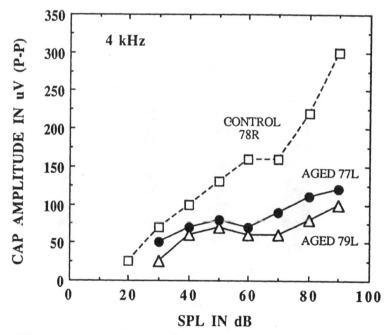

FIG. 6.4.   CAP input/output (I/O) functions for a young control (open squares) and two 36-month-old gerbils to a 4-kHz tone pip. The CAP response was obtained with a 4-kHz probe tone. Note that even though the threshold of the CAP is only shifted about 10 dB, there are significant declines in the slope of the I/O function and in the maximum amplitudes in the older animals.

significant than the overall reduction in CAP amplitude at high SPLs would suggest.

In contrast to the CAP response, there is little difference in the RW CM among young and old gerbils. Indeed, there is a trend for the CM amplitudes to be slightly *higher* in the older animals as shown in Fig. 6.5. While the difference in mean values does not reach statistical significance between the young and old gerbils in Fig. 6.5, some of the greatest CM values have been recorded in old gerbils, animals with a significant decline in their EP.

Examples of lowered EP coupled with greater than normal CM amplitudes in two quiet-aged gerbils are shown in Fig. 6.6. Especially puzzling is the fact that animal RS-108 shows the largest CM amplitude coupled with a significant EP loss (of about 40 mV at the RW). How is it possible for the EP to decrease with a concomitant increase in the CM?

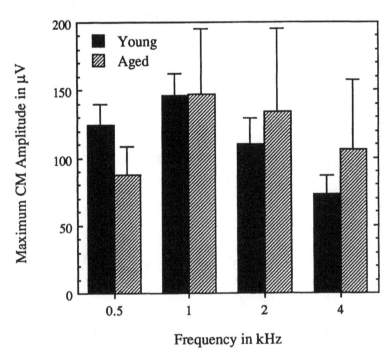

FIG. 6.5. Bar graph showing mean maximum amplitudes and SEMs of the CM recorded from RW electrodes in young ($n = 9$) and quiet-aged ($n = 11$) animals. Differences are not significant between the two populations at any frequency. The CM remains constant, or may even be larger, in the older animals, despite significant declines in the EP.

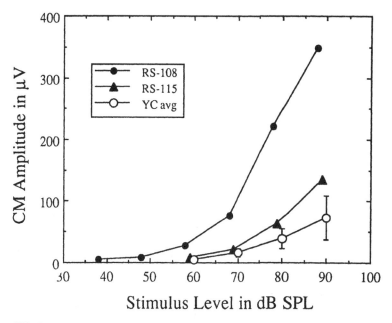

FIG. 6.6.   CMI/O functions recorded at the round window for 2 quiet-aged animals compared to average values from 9 young controls. Error bars represent 1 standard deviation. EP measured at the RW, T1, T2, and T3 for RS-108 was 49, 60, 56, and 55 mV, respectively. Gerbil RS-115 had EP values of 68, 76, and 69 mV at T1, T2, nd T3, respectively. It is clear that reduced EP does not necessarily diminish the CM.

The Dead Battery Theory

A simple way to understand what may be happening in these old cochleas with regard to declining EP coupled with an excessive CM follows from the reduction of the resistance pathways in the cochlea to their Thevenin equivalent (Cannon, 1976; Dallos, 1983). The resulting model, shown as the inset in Fig. 6.7, consists of a Thevenin battery (V_T) and source resistance (V_T) coupled to a hair cell-resistance split into a fixed (R_H) and a variable (ΔR) portion.

Decreased EP can be modeled as either a decrease in the battery voltage, an increase in the series Thevenin resistance, or both. Treating the network as a simple voltage divider, we see that the CM peak–peak (p–p) voltage can be expressed as:

$$V_{CM} = V_T \left\{ \left[\frac{R_H + \Delta R}{R_T + R_H + \Delta R} \right] - \left[\frac{R_H - \Delta R}{R_T + R_H - \Delta R} \right] \right\} \qquad (1)$$

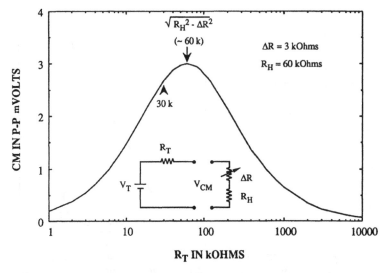

FIG. 6.7.   A simple model that can explain how the CM in older animals can be larger than normal despite significant declines in the EP. Inset: A Thevenin equivalent circuit representing the strial battery and the various resistance pathways in the cochlear electroanatomy. The load represents the basal (fixed, R_H) and the apical (varying, resistances of the hair cells. The CM is assumed to be measured across both load resistors. Curve: V_{CM} as a function of the Thevenin resistance, R_T. The curve was calculated for the indicated values of R_H and R, with $V_T = 120$ mV. The arrowhead at R_H kohms represents the quiescent value of the circuit in a young animal. It is assumed that R_T increases with age (see text).

From Equation 1 it is clear that a decrease in V_T will directly decrease the CM voltage. However, the effect of changing the series resistance R_T is not as intuitive. Assuming values as shown in Fig. 6.6 and that $V_T = 120$ mV, graphing V_{CM} versus R_T shows that there is a clear maximum in the CM voltage when R_T is changed. Note that by using these values the EP is 80 mV when $\Delta R = 0$, and the CM voltage is around 2.7 mV p-p (arrowhead). By setting the first derivative to zero, we see that the maximum CM voltage occurs when:

$$R_T = \sqrt{(R_H)^2 - (\Delta R)^2} \tag{2}$$

or, in this example, when $R_T = 59.98$ kohms and $V_{CM} = 3.0$ mV p-p.

The above equation is intuitively satisfying, because it is well known that maximum power transfer is obtained when the load resistance equals the source resistance, which is what Equation 2 reduces to when $\Delta R = 0$.

In this scenario, the normal equivalent source resistance in the cochlea is much less than its load resistance, creating a condition that would lie to the left of the maximum on the curve of Fig. 6.6. The effect of age would be to gradually increase the source resistance. Of course, if the source resistance becomes greater than the load, the CM amplitudes will begin to diminish.

The reference to a "dead battery" comes from the fact that the equivalent series resistance in a battery also increases with age, until a point is reached where the voltage drop across the series resistance is great enough to adversely affect the function of the battery. The obvious analogy here is best invoked by my remembrance of the cold nights during the Syracuse winter. After working in the lab until the wee hours of the morning, there were times when I came out to a car made inoperative by a dead battery. Note that the series resistance of a battery increases with decreasing temperature, a fact that is usually not dwelled on when one is faced with a cold walk home.

Jump-Starting the Dead Battery

An obvious solution to a dead battery is to provide another voltage source to effectively reduce the high source resistance. While not a true test of the above model, an attempt was made to "bypass" the dead strial battery in some quiet-aged gerbils to attempt to acutely restore some of the chronic loss of function. Cochlear function was monitored by means of CAP I/O functions, and current was injected with a double-barreled electrode in scala media; one barrel measured EP, the other was used to inject current from a constant current source. The electrodes were filled with 0.5 M KCl, and the return path of the current was through a Ag–AgCl pellet buried in the neck muscles.

Figure 6.8 shows the results from one animal. The initial CAP I/O function was obtained with an EP of 41 mV at T1. Current injection of $10\mu A$ resulted in a threshold decrease of about 20 dB and a maximum amplitude increase from 20 to 50 mV. The CAP response remained more sensitive for several minutes after the current injection. This residual sensitivity may have been caused by the extra K^+ pushed out electrophoretically by the current injection or by the acutely increased EP.

So it is apparently possible to jump-start old cochleas. The problem with this sort of prothesis is that a DC current is needed in scala media. DC currents in fluid environments are electrolytically difficult to manage and the violation of the scala media environment is almost certain to be detrimental to cells lining that compartment. Thus, the best scenario will be to somehow replace the pumps in the appropriate cells which maintain the EP in the first place. This will be a job for future molecular biologists.

ACKNOWLEDGMENTS

The author wishes to thank L. I. Hellstrom, F. S. Lee, and J. H. Mills for their help with this chapter. Implicit in all my research is the appreciation for Zwislocki's

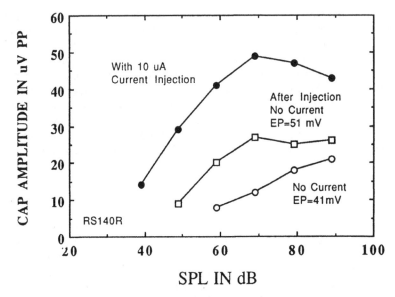

FIG. 6.8. Effects of current injection into scala media of T1 on the CAP response to a 4-kHz tone pip in a quiet-aged gerbil. The no-current I/O function was obtained initially with the electrode in place without current injection. Ten μA of current were injected, and the upper I/O function was obtained during the current injection. The middle I/O function was obtained several minutes after the current injection had ceased (see text).

contribution to my education. This work was supported by program grant DC00422-06 from NIDCD, National Institutes of Health, U.S. Department of Health and Human Services.

REFERENCES

Cannon, M. W., Jr. (1976). *Electrical impedances, current pathways, and voltage sources in the guinea pig cochlea* (Rep. ISR-14). Syracuse, NY: Institute for Sensory Research, Syracuse University.

Chamberlain, S. C. (1977). Neuroanatomical aspects of the gerbils inner ear: Light microscopic observations. *Journal of Comparative Neurology, 171*, 193–204.

Dallos, P. (1983). Some electrical circuit properties of the organ of Corti. I. Analysis without reactive elements. *Hearing Research, 12*, 89–119.

Hellstrom, L. I., & Schmiedt, R. A. (1990). Compound action potential input/output functions in young and quiet-aged gerbils. *Hearing Research, 50*, 163–174.

Hellstrom, L. I., & Schmiedt, R. A. (1991). Rate/level functions of auditory-nerve fibers in young and quiet-aged gerbils. *Hearing Research, 53*, 217–222.

Mills, J. H., Schmiedt, R. A., & Kulish, L. F. (1990). Age-related changes in auditory potentials of Mongolian gerbils. *Hearing Research, 46*, 201–210.

Schmiedt, R. A., & Schulte, B. A. (1992). Physiologic and histopathologic changes in quiet- and noise-aged gerbil cochleas. In A. L. Dancer, D. Henderson, R. J. Salvi, & R. P. Hamernik (Eds.), *Noise-induced hearing loss* (pp. 246–256). St. Louis, MO: Mosby—Year Book.

Schmiedt, R. A., & Zwislocki, J. J. (1977). Comparison of sound-transmission and cochlear-microphonic characteristics in Mongolian gerbil and guinea pig. *Journal of the Acoustical Society of America, 61*, 133–149.

Schmiedt, R. A., Mills, J. H., & Adams, J. C. (1990). Tuning and suppression in auditory nerve fibers of aged gerbils raised in quiet or noise. *Hearing Research, 45*, 221–236.

Schulte, B. A., & Adams, J. C. (1989). Distribution of immunoreactive Na^+, K^+ -ATPase in gerbil cochlea. *Journal of Histochemistry & Cytochemistry, 37*, 127–134.

Schulte, B. A., & Schmiedt, R. A. (1992). Lateral wall Na, -K-ATPase and endocochlear potentials decline with age in quiet-reared gerbils. *Hearing Research, 61*, 35–46.

Sewell, W. (1984). The effects of furosemide on the endocochlear potential and auditory-nerve fiber tuning curves in cats. *Hearing Research, 14*, 305–314.

Tarnowski, B. I., Schmiedt, R. A., Hellstrom, L. I., Lee, F. S., & Adams, J. C. (1991). Age-related changes in cochleas of mongolian gerbils. *Hearing Research, 54*, 123–134.

7
Photoreceptors, Black Smokers, and Seasonal Affective Disorder: Evidence for Photostasis

Steven C. Chamberlain
Eric P. Hornstein
Syracuse University

INTRODUCTION

Increasingly we are realizing that neurons and their various components are dynamic entities. The turnover of the cell membrane and remodeling of synapses, for example, may be commonplace. The daily shedding and renewal of light-sensitive membrane is a prominent feature of photoreceptors in both vertebrates and invertebrates, despite their rather different schemes for assembling arrays of such membrane. Until recently, massive cycling of photosensitive membrane was thought to be a universal process that presumably replaced light-damaged, or time-dated, components in the discs of rods and cones and the microvilli of rhabdoms. The effort to demonstrate the need for daily photoreceptor membrane shedding has proved difficult, however, and the creeping realization that some animals may lack this fundamental retinal process requires a reexamination of our assumptions about membrane turnover in photoreceptors. The basic question is why daily cycling of photosensitive membrane occurs at all.

In 1986, Penn and Williams reported homeostasis of quantum catch in albino rats raised in cyclic lighting of several different intensities. The mechanism for maintaining quantum catch involved changing the size and efficacy of the retinal photoreceptors. They named this constancy in quantum catch *photostasis* and suggested that the purpose of disc shedding and synthesis in rods was to maintain photostasis. If so, then the daily cycling of photosensitive membrane is made necessary by the seasonal variation in daily light exposure. Furthermore, animals living in lighting environments lacking seasons might not need such a metabolically demanding daily process. In this chapter, we compare the photoreceptors of four diverse species of invertebrates—the horseshoe crab which lives in seasonally changing cyclic lighting and three species of deep sea crustaceans which live in constant-light environments without seasons. Our objective is to evaluate photosensitive membrane turnover as a homeostatic mechanism for photostasis.

PHOTORECEPTORS OF THE HORSESHOE CRAB—*LIMULUS POLYPHEMUS*

The horseshoe crab (color plate, upper left) lives in shallow water along the east coast of North America. Its lighting environment is therefore both cyclic and seasonal. Two compound lateral eyes (Fig. 7.1) provide a rich model system for investigating all manner of retinal processes, including the daily shedding of photosensitive membrane (Chamberlain & Barlow, 1979, 1984).

In a mature adult, each eye is an array of about 1,000 modular assemblies—the ommatidia. In each ommatidium, about a dozen photoreceptors are arranged like the segments of a lemon about the central dendrite of the eccentric cell (see Fahrenbach, 1975, for an extensive review of the anatomy). The cuticular cone gathers light by internal refraction and directs it through the aperture to the rhabdom. Each photoreceptor contributes to the rhabdom with a specialized microvillar array along the central surface of its rhabdomeral segment (Fig. 7.2) whose cytoplasm is also specialized for its role in supporting phototransduction. The majority of the cytoplasm, however, is contained in the A-segment where most of the activities common to all neurons occur.

Each ommatidium is extensively innervated by efferent fibers from the brain (Fahrenbach, 1981). These fibers arise from neurons in the cheliceral ganglion (Calman & Battelle, 1991; Lee & Wyse, 1991) and appear to use octopamine as a neurotransmitter (e.g., Battelle, Evans, & Chamberlain, 1982; Evans, Chamberlain, & Battelle, 1983; Kass & Barlow, 1984). The efferents are driven by a circadian clock such that they are active at night and silent during the day (Barlow, 1983; Barlow, Bolanowski, & Brachman, 1977). The results of this cyclic efferent drive are diverse (see Barlow, Chamberlain, & Lehman, 1989, and Battelle, 1991, for recent reviews). Efferent activity increases the sensitivity of the lateral eye (Barlow et al., 1977), changes the strength of lateral inhibition between ommatidia (Batra & Barlow, 1990), reduces photoreceptor noise (Kaplan & Barlow, 1980), moves screening pigment (Kier & Chamberlain, 1990), and primes photomechanical movements (Chamberlain & Barlow, 1987), to mention just a few. The most obvious morphological reflection of circadian efferent input

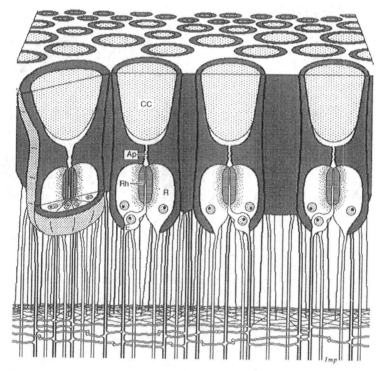

FIG. 7.1. Diagrammatic view of the horseshoe crab compound eye. Refractive cuticular cones (CC) gather light for each ommatidium and aim it through the aperture (AP). Photons are absorbed in the rhabdom (Rh) of the photoreceptors (retinular cells, R) where transduction to a depolarization in membrane potential occurs. The eccentric cell (E) is electrically coupled to the photoreceptors and generates nerve impulses which travel to the brain. The extensive plexus of eccentric cell lateral processes underlying the retina serves to mediate lateral inhibition.

is the daily remodeling of the ommatidium (color plate, upper right) which includes changes in the aperture and the arrangement of the rhabdom (Barlow, Chamberlain, & Levinson, 1980; Chamberlain & Barlow, 1987) and almost certainly involves actin and microtubules (Calman & Chamberlain, 1992).

The effect of circadian efferent drive most germane to this discussion, however, is the priming of daily rhabdom shedding (Chamberlain & Barlow, 1979, 1984). Figure 7.3 shows the ultrastructure of the process. Efferent activity during the darkness of night is necessary to prime the light-initiated shedding of rhabdomeral membrane in the morning. During the night (Fig. 7.3A) the microvilli are long, thin, and well organized in the rhabdom. The light of dawn causes a seemingly catastrophic disruption of

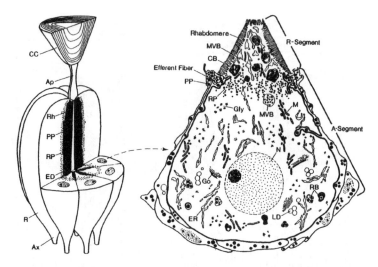

FIG. 7.2.   Structure and ultrastructure of photoreceptors in the horseshoe crab lateral
eye. The drawing on the left shows eight photoreceptors cells arranged like the segments
of a lemon around the central dendrite of the eccentric cell. On the cutaway surface the
rhabdom appears as rays along the photoreceptor–photoreceptor boundaries. The
drawing on the right shows a cross section of one photoreceptor. The surface
rhabdomeral segment (R-segment) is completely covered by the microvillar rhabdomere
where photons are absorbed. Most of the organelles normally found in neurons are
contained in the arhabdomeral segment (A-segment). The efferent fibers which
innervate the retina from the brain run along the peripheral ends of the rhabdom rays
as shown. Ap—aperture; Ax—photoreceptor axon; CB—combination bodies; CC—
cuticular cone; ED—eccentric cell dendrite; ER—endoplasmic reticulum; Gly—gly-
cogen rosettes; Go—Golgi complex; LD—lipid droplets; M—mitochondrion; MVB—
multivesicular bodies; N—nucleus; PP—screening pigment in pigment cells; R—
retinular cell (photoreceptor); RB—residual bodies; Rh—rhabdom; RP—screening
pigment in retinular cells.

the microvilli (Fig. 7.3B) with large amounts of microvillar membrane
thrown out into the R-segment cytoplasm as whorls, thereby reducing the
microvilli to short, fat stumps in a disorganized array. Within an hour of
this shedding event, however, the rhabdom is reconstituted and a cloud of
small multivesicular bodies lines the inner surface of the rhabdom (Fig.
7.3C). These multivesicular bodies gradually coalesce and move from the
R-segment cytoplasm into the A-segment cytoplasm (Figs. 7.3D,E). Figure
7.4 summarizes the sequence of cytoplasmic structures that constitute
transient rhabdom shedding and subsequent degradation in the photoreceptors of the horseshoe crab lateral eye.

The daily, efferent-primed, light-initiated transient shedding of the
microvillar membrane in *Limulus* photoreceptors is a robust phenomenon
which must be metabolically costly to the retina. Although the details vary,
in overall strategy it is typical of cyclic photosensitive membrane turnover

Upper Left: Dorsal views of an adult and a juvenile horseshoe crab, *Limulus polyphemus.* The lateral compound eyes of this animal are a well-studied model system for investigating the effects of circadian neural feedback from the brain to the eye. *Upper Right:* Circadian changes in retinal structure in the horseshoe crab. These 1-micron plastic sections stained with toluidine blue were cut along the optic axis of ommatidia from animals maintained in darkness. On the left is the structure typical of daytime. The aperture below the dark blue cuticular cone is narrowed and long, and the purple rays of the rhabdom are stretched away from the aperture. On the right is the structure typical of nighttime. The aperture below the cuticular cone is short and wide, and the purple rays of the rhabdom are pushed into the best position to catch light. These changes produce the circadian rhythm in the eye's sensitivity and resolution.

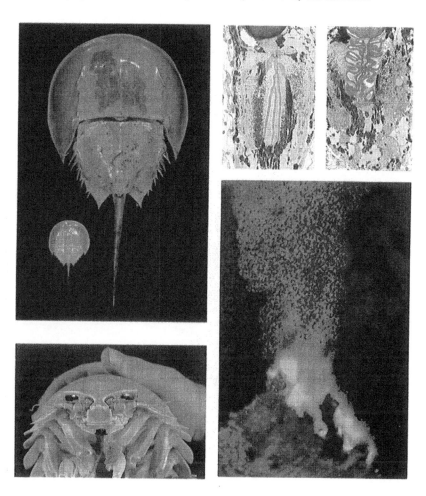

Lower left: Head on view of the giant deep sea isopod, *Bathynomus giganteus. Lower right:* Image-processed photograph of light emitted by a deep sea hydrothermal vent. This photograph was taken in 1988 during a series of ALVIN dives by Smith, Delaney, and Van Dover on the Endeavour Segment of the Juan de Fuca Ridge off the coast of the Pacific Northwest. Photograph courtesy of Milt Smith, University of Washington.

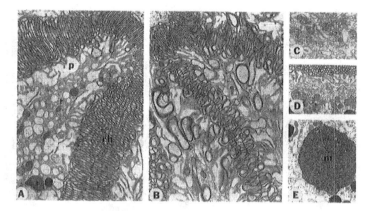

FIG. 7.3.   Rhabdom shedding in the horseshoe crab lateral eye. A. Ultrastructure of normal, dark-adapted retina before the light of dawn initiates membrane shedding. The microvilli of the rhabdom (rh) are long and well organized. Subrhabdomeral palisades (p) line the edges of the rhabdom rays. r—retinular cell cytoplasm; e—eccentric cell dendrite. B. Fifteen to 30 minutes after light exposure, much rhabdomeral membrane is incorporated into whorls, and the remaining microvilli are short and thick. The central ring between the retinular cells and the eccentric cell dendrite at upper left is largely spared. C. One hour after light-initiated rhabdom shedding, the microvilli are again well organized, and a cloud of small multivesicular bodies occupies the space formerly consisting of subrhabdomeral palisade. D. Two hours after shedding commences, smaller multivesicular bodies are aggregating into larger ones, and the whole array is moving away from the rhabdom. E. Four hours after shedding onset, aggregation has produced large multivesicular bodies (m) which have moved peripherally toward the A-segment.

in a wide range of vertebrates and invertebrates. Absent maintenance of photostasis, the purpose of this massive daily event has proved hard to elucidate. For example, a recent study (Smith, Friedman, & Goldsmith, 1991) failed to find any change in retinoids as a result of the shedding and rebuilding of the rhabdom. On the other hand, a preliminary study (Hoenig & Chamberlain, 1989), wherein animals were adapted to lowered intensities of natural cyclic lighting, yielded results consistent with the photostasis hypothesis, although it was not demonstrated that membrane turnover was involved. The role of photosensitive membrane turnover in *Limulus* remains unclear.

PHOTORECEPTORS OF THE DEEP SEA ISOPOD— *BATHYNOMUS GIGANTEUS*

Bathynomus giganteus, a rarely encountered abyssal species, is the largest known isopod (color plate, lower left). Its frontally directed triangular eyes are well adapted for its lifestyle as a predator of bioluminescing species

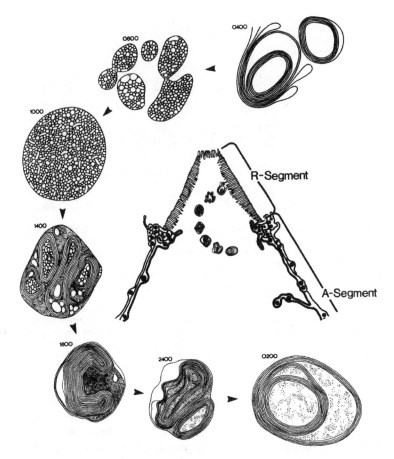

FIG. 7.4. Summary of rhabdom shedding in the photoreceptors of the lateral eye of the horseshoe crab. In summer, dawn triggers rhabdom shedding around 4 a.m. with the formation of membrane whorls. These whorls break into multivesicular bodies, which then coalesce and gradually convert to combination bodies and lamellar bodies. By 2 a.m. the following day, the lamellar bodies have moved well into the A-segment cytoplasm and have lost most of their contents to the surrounding cytoplasm. At other times of the year, the initiation of shedding, like dawn, occurs somewhat later in the day.

(Chamberlain, Meyer-Rochow, & Dossert, 1986). *B. giganteus* lives at a depth of 500–600 m, where no significant cyclic light penetrates from the surface, and the ambient light is largely derived from bioluminescence.

Figure 7.5 summarizes the retinal structure of *B. giganteus*. For the present discussion, a significant difference between this species and *Limulus* is that the proximal core of each ommatidium is occupied by interstitial cells which serve as a mirror. Microvilli concentrated in the hypertrophied

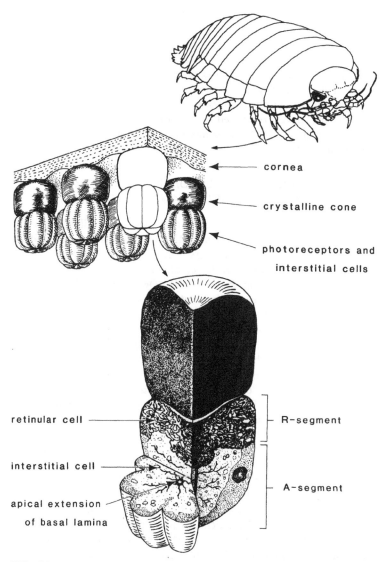

cornea

crystalline cone

photoreceptors and
interstitial cells

retinular cell ———————— R-segment

interstitial cell ————————

apical extension
of basal lamina — A-segment

FIG. 7.5. Summary of retinal structure in the deep sea isopod, *Bathynomus
giganteus*. The retinal structure is typical of crustaceans except that the photoreceptors
(retinular cells) have attenuated A-segments to make room for the reflective interstitial
cells at the core of each ommatidium. The elaborated R-segment increases the eye's
sensitivity and the diminished A-segment reduces its ability to process shed rhabdom.

R-segment thus have two chances to catch incident photons. Space for the interstitial cells is provided by a marked attenuation of the A-segment of each photoreceptor. Based on the size of the A-segment required in other species for rhabdom turnover, it seems unlikely that the diminished A-segment in these photoreceptors could be involved in daily cycling of microvillar membrane from the expanded R-segment. Indeed, the disruption of retinal structure caused by exposure to sunlight when the animals were collected never recovered, even after three months in darkness (Chamberlain et al., 1986). It seems unlikely that this species has daily rhabdom turnover.

PHOTORECEPTORS OF DEEP SEA SHRIMPS — *RIMICARIS EXOCULATA* AND *R. CHACEI*

Two new species of Caridean shrimp were recently described from hydrothermal vents along the Mid-Atlantic Ridge (Williams & Rona, 1986). As shown in Fig. 7.6, the black smokers occur along the Ridge at 23°N and 26°N latitude (Rona, 1980; Rona et al., 1984; Thompson, Humphris, Schroeder, Sulanowska, & Rona, 1988). Dense populations of shrimp inhabit the base and sides of the vent chimneys presumably feeding on sulfide oxidizing bacteria, which in turn feed on the minute sulfide particles released from the vents as black "smoke." Both *Rimicaris exoculata* and *R. chacei* have specialized visual organs that appear to be used by the animals both to orient toward the food source and to avoid swimming into the 350°C water jets by using the light emitted from the smoker itself (color plate, lower right). The "eye" of *R. exoculata* has been described before (Pelli & Chamberlain, 1989; Van Dover, Szuts, Chamberlain, & Cann, 1989); the eye of *R. chacei* is described here for the first time (Fig. 7.7). Both species have evolved a specialization of the normal decapod compound eye which is characterized by a dense array of photosensitive membrane backed up by a biological mirror. In *R. exoculata* the array is on the dorsal surface on either of the midline. In *R. chacei* the array is in the normal anterior position for the eyes, but is covered by a smooth cornea devoid of any dioptric apparatus. In both cases, the membrane array is formed from the massed R-segments of photoreceptors whose A-segments are severely attenuated (Fig. 7.7). It is extremely unlikely that any shedding or renewal of the rhabdom of the R-segments can take place in the thin strand of A-segment of either of these species.

PHOTOSTASIS, PHOTORECEPTOR STRUCTURE, AND LIGHTING ENVIRONMENT

If the maintenance of constant quantum catch by photostasis is characteristic of photoreceptors, then the shedding and synthesis of photosensitive

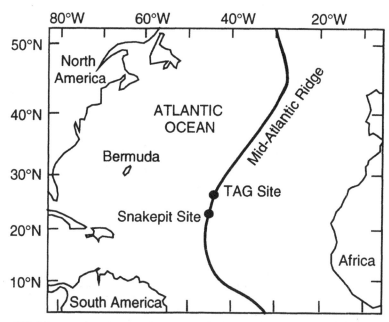

FIG. 7.6.   Location of deep sea shrimp habitats. The map shows the Mid-Atlantic Ridge and the location of two fields of hydrothermal black smoker vents along the ridge. The new Caridean shrimps, *Rimicaris exoculata* and *R. chacei*, were discovered and described from the base of black smoker chimneys at the TAG site and Snakepit site.

membrane could be the mechanism by which photostasis is maintained in the face of seasonally changing cyclic lighting. Animals living in noncyclic lighting free of seasonal variation might, therefore, not need extensive daily turnover of photosensitive membrane. Indeed our survey of these four species shows that the three animals living in constant-light environments probably do not have the large-scale daily turnover of rhabdomeral membrane characteristic of animals living in cyclic lighting. (Note that while the black-body radiation in the environment of *R. exoculata* and *R. chacei* is exceedingly dim, the bioluminescence environment of *B. giganteus* is not.)

The specific differences between the deep sea species and *Limulus* in the structure of photoreceptors are that in the deep sea species, the R-segment is enlarged with more densely packed rhabdom, and the A-segment is attenuated compared to *Limulus*. If one calculates the ratio of the volume of the R-segment to the volume of the A-segment, then the deep sea forms have volume ratios significantly greater than 1, and *Limulus* has a volume ratio significantly less than 1 (Hornstein & Chamberlain, 1991). We therefore calculated these volume ratios for a few species from constant-light environments (Chamberlain et al., 1986; Meyer-Rochow & Walsh, 1977; Van Dover et al., 1989) and some species from typical cyclic-lighting environ-

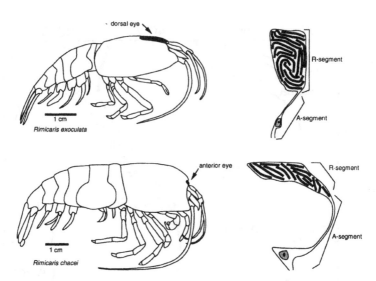

FIG. 7.7.   The eyes and photoreceptors of two deep sea shrimp. In *Rimicaris exoculata* the compound eyes have migrated to the dorsal surface to form a high-sensitivity array. In *Rimicaris chacei* the compound eyes remain in the normal anterior position; however, the dioptric array has degenerated, and the photoreceptors have elaborated to form a high-sensitivity array. The sketches of photoreceptors on the right show that in both species, the R-segment is replete with rhabdom, and the A-segment is exceedingly attenuated. There is no space to support daily membrane turnover on the scale seen in a surface species such as the horseshoe crab.

ments (Blest, Stowe, & Price, 1980; Calman & Chamberlain, 1982; Eguchi, 1976; Eguchi & Waterman, 1967; Home, 1975, 1976; Meyer-Rochow & Walsh, 1978; Schönenberger, 1977; Skalska-Rakowska & Baumgartner, 1985; Williams, 1982). These ratios are plotted versus total photoreceptor volume in Fig. 7.8. Over more than two decades of photoreceptor volume, the correlation seems to hold between light environment and R-segment/A-segment ratio. For species from constant-light environments, the R-segment is hypertrophied and much larger than the A-segment which is attenuated. For species from cyclic lighting, the R-segment is much smaller than the A-segment. This correlation is consistent with the hypothesis that rhabdom turnover serves to maintain photostasis in the face of seasonally varying cyclic lighting. Species living in constant lighting have no need for rhabdom turnover and consequently are free to shrink their A-segments.

WHY PHOTOSTASIS? SEASONAL AFFECTIVE DISORDER

Even if one accepts that photosensitive membrane turnover is a homeostatic mechanism for photostasis, the question remains as to why a constant daily

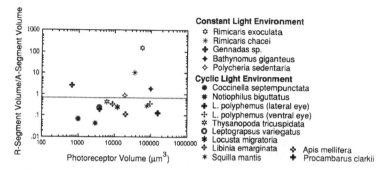

FIG. 7.8. Correlation of photoreceptor structure and lighting environment. The ratio of the R-segment volume to the A-segment volume is plotted on the vertical axis against the total volume of the photoreceptor on the horizontal axis for a variety of invertebrate species. Species from a constant-light environment have larger R-segments than A-segments. The reverse is true for species from cyclic-lighting environments. The horizontal dotted line divides the separate domains.

photon catch should be so desirable to the organism. Some hints may lie in an investigation of Seasonal Affective Disorder (SAD). SAD is an annual depression that occurs in the late fall and winter which may be accompanied by hypersomnia and increased appetite and weight gain (Rosenthal et al., 1984). Remé and others have suggested that SAD is caused by a failure of photostasis (Remé, Terman, & Wirz-Justice, 1990a) due to deficient photosensitive membrane turnover (Remé, Terman, & Wirz-Justice, 1990b). The argument is that membrane turnover in photoreceptors acts to compensate for the reduced light flux and day length of winter and that insufficient compensation leads to a failure of photostasis and consequently SAD. The finding that phototherapy can ameliorate SAD (e.g., Terman, Remé, Rafferty, Gallin, & Terman, 1990) is consistent with this scenario. Thus, the incidence of SAD should be more severe in more northern latitudes where seasonal changes in daily light flux are greater, and indeed this is the case (Rosen et al., 1990). In addition, the degree to which photostasis fails might be expected to vary from individual to individual, so that a continuum might be expected to exist between normal individuals and those with complete SAD, which also seems to be the case (Terman et al., 1989).

SAD would seem to be a rather global result for a deficiency in a cellular mechanism in peripheral photoreceptors, and the relationships between cause and effect in mammals may prove rather complex. Our finding that photostasis may be a general principle for all organisms, not just mammals, suggests that investigations of model systems such as *Limulus* may facilitate our understanding of the nature and purpose of photosensitive membrane turnover and the significance of photostasis.

ACKNOWLEDGMENTS

We thank Drs. J. Hoenig and E. Stopa for helpful discussions and W. P. Dossert and R. N. Jinks for technical assistance. Supported by NIH grant EY03446 and the Department of Bioengineering and Neuroscience, Syracuse University.

REFERENCES

Barlow, R. B., Jr. (1983). Circadian rhythms in the *Limulus* visual system. *Journal of Neuroscience, 3,* 856–870.

Barlow, R. B., Jr., Bolanowski, S. J., Jr., & Brachman, M. L. (1977). Efferent optic nerve fibers mediate circadian rhythms in the Limulus eye. *Science, 197,* 86–89.

Barlow, R. B., Jr., Chamberlain, S. C., & Lehman, H. K. (1989). Circadian rhythms in the invertebrate retina. In D. Stavenga & R. Hardie (Eds.), *Facets of vision* (pp. 257–280). Berlin: Springer-Verlag.

Barlow, R. B., Jr., Chamberlain, S. C., & Levinson, J. Z. (1980). *Limulus* brain modulates the structure and function of the lateral eye. *Science, 210,* 1037–1039.

Batra, R., & Barlow, R. B., Jr. (1990). Efferent control of temporal response properties of the *Limulus* lateral eye. *Journal of General Physiology, 95,* 229–244.

Battelle, B-A. (1991). Regulation of retinal functions by octopaminergic efferent neurons in *Limulus.* In N. Osborne & J. Chader (Eds.), *Progress in retinal research* Vol. 10, (pp. 333–355). Oxford: Pergamon Press.

Battelle, B-A., Evans, J. A., & Chamberlain, S. C. (1982). Efferent fibers to *Limulus* eyes synthesize and release octopamine. *Science, 216,* 1250–1252.

Blest, A. D., Stowe, S., & Price, D. G. (1980). The sources of acid hydrolases for photoreceptor membrane degradation in a grapsid crab. *Cell and Tissue Research, 205,* 229–244.

Calman, B. G., & Battelle, B-A. (1991). Central origin of the efferent neurons projecting to the eyes of *Limulus polyphemus. Visual Neuroscience, 6,* 481–495.

Calman, B.G., & Chamberlain, S. C. (1982). Distinct lobes of *Limulus* ventral photoreceptors. II. Structure and ultrastructure. *Journal of General Physiology, 80,* 839–862.

Calman, B. G., & Chamberlain, S. C. (1992). Control of motility in the cells of the *Limulus* lateral eye: Localization of actin filaments and microtubules. *Visual Neuroscience, 9,* 365–375.

Chamberlain, S. C., & Barlow, R. B., Jr. (1979). Light and efferent activity control rhabdom turnover in *Limulus* photoreceptors. *Science, 206,* 361–363.

Chamberlain, S. C., & Barlow, R. B., Jr. (1984). Transient membrane shedding in *Limulus* photoreceptors: Control mechanisms under natural lighting. *Journal of Neuroscience, 4,* 2792–2810.

Chamberlain, S. C., & Barlow, R. B., Jr. (1987). Control of structural rhythms in the lateral eye of *Limulus:* Interactions of natural lighting and circadian efferent activity. *Journal of Neuroscience, 7,* 2135–2144.

Chamberlain, S. C., Meyer-Rochow, V. B., & Dossert, W. P. (1986). Morphology of the compound eye of the giant deep-sea isopod *Bathynomus giganteus. Journal of Morphology, 189,* 145–156.

Eguchi, E. (1976). Rhabdom structure and receptor potentials in single crayfish retinular cells. *Journal of Cellular and Comparative Physiology, 66,* 411–430.

Eguchi, E., & Waterman, T. H. (1967). Changes in retinal fine structure induced in the crab *Libinia* by light and dark adaptation. *Zeitschrift für Zellforschung, 79,* 209–229.

Evans, J. A., Chamberlain, S. C., & Battelle, B-A. (1983). Autoradiographic localization of newly synthesized octopamine to retinal efferents in the *Limulus* visual system. *Journal of Comparative Neurology, 219,* 369–383.

Fahrenbach, W. H. (1975). The visual system of the horseshoe crab *Limulus polyphemus. International Review of Cytology, 41,* 285–349.

Fahrenbach, W. H. (1981). The morphology of the *Limulus* visual system VII. Innervation of photoreceptor neurons by neurosecretory efferents. *Cell and Tissue Research, 216,* 655–659.

Hoenig, H., & Chamberlain, S. C. (1989). Testing the "photostasis" hypothesis in the *Limulus* lateral eye. *Investigative Ophthalmology and Visual Science, 30,* (suppl.) 291.

Home, E. M. (1975). Ultrastructural studies of development and light-dark adaptation of the eye of *Coccinella septempunctata* L., with particular reference to ciliary structures. *Tissue and Cell, 7,* 703–722.

Home, E. M. (1976). The fine structure of some carabid beetle eyes, with particular reference to ciliary structures in the retinula cells. *Tissue and Cell, 8,* 311–333.

Hornstein, E. P., & Chamberlain, S. C. (1991). Correlation of photoreceptor structure and lighting environment: Implications for photostasis. *Society for Neuroscience Abstracts, 17,* 298.

Kaplan, E., & Barlow, R. B., Jr. (1980). Circadian clock in *Limulus* brain increases response and decreases noise of retinal photoreceptors. *Nature, 286,* 393–395.

Kass, L., & Barlow, R. B., Jr. (1984). Efferent neurotransmission of circadian rhythms in *Limulus* lateral eye. I. Octopamine-induced increases in retinal sensitivity. *Journal of Neuroscience, 4,* 904–917.

Kier, C. K., & Chamberlain, S. C. (1990). Dual controls for screening pigment movement in photoreceptors of the *Limulus* lateral eye: Circadian efferent input and light. *Visual Neuroscience, 4,* 237–255.

Lee, H. E., & Wyse, G. A. (1991). Immunocytochemical localization of octopmaine in the central nervous system of *Limulus polyphemus*: A light and electron microscopic study. *Journal of Comparative Neurology, 307,* 683–694.

Meyer-Rochow, V. B., & Walsh, S. (1977). The eyes of mesopelagic crustaceans. I. *Gennadas* sp. (Penaeidae). *Cell and Tissue Research, 184,* 87–101.

Meyer-Rochow, V. B., & Walsh, S. (1978). The eyes of mesopelagic crustaceans. III. *Thysanopoda tricuspidata* (Euphausiacea). *Cell and Tissue Research, 195,* 59–79.

Pelli, D. G., & Chamberlain, S. C. (1989). On the visibility of 350°C blackbody radiation by the shrimp *Rimicaris exoculata* and man. *Nature, 337,* 460–461.

Penn, J. S., & Williams, T. P. (1986). Photostasis: Regulation of daily photon-catch by rat retinas in response to various cyclic illuminances. *Experimental Eye Research, 43,* 915–928.

Remé, C. E., Terman, M., & Wirz-Justice, A. (1990a). The visual input stage of the mammalian circadian pacemaking system: I. Is there a clock in the mammalian eye? *Journal of Biological Rhythms, 6,* 5–29.

Remé, C. E., Terman, M., & Wirz-Justice, A. (1990b). Are deficient retinal photoreceptor renewal mechanisms involved in the pathogenesis of winter depression? *Archives of General Psychiatry, 47,* 878–879.

Rona, P. A. (1980). TAG hydrothermal field: Mid-Atlantic Ridge crest at latitude 26°N. *Journal of the Geological Society of London, 137,* 385–402.

Rona, P. A., Thompson, G., Mottl, M. J., Karson, J. A., Jenkins, W. J., Graham, D., Mallette, M., Von Damm, K., & Edmond, J. M. (1984). Hydrothermal activity at the Trans-Atlantic Geotraverse hydrothermal field, Mid-Atlantic Ridge crest at 26°N. *Journal of Geophysical Research, 89,* 11,365–11,377.

Rosen, L. N., Targam, S. D., Terman, M., Bryant, M. J., Hoffman, H., Kasper, S. F., Hamovit, J. R., Docherty, J. P., Welch, B., & Rosenthal, N. E. (1990). Prevalence of seasonal affective disorder at four latitudes. *Psychiatry Research, 31,* 131–144.

Rosenthal, N. E., Sack, D. A., Gillin, J. C., Lewy, A. J., Goodwin, F. K., Davenport, Y.,

Mueller, D. S., Newsome, D. A., & Wehr, T. A. (1984). Seasonal affective disorder. A description of the syndrome and preliminary findings with light therapy. *Archives of General Psychiatry, 41,* 72–80.

Schönenberger, N. (1977). The fine structure of the compound eye of *Squilla mantis* (Crustacea, Stomatopoda). *Cell and Tissue Research, 176,* 205–233.

Skalska-Rakowska, M., & Baumgartner, B. (1985). Longitudinal continuity of the subrhabdomeric cisternae in the photoreceptors of the compound eye of the drone, *Apis mellifera. Experentia, 41,* 43–45.

Smith, W. C., Friedman, M. A., & Goldsmith, T. H. (1991). Retinoids in the lateral eye of *Limulus:* Evidence for a retinal photoisomerase. *Visual Neuroscience, 8,* 329–336.

Terman, M., Botticelli, S. R., Link, B. G., Link, M. J., Quitkin, F. W., Hardin, T. E., & Rosenthal, N. E. (1989). Seasonal symptom patterns in New York: Patients and population. In C. Thompson & T. Silverstone (Eds.), *Seasonal affective disorder* (pp. 77–95). London: Clinical Neuroscience Publishers.

Terman, M., Remé, C. E., Rafferty, B., Gallin, P. F., & Terman, J. S. (1990). Bright light therapy for winter depression: Potential ocular effects and theoretical implications. *Photochemistry and Photobiology, 51,* 781–792.

Thompson, G., Humphris, S. E., Schroeder, B., Sulanowska, M., & Rona, P. A. (1988). Active vents and massive sulfides at 26°N (TAG) and 23°N (Snakepit) on the Mid-Atlantic Ridge. *Canadian Mineralogist, 26,* 697–711.

Van Dover, C. L., Szuts, E., Chamberlain, S. C., & Cann, J. R. (1989). A novel eye in "eyeless" shrimp from hydrothermal vents of the Mid-Atlantic Ridge. *Nature, 337,* 458–460.

Williams, D. S. (1982). Ommatidial structure in relation to turnover of photoreceptor membrane in the locust. *Cell and Tissue Research, 225,* 595–617.

Williams, A. B., & Rona, P. A. (1986). Two new Caridean shrimps (Bresiliidae) from a hydrothermal field on the Mid-Atlantic Ridge. *Journal of Crustacean Biology, 6,* 446–463.

8 And Now, for Our Two Senses

Stanley J. Bolanowski
Christine M. Checkosky
Syracuse University

Thomas M. Wengenack
University of Rochester School of Medicine and Dentistry

INTRODUCTION

Much is being said in this volume regarding Dr. Zwislocki's influence, both personally and scientifically, by all of the contributing authors. One particularly influential view that he champions is the importance of being aware of new technical advancements and developments in all of the sensory sciences. The basis of such a philosophy is that the understanding of neural processes used by one sense modality may have significance for the understanding of others. Further, it engenders the idea that awareness of the observations and discoveries in one sensory system may foster new approaches or views for the understanding of a different modality. Some would argue that to divide one's time researching more than one sense modality is counterproductive, simply because of time constraints. They would argue that all effort should be intensely focused. Others posit that variety is indeed "the spice of life." In a real sense, one's position on this issue is dictated by one's personality and where one wants to go scientifically. The impact that we have on our respective fields will be assessed, in the final analysis, only by our successors. It is not our intent here to philosophize about these issues, but merely to show how research in the field of sensory sciences has progressed in the first author's laboratories and how Professor Zwislocki directly influenced him, and indirectly the co-authors. In particular, we have continued to perform research on two sensory systems — vision and touch — and much of what is presented in this chapter are recent, and in certain instances unpublished, findings.

VISION

It had long been known, since the time of the early Gestaltists, that viewing a totally homogeneous and diffuse visual field or Ganzfeld results in a dramatic vanishing of visual sensation, despite continuing stimulation. A similar observation has also been obtained with stimuli stabilized on the retina (e.g., Ditchburn, 1973; Yarbus, 1967). This loss of vision called *fading* or *blankout* is significant in that it has been the basis for the idea that spatiotemporal information is essential for the maintenance of visual perception. Furthermore, it has been argued that the loss of vision that occurs in the absence of spatiotemporal variations is attributable to attenuation of the retinal signal (see, e.g. Ditchburn, 1973; Gregory, 1971; Riggs, 1965). We confirmed the consistent loss of visual sensation when the Ganzfeld is viewed monocularly (Bolanowski & Doty, 1982a, 1982b, 1987). However, because we have also found that there is no such loss when the Ganzfeld is viewed binocularly, the locus of the effect cannot be retinal, and spatiotemporal change may not be required for the continuous maintenance of visual perception. Also, because we have found that the entire process of blankout can be prevented by pressure blocking the eye viewing darkness, the phenomenon may actually be a manifestation of binocular rivalry/suppression (Levelt, 1965; Wheatstone, 1938). In other words, the percept of blankout is probably the result of the eye in darkness becoming dominant, suppressing the eye viewing the Ganzfeld (Bolanowski & Doty, 1987; Bolanowski, King, & Doty, 1985; Bolanowski, Makous, & Raman, 1987). A similar conclusion has been reached by others using binocularly presented, stabilized retinal images (Rozhkova, Nickolayev, & Shchadrin, 1982).

Phenomenologically, the blankout process is always reported to resemble a perceptual curtain originating nasally and being drawn nasotemporally across the visual field. Always present, however, is the persistence of perception in the far temporal visual field, an area that seems to correspond to the region of visual space seen by only one eye (temporal crescent). Generally speaking, 1 to 5 blankout periods can occur during 1 minute of Ganzfeld viewing, depending on the observer, eye dominance, hue, and luminance level. Because the blankout periods occur intermittently during test presentations, Bolanowski and Doty (1987) measured four blankout parameters: (a) the latency to first blankout, (b) the percentage of time spent in blankout, (c) the number of blankout events occurring during the stimulation period, and (d) the probability that blankout will occur for a given stimulus condition calculated by dividing the number of stimulus presentations producing blankout by the total number of these presentations. Figure 8.1, taken from Bolanowski and Doty (1987), shows typical results obtained on three observers (columns) in response to 1-min-long, binocularly presented, achromatic Ganzfelder. The lower four rows of the figure show the results for the parameters previously described. The values

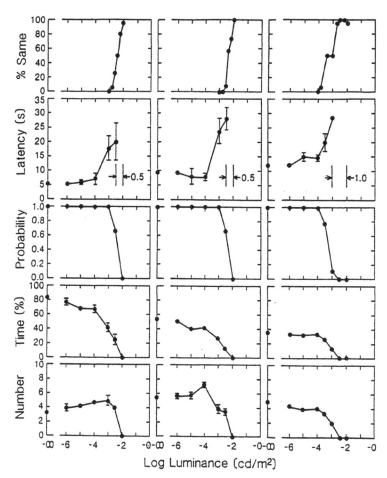

FIG. 8.1.   Effects of luminance disparity between the two eyes on four parametric measures (lowest four rows) of the phenomenon of blankout induced by viewing 1-min Ganzfelder. The intensity of light presented to the right was held constant at 16.2 cd/m² (−2.0-log luminance), and the horizontal axes plot the light intensity presented to the left eye. Plotted in the columns are results obtained on three different observers. To obtain the results shown in the topmost panels, the observers were required to state whether binocularly presented Ganzfelder of 1-sec duration were the same in intensity, stimulus parameters being otherwise as for the lower panels. (From Bolanowski, S. J., Jr., & Doty, R. W., 1987. Reprinted with permission from Vision Research).

along the horizontal axes signify the intensity of light presented to the left eye, while the right eye was presented a fixed intensity of light (−2.0-log luminance). The monocular condition is given at −∞ log luminance. For every subject tested, as the luminance levels between the two eyes becomes less disparate, the number of blankouts, the probability of blankout occurrence, and the amount of time spent in blankout decrease. The latency to first blankout, on the other hand, increases. At about 0.5–1.0-log luminance disparity, as shown in the inserts in the latency plots, no blankout occurs. On average, the disparity in light intensity presented to the two eyes for blankout to be signaled is approximately 0.75-log units. As shown in the panels of the upper row of this figure, this value corresponds to the point where subjects can, at chance levels, discern differences in Ganzfeld luminances briefly (1 sec) presented simultaneously to the two eyes. In the latter case, the vertical axes of the graphs show the percentage of time that the Ganzfelder were called "same."

Because the phenomenon of blankout and its absence cannot be of retinal origin, and because the neuronal substrate for binocular vision is present in striate (V1) cortex of the macaque (e.g., Poggio & Fischer, 1977; Walker, 1978), we performed a series of functional-anatomy (Bolanowski, Demeter, & Doty, 1984; Bolanowski, Demeter, & Doty, in preparation) and physiological–anatomical studies (Wengenack, 1991; Wengenack & Bolanowski, 1990a, 1990b; Wengenack, Checkosky, & Bolanowski, 1988) on this region of visual cortex to help determine the loci of the Ganzfeld-induced perceptual effects. All of these studies used the unanesthetized monkey (*Macaca fasicularis*) as a model for man, because anesthesia and even mild sedation has been shown to adversely affect several aspects of binocular vision (e.g., Bárány & Halldén, 1948). The functional-anatomy studies used the metabolic marker techniques of 2-[1-^{14}C] deoxy-D-glucose (2-DG; Sokoloff et al., 1977) and cytochrome oxidase (CO; Seligman, Karnovsky, Wasserkrug,&Hanker,1968;Wong-Riley,1976,1979),whilethephysiological/anatomical studies used standard chronic-recording techniques: a permanently mounted recording chamber affixed to the skull overlying the opercular cortex; elgiloy metal microelectrodes used for monitoring single-unit activity and for making electrolytic microlesions; and subsequent histological processing of adjacent brain sections for CO and for the Prussian blue reaction to identify electrode track trajectory and location of unit activity of interest.

The binocular Ganzfeld used in all of the studies involving macaques was fashioned after the one used in our previous human psychophysical studies (Bolanowski, 1987; Bolanowski & Doty, 1987), the arrangement suitably modified to accommodate the monkey's face and head. A topical anesthetic and a cycloplegic were also administered into each eye and translucent contact lenses inserted to ensure that the animals were presented fully diffuse stimuli. A head bolt, implanted previously under general anesthesia, permitted precise alignment of the monkey's head with respect to the visual stimulator while ensuring comfortable yet firm restraint.

For the functional anatomy experiments (Bolanowski et al., 1984, in preparation), each animal was placed in the apparatus and an intravenous catheter inserted to allow infusion of the 2-DG at the onset of visual stimulation. For monocular stimulation, an opaque contact lens was placed over the eye not stimulated, and the eye was taped shut with black tape. All stimuli were presented at 20.0 cd/m^2 for a duration of 45 min. For the stimulus parameters used, and assuming correspondence between macaque and man, we suspect that the animals presented the continuous monocular Ganzfeld were probably blanked-out approximately 55% of the time. At the conclusion of the experiment the animal was given a lethal dose of anesthetic, perfused transcardially, the brain removed and prepared for frozen sectioning and subsequent autoradiography and CO histochemistry. The experiments were performed on 14 animals, some receiving binocular ($n = 8$), others receiving monocular, stimulation ($n = 6$).

Regardless of whether the Ganzfelder were presented continuously or were flashed, the binocular cases all showed homogeneous uptake of 2-DG in layers 4c and 4a with 4b weakly labeled. When viewed in tangential sections, the supragranular layers showed patch-like uptake which displayed an arrangement reminiscent to that seen on adjacent sections reacted for CO; the CO patterns in these layers described previously by many other investigators (e.g., Horton, 1984; Horton & Hubel, 1981; Humphrey & Hendrickson, 1983; Tootell, Hamilton, Silverman, & Switkes, 1988). Under flashed Ganzfeld conditions, layers 5–6 also showed a patchy array of 2-DG uptake, again seeming to correspond to the CO array seen in these lower layers. Transiently presented, monocular Ganzfelder also produced patchy 2-DG uptake in layers 2–3 and 5–6, with half the density as seen for the binocular cases. Furthermore, alternating rows of uptake, indicative of ocular dominance columns, were present in layer 4 with the patches of 2-DG in the upper and lower layers laminarly coincident with them. This result was expected, based on the work of Horton and Hubel (1981), Humphrey and Hendrickson (1983), and Kennedy, Des Rosiers, Reivich, Sharpe, and Sokoloff (1975). Suprisingly, however, when the monocular Ganzfelder were continuously presented, no patch-like uptake of 2-DG was found in any layer. Indeed, in layer 4 one-half of the cases showed rows of uptake signifying ocular dominance columns, supporting the fact that the Ganzfeld stimuli were actually producing activity in striate cortex and consistent with the electrophysiological results of Kayama, Riso, Bartlett, and Doty (1979) and our own observations (see later in the chapter).

Thus, the results confirm that contours and temporal transients are unnecessary for the activation of neurons in V1, a fact concordant with the psychophysical observations described previously. The results also suggest a physiological basis for the loss of vision produced by monocular Ganzfelder and its prevention under binocular Ganzfeld conditions. That is, the fact that discrete regions in layers 2–3 can be differentially activated using steady-binocular as opposed to steady-monocular Ganzfelder suggests that these regions are somehow involved in the processes responsible for blankout/rivalry and binocular vision in general. While we have not as yet attempted to precisely correlate the CO and the 2-DG patterns that we obtained, it is possible that the uptake of 2-DG is occurring in the CO patches. This would be wholly consistent with the fact that the CO regions can be excited by diffuse (low spatial frequency) illumination (Humphrey & Hendrickson, 1983; Tootell, Silverman, Switkes, & DeValois, 1982), but perhaps at odds with the fact that they are strongly ocularly dominant and presumably involved in color vision (Livingstone & Hubel, 1984).

To determine how V1 neurons respond to Ganzfeld illumination and to ascertain if these units are located in CO patches, we (Wengenack, 1991; Wengenack & Bolanowski, 1990a, 1990b; Wengenack & Bolanowski, in preparation; Wengenack et al., 1988) recorded single-unit activity in the awake macaque. Activity was obtained in response to Ganzfelder, and the units were correlated with anatomical location, both with respect to the CO patches and to the various cortical layers. Out of the 704 units studied, 51.1% ($n=360$) responded to Ganzfeld illumination. There were three major types of responses: transient, slowly adapting, and sustained, with a small proportion yielding "mixed" responses. Figure 8.2 shows typical response profiles to the Ganzfeld illumination, the data displayed in the form of peri-stimulus-time (PST) histograms.

The stimulus paradigm used in generating the responses is given at the bottom of the figure. Activity was first obtained in the absence of any stimulation for a period of 5 sec. After this time, the right Ganzfeld was activated. After 5 sec of right-eye-alone stimulation, the left Ganzfeld was also turned on producing binocular stimulation for 5 sec. After an elapsed time of 10 sec, the right Ganzfeld was extinguished allowing for monocular, left-eye stimulation lasting 5 sec. A period of 5 sec post-left-eye stimulation followed to determine again the baseline response. Each histogram was generated over 10 presentations of the stimulus. Seen in Fig. 8.2A is a typical PST obtained from a transiently responding unit, transient responses being found in 8.4% ($n=59$) of the units recorded. The transient responses can occur at onset, offset, or both. This particular unit responded both at stimulus onset and offset as well as to stimuli presented to either eye. Approximately one-half the transient units responded to only monocular stimulation ($n=30$), while the other half responded to binocular, as well as monocular, stimuli ($n=29$).

Figure 8.2B shows a typical slowly adapting response: increase in activity at light onset, and a slow decrease towards baseline activity. This type of response was found in 8.2% ($n=56$) of the units. For this particular example, the unit responded only to right-eye illumination, although approximately one-third of these types of units also responded to binocular stimulation.

TACTION

n 1988, Bolanowski, Gescheider, Verrillo, and Checkosky (1988) proposed new model for the mechanical aspects of touch. Based on previous ychophysical, anatomical, and physiological experiments performed by (e.g., Bolanowski & Verrillo, 1982; Bolanowski & Zwislocki, 1984; praro, Verrillo, & Zwislocki, 1979; Gescheider, Frisina, & Verrillo, 1979; scheider, O'Malley, & Verrillo, 1983; Gescheider, Sklar, Van Doren, & rrillo, 1985; Gescheider, Verrillo, & Van Doren, 1982; Verrillo, 1962, 3, 1965, 1966a, 1966b, 1966c; Verrillo & Bolanowski, 1986) and others ., Freeman & Johnson, 1982; Iggo & Ogawa, 1977; Johansson, 1976, 8; Johansson, Landström, & Lundström, 1982; Johansson & Vallbo, ; Merzenich & Harrington, 1969; Mountcastle, LaMotte, & Carli, ; Ochoa & Torebjörk, 1983; Talbot, Darian-Smith, Kornhuber, & ntcastle, 1968), the new model proposes that there are four separate distinct channels of information that combine to signal threshold and threshold events occuring at the somatosensory periphery. The model based on various assumptions regarding how the nervous system

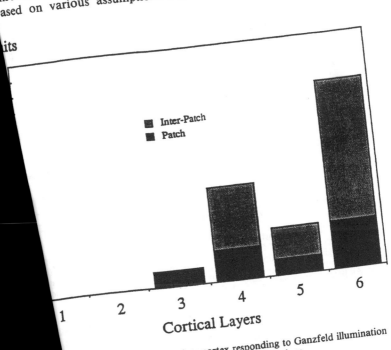

Distribution of units in striate cortex responding to Ganzfeld illumination to cortical layers and CO patch and interpatch regions.

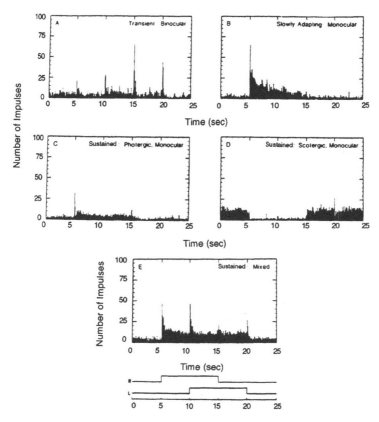

FIG. 8.2. Major types of unit responses to Ganzfeld illumination: (A) transient, (B) slowly adapting, (C) sustained–photergic, (D) sustained–scotergic, and (E) mixed. The results are shown in the form of peri-stimulus-time histograms (PST, binwidth = 50 ms) constructed by averaging the responses to 10 presentations of the stimulus. The stimulus paradigm is given at the bottom of the figure. The total number of spikes recorded per 5-sec epoch of the paradigm are also inserted beneath each PST. The intensity of the stimulus was equal for both eyes (11.3cd/m²).

Figures 8.2C and 8.2D show typical examples of units responding in a sustained manner, this response type being found for 32.3% ($n = 127$) of the units. For these types of units, two major classes of responses were found: *photergic* (Fig. 8.2C), those responding with increased activity to the Ganzfeld stimulus; and *scotergic* Fig. 8.2D), those responding with a decrease in activity (i.e., below baseline). The two examples shown are for units that responded monocularly to right-eye stimulation, purely monocular responders comprising 27.3% of all the sustained units. Fully 72.7% of the luxotonic units could be binocularly activated. Lastly, a few units (< 4%) responded with mixed responses; one example is shown in Fig. 8.2E. In this instance, the unit displayed a sustained response as well as transient responses at stimulus onsets. The unit responded to binocular as well as moncular stimuli.

The binocular-sustained units are of particular interest, because their responses most closely correspond to the psychophysical phenomena described earlier: blankout, it's absence under binocular Ganzfeld conditions, and the presence of patchy uptake of 2-DG. In-depth analysis of the binocular interactions found in the sustained units showed that they responded in four specific ways, the response types are given simple descriptive names here, although they have been categorized using probable neural mechanisms such as nonlinear summation (Wengenack, 1991; Wengenack & Bolanowski, in preparation). Figure 8.3 shows, by example, the four simple categories of responses. In the top row are examples of the response of *averaging* units. That is, the binocular response in either instance is approximately equal to or between either response obtained monocularly. Figure 8.3A shows a photergic response and Fig. 8.3, a scotergic response. The PSTs in the second row (Figs. 8.3C and 8.3D) show activity called *inhibitory*. That is, the binocular response is at a level equal to that found in the absence of stimulation, in spite of the fact that the units respond to illumination of either eye alone. The third row (Figs. 8.3E and 8.3F) shows examples of units displaying *summation*, the binocular response being greater than either monocular response. This type of response has direct implications regarding possible neural substrates for the psychophysically obtained results of Bolanowski (1987), who showed that there is perfect binocular brightness summation in the Ganzfeld. Lastly, the fourth row shows two PSTs of units responding in a *suppressive* way, the binocular response being less than the baseline response, even though the monocular responses are greater.

To determine if units responding to Ganzfeld illumination are located in the CO patches, we characterized them electrophysiologically, made electrolytic microlesion at the site, and then anatomically determined the lesion site in relation to the CO patches and cortical layers (Wengenack, 1991; Wengenack & Bolanowski, in preparation). Figure 8.4 shows the results obtained for 22 units, most of which were sustained ($n = 18$), although there were two each in the slowly adapting and transient categories. No differences in the results were found regarding location and response type. As shown in the figure, most of the units were localized in the subgranular layers 5–6. Six units were localized in layer 4 and only one in layer 3. Furthermore, there appears to be no relation between the CO patches and units responding to Ganzfeld illumination. That is, 15 units were located in interpatch regions, and 7 were located in the CO patches. This is surprising because of the fact that the CO regions can be excited by diffuse illumination (see prior discussion), and because our 2-DG results seemed to implicate the CO patches in the blankout/nonblankout perceptual phenomenon. We are presently

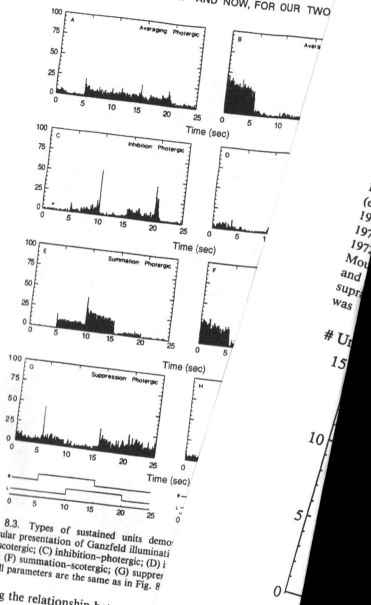

FIG. 8.3. Types of sustained units demo[...]
binocular presentation of Ganzfeld illuminati[...]
ging–scotergic; (C) inhibition–photergic; (D) i[...]
tergic; (F) summation–scotergic; (G) suppres[...]
gic. All parameters are the same as in Fig. 8[...]

analyzing the relationship between th[...]
have obtained in the 2-DG studies. B[...]
presented here, we suspect that the 2-[...]
Ganzfelder conditions should not f[...]
obtained in the supra-and subgran[...]

FIG. 8.4.
in relation

encodes tactile events, the so-called psychophysical–physiological-linking hypotheses, and we are continuing to test these assumptions using a variety of techniques and approaches for the purposes of expanding and, if necessary, modifying the model. We will briefly outline the model and then discuss one test which showed that the model requires modification regarding the neural code used to signal a threshold event in one of the four channels.

Figure 8.5 shows the model as based on psychophysical results and shows the averaged threshold-frequency characteristics of the four channels as measured on groups of observers. The results were obtained on the glabrous skin of the hand (thenar eminence) which was stimulated with bursts of sinusoidal displacements.

The Pacinian (P) channel, nominally operating with high sensitivity in the frequency range of 40 to < 500 Hz, has the properties of temporal (Verrillo, 1965; Zwislocki, 1960, 1969) and spatial (Verrillo, 1966b) summation, is temperature dependent (Bolanowski & Verrillo, 1982) and is responsible for the human perception of vibration. The non-Pacinian (NP) I channel operates in the midfrequency range (3–40 Hz), does not have the properties of temporal and spatial summation, is relatively temperature insensitive, and is responsible for the human perception of flutter. The NP II channel operates in the same frequency region as does the P channel, but at a reduced sensitivity with respect to the P channel. It is affected by

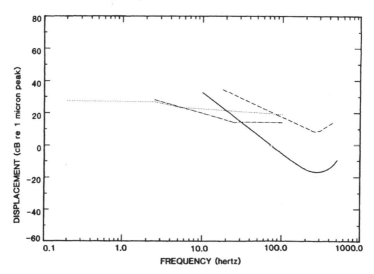

FIG. 8.5.   The four-channel model of the mechanical aspects of touch as measured by vibratory stimuli. Shown are the threshold-frequency characteristics of the various channels: _____ , PC; _ _ _ _ , NP I; _ _ _ _ _ , NP II; and _____ , NP III.

changes in skin-surface temperature and probably is not capable of temporal or spatial summation. Its perceptual attribute is a buzz. Finally, NP III operates over a wide range of stimulus frequencies extending to very low frequencies ($<$ 0.4 Hz). It is relatively temperature insensitive and has not been assessed regarding its capabilities of temporal and spatial summation. NP III is known to mediate the human perception of pressure.

The four channels were delineated by using a variety of techniques and manipulations in the stimulus domain: forward masking, variations in stimulus size and duration, variations in skin surface temperature, and locus of stimulation (e.g., hairy vs. glabrous skin). It should be pointed out that because of the various properties of the channels (e.g., spatial summation), the overall threshold-frequency response that is obtained in psychophysical experiments is strongly dependent on stimulus parameters. For example, using a large stimulus area will produce an overall threshold-frequency response from 0.4 to 500 Hz which follows the contour defined by NP III (low-frequency region), NP I (middle-frequency region), and P (high-frequency region). Stimulating smaller areas, however, will produce a threshold-frequency response contour which from low to high frequencies will follow NP III, NP I, and NP II. This is because the P channel exhibits the property of spatial summation and is insensitive to punctate stimuli.

The psychophysical–physiological link was based in part on the classification of four groups of low-threshold, mechanoreceptive fibers: rapidly adapting (RA) fibers; type I, slowly adapting (SA I) fibers; type II, slowly adapting fibers (SA II); and Pacinian corpuscle (PC) fibers (Johansson & Vallbo, 1979). These fibers were classified by microneurographic recordings from the glabrous skin of the human hand and were correlated with four end organs: PC fibers, Pacinian corpuscles; RA fibers, Meissner's corpuscles; SA I fibers, Merkel-cell neurite complexes; and SA II fibers, Ruffini endings (review by Vallbo & Johansson, 1984). The model that we proposed correlates the four physiological/anatomical types with the four psychophysical channels described in relation to Fig. 5.5. These correlations were made by fitting neurophysiological frequency-response curves, constructed by extrapolating and interpolating the averaged data of Johansson, et al. (1982), to the four psychophysical frequency-response curves. Figure 8.6 shows the results of that analysis and relates the four psychophysical functions, taken from Fig. 8.5, to the four physiological types. As can be seen in Fig. 8.6, NP I is correlated with RA fibers, P with PCs, NP II with SA IIs, and NP III with SA Is.

Of primary importance in establishing the psychophysical–physiological link was the need to select a neural code, based on various assumptions, that would be appropriate for use by each fiber group to signal stimulus detection. There are many kinds of firing patterns which could serve as the neural code: the average firing rate (spikes per sec), number of spikes-per-stimulus burst, or even *entrainment*, that is, a spike occuring at every cycle of a vibratory stimulus. As an example, Fig. 8.7 shows what happens to the shape of the frequency characteristics of PCs for several response criteria, the data replotted from Johansson et al. (1982). There is wide variation in the shape, sensitivity, and location along the frequency axis of the frequency-response functions so constructed emphasizing the impor-tance of choosing appropriate criteria when making correlations between physiology and psychophysics.

With regard to the P channel, we (Bolanowski et al., 1988) proposed that the neural code used to signal threshold was 4 spikes per stimulus burst occurring on a single PC fiber, this based on a variety of assumptions and the correspondence between the shapes of the psychophysical and physio-logical frequency-response functions.

One characteristic that can be used to test the 4-spike-per-burst proposi-tion is the capability of the P channel to temporally summate vibratory stimuli (Verrillo, 1965). Temporal summation refers to the psychophysical phenomenon in which the stimulus amplitude required for threshold detection decreases with increasing stimulus duration. Based on theoretical condiserations and experimental evidence, Zwislocki (1960) proposed that temporal summation could be modeled by an energy integrator having a time constant of 200 ms. Such a temporal integrator would produce summation at a rate of -3 dB/doubling of the duration of the stimulus from durations of 10 to approximately 100 ms. Based on other consider-ations, he concluded that for durations greater than 100 ms, the decrease in threshold would be asymptotic and complete at 1,000 ms. Figure 8.8 shows average psychophysical results obtained from five observers in a study measuring the effect of stimulus duration on threshold detection of a 100-Hz vibratory stimulus applied with a 2.9 cm^2 contactor to the thenar eminence (Checkosky, 1991). This stimulus activates only the P channel. The threshold shift is plotted in dB referenced to the threshold level obtained at 1,000 ms. The solid curve through the data points is the theoretical curve of Zwislocki (1960). As other investigators have found (Gescheider, 1976; Verrillo, 1965), the results presented in Fig. 8.8 show that the P channel is capable of temporal summation and that the effect is adequately predicted by the model.

A channel which exhibits temporal summation must use a peripheral neural code that signals information about the temporal aspects of the stimulus. Also, it has been established that the P channel is mediated by PC fibers and that temporal summation can be modeled by a temporal integrator (low-pass filter) with a time constant of 200 ms. Therefore, neural activity obtained from a PC responding to vibratory stimuli, when input to an integrating filter, should produce an output resembling the

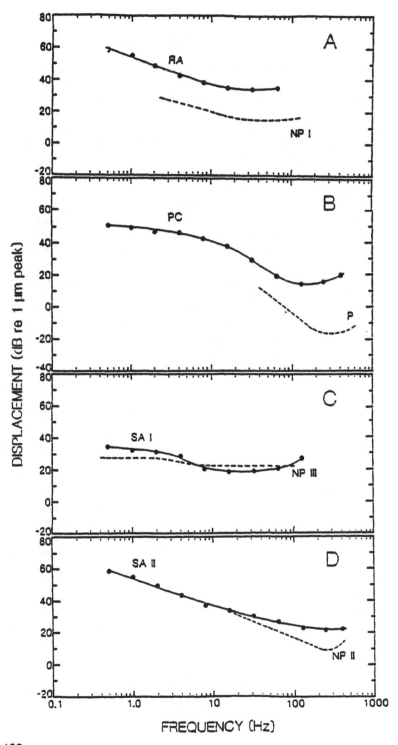

FIG. 8.6

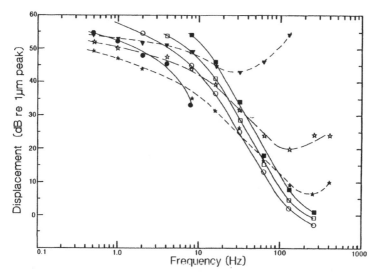

FIG. 8.7. Average frequency-response characteristics for PC fibers generated for different response criteria: firing rates (●, 2 spikes/sec; ○, 10 spikes/sec; □, 20 spikes/sec; ■, 40 spikes/sec) and spike occurences (★, 2 spikes/burst; ▼, 12 spikes/burst; ☆, 1 spike/cycle). The data were obtained by interpolating and extrapolating the results of Johansson et al. (1982).

temporal-summation function. Coding schemes (e.g., entrainment, 2 spikes/sec, etc) which do not produce an output that obeys temporal summation can be rejected as codes for the P channel. Checkosky (1991) and Checkosky and Bolanowski (1992) recorded neural-spike data from individual PCs ($n=7$) isolated from cat mesentery in response to bursts of 300-Hz displacement stimuli presented over a wide variety of stimulus amplitudes and durations. The level of amplitudes used ensured that activity from each PC spanned a range from very low activity (e.g., 1 spike per burst) to entrainment (i.e., 300 spikes per sec). The burst durations spanned the range from 10 to 1,000 ms. The real-time data were recorded on magnetic tape and later input into a low-pass filter modeling the temporal integrator. The output of the integrator was set at a threshold level that mimicked the psychophysical detection-threshold level. To test the criterion

---

FIG. 8.6. (Opposite page) Relationship between physiologically measured frequency characteristics for different fiber types [(a) RA; (b) PC; (c) SA I; and (d) SA II] and psychophysically obtained threshold-frequency characteristics [(a) NP I; (b) P; (c) NP III; and (d) NP II]. Neurophysiological data points are interpolations and extrapolations of the average results of Johansson et al., (1982) for selected response criteria: (a) 1 spike/stimulus burst; (b) 4 spikes/stimulus burst; (c) 0.8 spikes/sec; and (d) 5 spikes/sec. (From Bolanowski et al., 1988. Reprinted with permission from the *Journal of the Acoustical Society of America.*)

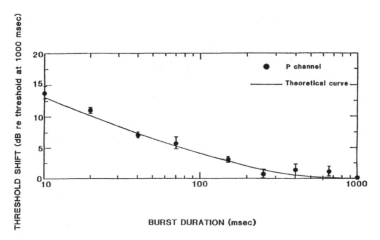

FIG. 8.8. Psychophysically measured average threshold-shift versus burst-duration function (●) obtained with a 100-Hz stimulus for 5 observers. The stimulus was presented to the thenar eminence with a 2.9 cm² contactor and the skin-surface temperature maintained at 30°C. Error bars signify the standard error of the means. The solid curve through the data points is Zwislocki's (1960) theoretical curve.

of 4 spikes per burst, the input to the model integrator consisted of a neural-spike train in response to a short-duration (<100 ms) stimulus that had an amplitude that produced 4 spikes. The voltage output level that corresponded to the resulting output amplitude of the model integrator was then used as the input criterion level for subsequent testing. Data for each duration were sampled in this manner for each stimulus amplitude, from the lowest amplitude to the higher ones, until an amplitude was reached in which 100% of the stimulus presentations produced an output that exceeded the criterion level. During the evaluations, the stimulus amplitude, at each duration, that produced a response exceeding the criterion level for 50% of the presentations was defined as a threshold event. The threshold amplitude was then found for all the other stimulus durations. The resulting data from all the PCs were averaged, and the results of the analysis are compared (Fig. 8.9) to the theoretical curve predicted by the theory of temporal summation and that found in psychophysical experiments (see Fig. 8.8).

The stimulus amplitudes necessary to produce the threshold response are shown plotted as a function of burst duration. As in Fig. 8.8, the amplitudes at each duration have been normalized, using the amplitude of the asymptotic value at 1,000 ms as the reference. The amplitudes correspond to stimulus amplitudes which produced approximately 4 spikes per burst for the shorter-duration stimuli (10–100 ms). To obtain an output sufficient to exceed the criterion level, however, longer durations required

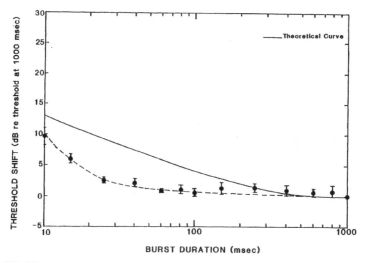

FIG. 8.9. The relationship between threshold shift and burst duration obtained using the temporal integrator with 200-msec time constant. The results are averaged across the tape-recorded responses of seven PCs maintained at 33°C. Error bars signify the standard error of the means. The amplitudes correspond to stimulus amplitudes which produced approximately 4 spikes/burst for the shorter duration stimuli (10–100 ms). Longer durations required amplitudes corresponding to a greater number of spikes/burst. The solid curve denotes the theoretical temporal-summation curve which is identical to that found psychophysically (see Fig. 8.8). The dashed curve drawn through the data points was fitted by eye. (From Checkosky & Bolanowski, 1992. Reprinted with permission from the *Journal of the Acoustical Society of America.)*

stimulus amplitudes which evoked far more spikes per burst. For example, a 250-ms stimulus required 6–12 spikes per burst to exceed the criterion level, and a 600-ms burst required 14–32 spikes per burst. The results show that stimuli of the longer duration require a number greater than 4 spikes per burst to produce an output from the temporal integrator that meets the criterion. This result was independent of the criterion level used and indicates that the number of spikes per burst, be it 4 or some other number, cannot be the code for threshold in the P channel. Furthermore, the analysis showed that regardless of the input to the lowpass filter, a function approximating that found psychophysically and predicted by the theory of temporal summation could not be obtained, indicating that the threshold event in the P channel cannot be mediated by the activity of a single PC.

ACKNOWLEDGMENTS

The authors wish to acknowledge support for research and writing from Grants DC00098, DC00380, and EY04354, National Institutes of Health, U.S. Department of Health and Human Services.

REFERENCES

Bárány, E. H., & Halldén, U. (1948). The influence of some central nervous depressants on the reciprocal inhibition between the two retinae as manifested in retinal rivalry. *Acta Psychologia Scandanavica, 14,* 296–316.

Bolanowski, S. J., Jr. (1987). Contourless stimuli produce binocular brightness summation. *Vision Research, 27,* 1943–1951.

Bolanowski, S. J., Jr., Demeter, S., & Doty, R. W. (1984). Monocular versus binocular Ganzfeld produces differential uptake of 2 – ¹⁴C-deoxyglucose in striate and prestriate cortex of awake macaque. *Society for Neuroscience Abstracts, 10,* 730.

Bolanowski, S. J., Jr., & Doty, R. W. (1982a). Psychophysics and physiology of Ganzfeld. *Perception, 11,* A26.

Bolanowski, S. J., Jr., & Doty, R. W. (1982b). Monocular loss, binocular maintenance of perception in Ganzfeld. *Society for Neuroscience Abstracts, 8,* 675.

Bolanowski, S. J., Jr., & Doty, R. W. (1987). Perceptual "blankout" of monocular homogeneous fields (Ganzfelder) is prevented with binocular viewing. *Vision Research, 27,* 967–982.

Bolanowski, S. J., Jr., Doty, R. W., & Demeter, S. (in preparation). *Binocular versus monocular Granzfeld stimulation produces differential uptake of 2-¹⁴C-deoxyglucose in striate and prestriate cortex of the macaque.*

Bolanowski, S. J., Jr., Gescheider, G. A., Verrillo, R. T., & Checkosky, C. M. (1988). Four channels mediate the mechanical aspects of touch. *Journal of the Acoustical Society of America, 84,* 1680–1694.

Bolanowski, S. J., Jr., King, O. S., & Doty, R. W. (1985). Loss of visual sensation in the monocular Ganzfeld follows rules comparable to binocular rivalry. *Society for Neuroscience Abstracts, 11,* 228.

Bolanowski, S. J., Jr., Makous, J. C., & Raman, D. R. (1987). The relationship among "blankout" of monocularly presented Ganzfelder, rivalry suppression and strabismic suppression. *Neuroscience, 22,* S422.

Bolanowski, S. J., Jr., & Verrillo, R. T. (1982). Temperature and criterion effects in a somatosensory subsystem: A neurophysiological and psychophysical study. *Journal of Neurophysiology, 48,* 836–855.

Bolanowski, S. J., Jr., & Zwislocki, J. J. (1984). Intensity and frequency characteristics of Pacinian corpuscles. I. Action potentials. *Journal of Neurophysiology, 51,* 793–811.

Capraro, A. J., Verrillo, R. T., & Zwislocki, J. J. (1979). Psychophysical evidence for a triplex system of mechanoreception. *Sensory Processes, 3,* 334–352.

Checkosky, C. M. (1991). *Temporal summation in the Pacinian channel: Implications for the neural code for detecting vibrotactile stimuli.* Unpublished doctoral dissertation, University of Rochester School of Medicine and Dentistry.

Checkosky, C. M., & Bolanowski, S. J. (1992). Effects of stimulus duration on the response properties of Pacinian corpuscles: Implications for the neural code. *Journal of the Acoustical Society of America, 91,* 3372–3380.

Ditchburn, R. W. (1973). *Eye movements and visual perception.* Oxford: Clarendon Press.

Freeman, A. W., & Johnson, K. O. (1982). A model accounting for effects of vibratory amplitude on responses of cutaneous mechanoreceptors in macaque monkey. *Journal of Physiology (London), 323,* 43–64.

Gescheider, G. A. (1976). Evidence in support of a duplex theory of mechanoreception. *Sensory Processses, 1,* 68–76.

Gescheider, G. A., Frisina, R. D., & Verrillo, R. T. (1979). Selective adaptation of vibrotactile thresholds. *Sensory Processes, 3,* 37–48.

Gescheider, G. A., O'Malley, M. J., & Verrillo, R. T. (1983). Vibrotactile forward masking: Evidence for channel independence. *Journal of the Acoustical Society of America, 74,* 474–485.

Gescheider, G. A., Sklar, B. F., Van Doren, C. L., & Verrillo, R. T. (1985). Vibrotactile forward masking: Psychophysical evidence for a triplex theory of cutaneous mechanoreception. *Journal of the Acoustical Society of America, 74,* 534–543.

Gescheider, G. A., Verrillo, R. T., & Van Doren, C. L. (1982). Predictions of vibrotactile masking functions. *Journal of the Acoustical Society of America, 72,* 1421–1426.

Gregory, R. L. (1971). *Eye and brain.* New York: MGraw-Hill.

Horton, J. C. (1984). Cytochrome oxidase patches: A new cytoarchitectonic feature of monkey visual cortex. *Philosophical Transactions of the Royal Society of London (B), 304,* 199–253.

Horton, J. C., & Hubel, D. H. (1981). A regular patchy distribution of cytochrome-oxidase staining in primary visual cortex of the macaque monkey. *Nature, 292,* 762–764.

Humphrey, A. L., & Hendrickson, A. E. (1983). Background and stimulus-induced patterns of high metabolic activity in the visual cortex (area 17) of the squirrel and macaque monkey. *Journal of Neuroscience, 3,* 345–358.

Iggo, A., & Ogawa, H. (1977). Correlative physiological and morphological studies of rapidly adapting mechanoreceptors in cat's glabrous skin. *Journal of Physiology (London), 266,* 275–296.

Johansson, R. S. (1976). Receptive sensitivity profile of mechanosensitive units innervating the glabrous skin of the human hand. *Brain Research, 104,* 330–334.

Johansson, R. S. (1978). Tactile sensibilty of the human hand: Receptive field characteristics of mechanoreceptive units in the glabrous skin. *Journal of Physiology, 281,* 101–123.

Johansson, R. S., Landström, U., & Lundström, R. (1982). Sensitivity to edges of mechanoreceptive afferent units innervating the glabrous skin of the human hand. *Brain Research,* 244, 27–32.

Johansson, R. S., & Vallbo, A. B. (1979). Tactile sensibility in the human hand: Relative and absolute densities of four types of mechanoreceptive units in glabrous skin. *Journal of Physiology (London), 286,* 283–300.

Kayama, Y., Riso, R. R., Bartlett, J. R., & Doty, R. W. (1979). Luxotonic responses of units in macaque striate cortex. *Journal of Neurophysiology, 42,* 1495–1517.

Kennedy, C., Des Rosiers, M. H., Reivich, M., Sharpe, F., & Sokoloff, L. (1975). Mapping of functional neural pathways by autoradiographic survey of local metabolic rate with [14C] deoxygluose. *Science, 187,* 850–853.

Levelt, W. J. M. (1965). *On binocular rivalry.* Unpublished doctoral dissertation, University of Utrecht, RVO-TNO, Soesterberg, The Netherlands.

Livingstone, M. S., & Hubel, D. H. (1984). Anatomy and physiology of a color system in the primate visual cortex. *Journal of Neuroscience, 4,* 309–356.

Merzenich, M. M., & Harrington, T. (1969). The sense of flutter-vibration evoked by stimulation of the hairy skin of primates: Comparisons of human sensory capacity with the responses of mechanoreceptive afferents innervating the hairy skin of monkeys. *Experimental Brain Research, 9,* 236–260.

Mountcastle, V. B., LaMotte, R. H., & Carli, G. (1972). Detection thresholds for stimuli in humans and monkeys: Comparison with threshold events in mechanoreceptive afferent nerve fibers innervating the monkey hand. *Journal of Neurophysiology, 35,* 122–136.

Ochoa, J. L., & Torebjörk, H. E. (1983). Sensations evoked by intraneural microstimulation of single mechanoreceptor units innervating the human hand. *Journal of Physiology, 342,* 633–653.

Poggio, G. F., & Fisher, B. (1977). Binocular interactions and depth sensitivity in striate and prestriate cortex of behaving rhesus monkey. *Journal of Neurophysiology, 40,* 1392–1405.

Riggs, L. A. (1965) Visual acuity. In C. H. Graham (Ed.), *Vision and visual perception* (pp. 321–345). New York: Wiley.

Rozhkova, G. I., Nickolayev, P. P., & Shchadrin, V. E. (1982). Perception of stabilized retinal stimuli in dichoptic viewing conditions. *Vision Research, 22,* 293–302.

Seligman, A. M., Karnovsky, M. J., Wasserkrug, H. L., & Hanker, J. S. (1968). Nondroplet ultrastructural demonstration of cytochrome oxidase activity with a polymerizing osmiophilic reagent, diaminobenzidine (DAB). *Journal of Cellular Biology, 38,* 1–14.

Sokoloff, L., Reivich, M., Kennedy, C., Des Rosiers, M. H., Patlak, C. S., Pettigrew, K. D., Sakurada, O., & Shinohara, M. (1977). The [14C]deoxyglucose method for the measurement of local cerebral glucose utilization: Theory, procedure, and normal values in the conscious and anesthetized albino rat. *Journal of Neurochemistry, 28,* 897–916.

Talbot, W. H., Darian-Smith, I., Kornhuber, H. H., & Mountcastle, V. B. (1968). The sense of flutter-vibration: Comparison of the human capacity with response patterns of mechanoreceptive afferents from the monkey hand. *Journal of Neurophysiology, 31,* 301–334.

Tootell, R. B. H., Hamilton, S. L., Silverman, M. S., & Switkes, E. (1988). Functional anatomy of macaque striate cortex. I. Ocular dominance, binocular interactions, and baseline conditions. *Journal of Neuroscience, 8,* 1500–1530.

Tootell, R. B., Silverman, M. S., Switkes, E., & DeValois, R. L. (1982). The organization of cortical modules in primate striate cortex. *Society for Neuroscience Abstracts, 8,* 707.

Vallbo, A. B., & Johansson, R. S. (1984). Properties of cutaneous mechanoreceptors in the hand related to touch sensations. *Human Neurobiology, 3,* 3–14.

Verrillo, R. T. (1962). Investigation of some parameters of the cutaneous threshold for vibration. *Journal of the Acoustical Society of America, 34,* 1768–1773.

Verrillo, R. T. (1963). Effect of contactor area on the vibrotactile threshold. *Journal of the Acoustical Society of America, 35,* 1962–1966.

Verrillo, R. T. (1965). Temporal summation in vibrotactile sensitivity. *Journal of the Acoustical Society of America, 37,* 843–846.

Verrillo, R. T. (1966a). Vibrotactile sensitivity and the frequency response of the Pacinian corpuscle. *Psychonomic Science, 4,* 135–136.

Verrillo, R. T. (1966b). Effects of spatial parameters on the vibrotactile threshold. *Journal of Experimental Psychology, 71,* 570–574.

Verrillo, R. T. (1966c). Vibrotactile thresholds for hairy skin. *Journal of Experimental Psychology, 72,* 47–50.

Verrillo, R. T., & Bolanowski, S. J., Jr. (1986). The effects of skin temperature on the psychophysical responses to vibration on glabrous and hairy skin. *Journal of the Acoustical Society of America, 80,* 528–532.

Walker, P. (1978). Binocular rivalry: Central or peripheral selective processes. *Psychological Bulletin, 85,* 376–389.

Wengenack, T. M. (1991). *Characterization and localization of units responding to diffuse illumination in visual cortex of the awake macaque.* Unpublished doctoral dissertation, University of Rochester School of Medicine and Dentistry.

Wengenack, T. M., & Bolanowski, S. J., Jr. (1990a). Classification of neural activity in V1 of the awake macaque as produced by Ganzfeld illumination. *Investigative Ophthalmology and Visual Science, 31,* 92.

Wengenack, T. M., & Bolanowski, S. J., Jr. (1990b). Localization of units in V1 of the awake macaque responding to diffuse illumination. *Society for Neuroscience Abstracts, 16,* 1219.

Wengenack, T. M., & Bolanowski, S. J., Jr. (in preparation). *Localization of units in striate cortex of the awake macaque responding to diffuse illumination.*

Wengenack, T. M., Checkosky, C. M., & Bolanowski, S. J., Jr (1988). Classification of neural activity in V1 of the awake macaque as produced by Ganzfeld illumination. *Society for Neuroscience Abstracts, 14,* 201.

Wheatstone, C. (1938). On some remarkable, and hitherto unobserved, phenomena of binocular vision. *Philosophical Transactions of the Royal Society of London, 128,* 371–394.

Wong-Riley, M. T. T. (1976). Endogenous peroxidatic activity in brain stem neurons as demonstrated by their staining with diaminobenzidine in normal squirrel monkeys. *Brain Research, 108,* 257–277.

Wong-Riley, M. T. T. (1979). Changes in the visual system of monocularly sutured or enucleated cats demonstrable with cytochrome oxidase histochemistry. *Brain Research, 171,* 11–28.

Yarbus, A. L. (1967). *Eye movements in vision* (trans. ed., L. A. Riggs; trans. by B. Haigh). New York: Plenum Press.

Zwislocki, J. J. (1960). Theory of temporal auditory summation. *Journal of the Acoustical society of America, 32,* 1046–1060.

Zwislocki, J. J. (1969). Temporal summation of loudness: An analysis. *Journal of the Acoustical Society of America, 46,* 431–441.

9 Interaural Temporal Coding of Complex High-Frequency Sounds: A Transformation in the Inferior Colliculus?

Ranjan Batra
University of Connecticut Health Center

At the Institute for Sensory Research I studied the responses of neurons in the visual system to patterned visual stimuli. Upon leaving the Institute, I continued to study the responses of neurons to patterned stimuli. The difference is that now the neurons are auditory and the stimuli are acoustic.

One particular kind of patterned acoustic stimulus has proven extremely useful: the sinusoidally amplitude-modulated (SAM) tone (Fig. 9.1). SAM tones have many of the features of more complex sounds, and yet are relatively simple to manipulate. A SAM tone is a pure tone except, that its amplitude is modulated at a rate that is slow compared to the frequency of the tone. Thus, it can be used to test the properties of a neuron near a particular frequency. Neurons in the auditory nerve synchronize to the envelopes of SAM tones (Frisina, Smith, & Chamberlain, 1985; Javel, 1980; Joris & Yin; 1992; Kim, 1990; Møller, 1976; Palmer, 1982; Smith &

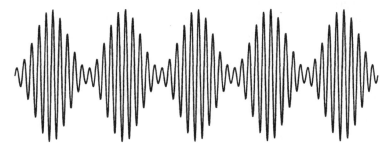

FIG. 9.1. A sinusoidally amplitude-modulated (SAM) tone. The SAM tone was modulated to a depth of 80%.

Brachman, 1980) and convey the pattern of amplitude variation to higher auditory centers.

Sounds with envelopes, such as SAM tones, are interesting for two reasons. First, such sounds are important in investigating the processing of complex patterned stimuli such as speech. Second, and less well known, the envelopes of such sounds can be used in locating the sound's source.

Unlike the visual and somatosensory systems, in which space is mapped directly onto the receptor surface, no map of auditory space exists in the cochlea, which is instead mapped according to frequency. Consequently, our ability to localize sounds must rest on neuronal computations performed by the central auditory system. Localization along the azimuth, that is, in the horizontal plane, is based largely on our ability to interpret minute differences in the intensity and the time of arrival of a sound at either ear. Traditionally, interaural temporal differences (ITDs) have been thought to be used only at lower frequencies where neurons of the auditory nerve can synchronize to the periodic pressure variations. However, if a sound of higher frequency is amplitude-modulated, then peripheral neurons can synchronize to the modulation envelope and convey the pattern of modulation to a central comparator. The ITDs of complex, high-frequency sounds can be detected by human listeners (Bernstein & Trahiotis, 1985; David, Guttman, & van Bergeijk, 1959; Henning, 1974; Leakey, Sayers, & Cherry, 1958; McFadden & Pasanen, 1976; Neutzel & Hafter, 1976) and may serve as a cue for sound localization.

The initial sites for encoding ITDs appear to be the medial and lateral superior olives (Fig. 9.2). These two nuclei encode ITDs in different ways. Neurons of the medial superior olive (MSO) discharge maximally to a particular ITD, irrespective of the modulation frequency (Yin & Chan, 1990). Neurons of the MSO are typically excited by stimulation of either ear (Caird & Klinke, 1983; Goldberg & Brown, 1968; Guinan, Norris, & Guinan, 1972; Langford, 1984; Yin & Chan, 1990). The graph (Fig. 9.2A) shows the expected response of a neuron in the MSO to SAM tones as the ITD is varied. Each curve depicts the response to a different modulation frequency. As the ITD changes, the response at a particular modulation frequency undergoes a periodic change, as consecutive periods of the modulation come in and out of coincidence. However, the ITD at which the central maximum occurs is the same for all modulation frequencies.

In contrast, neurons of the lateral superior olive (LSO) are maximally suppressed at a particular ITD (Joris & Yin, 1990; Kuwada & Batra, 1991). These neurons receive excitatory input from the ipsilateral side, but inhibitory inputs from the contralateral side (Boudreau & Tsuchitani, 1968; Caird & Klinke, 1983; Covey, Vater, & Casseday, 1991; Finlayson & Caspary, 1991; Guinan et al., 1972; Harnischfeger, Neuweiler, & Schlegel, 1985; Moore & Caspary, 1983; Tsuchitani, 1977; Wu & Kelly, 1991). As

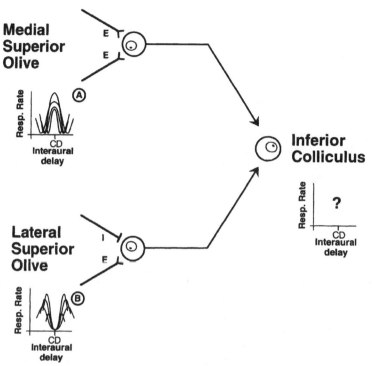

FIG. 9.2.   Encoding interaural temporal differences (ITDs) in the mammalian brain-stem. Encoding of ITDs begins in the medial and lateral superior olives (MSO and LSO), but these two nuclei encode ITDs in different ways. Neurons of the MSO encode a preferred ITD by discharging maximally (graph A, CD). When tested with SAM tones, this preferred ITD is the same regardless of the modulation frequency. This code is a consequence of the bilateral excitatory input that neurons of the MSO receive. In contrast, neurons of the LSO encode a preferred ITD by maximal suppression (graph B). This preferred ITD is also independent of the modulation frequency of a SAM tone. The code used by the LSO is a consequence of the convergence of an ipsilateral excitatory input with a contralateral inhibitory input. The outputs of the MSO and the LSO converge on the inferior colliculus. What kind of sensitivity to ITDs is observed there?

with neurons of the MSO, the response undergoes a periodic change as the ITD is varied. However, there is now a central minimum, which is the same at all modulation frequencies (Fig. 9.2B).

The MSO and LSO send their output to the inferior colliculus. Our question is: What kind of sensitivity to ITDs do neurons in the inferior colliculus exhibit, and what inputs do they receive from either side?

My colleagues and I are studying how neurons of the auditory system encode ITDs in the envelopes of high-frequency sounds. As our experimental subject we chose the dutch-belted rabbit. The rabbit provides one key advantage over other preparations. Single neurons can be studied without the use of anesthesia, an important advantage, because our ability to localize sounds is based on neural computations that could be sensitive to anesthetics. In the inferior colliculus, we know that barbiturate anesthesia does affect the sensitivity of neurons that process ITDs of low-frequency sounds (Kuwada, Batra, & Stanford, 1989).

Details of our methodology have been described elsewhere (Batra, Kuwada, & Stanford, 1989; Kuwada, Stanford, & Batra, 1987). The rabbits were prepared for recording under surgical anesthesia. The skull was exposed, and a short rod anchored to it with small screws and cement. A few days or weeks after the rabbit had recovered from this surgery it was again anesthetized, and a small hole was drilled in the skull over the inferior colliculus. The hole was capped with elastopolymer.

During a recording session, the rabbit was seated in a padded couch, and restrained with nylon straps. The restraint was for the rabbit's own protection, because any substantial movement during the recording might cause it harm. The rod on the head was firmly clamped. The elastopolymer cap was removed, the dura desensitized with lidocaine, and a metal electrode advanced into the brain. All recordings were made extracellularly.

Sounds were delivered to either ear through a sealed system, which was coupled to the ear canal via custom-fitted ear molds. The acoustic system was calibrated after the last recording session, either under deep anesthesia or after the animal had been killed

During the recording session the rabbit was monitored using a video camera. Recording session typically lasted 2 hours. If the rabbit fidgeted, the session was terminated, because even small movements of the rabbit made it difficult to record from single neurons.

Neurons in the inferior colliculus that were sensitive to ITDs of SAM tones largely fell into two categories: those that showed MSO-like sensitivity to ITDs at the higher modulation frequencies (>200–250 Hz), that is, frequencies that would be expected to be useful for sound localization, and those that showed LSO-like sensitivity at these frequencies. Figure 9.3 illustrates the responses of two neurons in the inferior colliculus: one that had responses consistent with those expected in the MSO (Fig. 9.3A), and the other that had responses consistent with those expected in the LSO (Fig. 9.3B). The left column shows the response to binaurally presented SAM tones at several modulation frequencies as a function of the ITD. For the MSO-like neuron, a central maximum occurs at the same ITD at all modulation frequencies, while for the LSO-like neuron, it is a central minimum that is common across modulation frequencies.

The next two columns demonstrate the kind of input each neuron receives from either ear. The middle column shows the response to contralateral stimulation with pure tones, in the form of a peri-stimulus-time (PST)

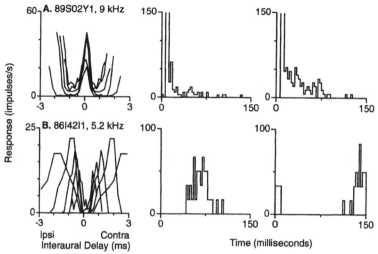

FIG. 9.3.   Responses of a MSO-like and a LSO-like neuron in the inferior colliculus. Each row depicts the response of a different neuron at its best frequency. Left Column: Responses to ITDs of SAM tones. The ITD of the envelope was varied continuously by presenting the same carrier frequency to both ears, and introducing a 1-Hz difference between the left and right modulation frequencies. The delay curves of each neuron at different modulation frequencies were calculated from the response to this "binaural SAM" stimulus. For the neuron in A, delay curves at different modulation frequencies align near their peaks, as is the case for neurons of the MSO. For the neuron in B, delay curves at different modulation frequencies align near their troughs, as is the case for neurons of the LSO. Durations of stimuli were 3–5.1 sec. Carrier frequencies as shown. Intensity levels (contra/ipsi dB SPL): A – 57/48 dB; B – 41/45 dB. Modulation depth was 80% in all cases. Middle column: Responses to contralateral stimulation with pure tones, shown as PST histograms. In A, the initial transient has been truncated to show changes in the sustained response. Frequency and intensity level were the same as for stimulation with SAM tones. Stimulus duration was 75ms. Right column: Responses to binaural stimulation. Frequencies, stimulus durations, and contralateral intensity levels were the same as before. Ipsilateral intensity levels: A – 58 dB; B – 65 dB.

histogram. The right column shows the change in response when both contralateral and ipsilateral stimuli were delivered simultaneously. The MSO-like neuron (Fig. 9.3A) was excited by contralateral stimulation, and this response was enhanced by concurrent ipsilateral stimulation, indicating that this neuron received excitatory input from both sides, much as is seen in the MSO. The LSO-like neuron (Fig. 9.3B) was excited by contralateral stimulation, but this response was inhibited by concurrent ipsilateral stimulation, indicating that ipsilateral input was inhibitory. The responses of the LSO-like neuron correspond to what would be expected of a neuron in the contralateral LSO. There is, in fact, a projection from the contralateral LSO to the inferior colliculus (e.g., Brunso-Bechtold, Thompson, &

Masterton, 1981; Roth, Aitkin, Andersen, & Merzenich, 1978; Stotler, 1953), which appears to be excitatory (Glendenning, Baker, Hutson, & Masterton, 1992).

Almost all neurons in the inferior colliculus that showed LSO-like sensitivity to ITDs were excited contralaterally and inhibited ipsilaterally when tested with pure tones. In contrast, only a few neurons that possessed MSO-like sensitivity were excited by stimulation of either ear—rather surprisingly, a large proportion were not.

In the inferior colliculus, neurons with a MSO-like sensitivity to ITDs were frequently excited by contralateral stimulation and inhibited by ipsilateral stimulation. The responses of three neurons of this type are shown in Fig. 9.4, in a format similar to Fig. 9.3. Again, each row depicts the response of a different neuron. The panels in the left column show the responses to interaurally delayed SAM tones. These responses indicate MSO-like sensitivity to ITDs. In Figs. 9.4A and Figs. 9.4B, the middle panel shows the response to contralateral stimulation alone. In both cases, contralateral stimulation evoked an excitatory response. The rightmost panels of Figs. 9.4A and 9.4B show the response of each neuron when the ipsilateral ear was concurrently stimulated. In both cases, the level of response is reduced relative to contralateral stimulation alone, indicating that the ipsilateral input was inhibitory. The individual inputs were tested somewhat differently in the neuron of Fig. 9.4C (right panel). In this case, during ongoing contralateral stimulation (hatched bar), the ipsilateral ear was concurrently stimulated for a brief period (solid bar). The suppression of the response to contralateral stimulation indicates the inhibitory nature of the ipsilateral input.

Thus, in the inferior colliculus, neurons with MSO-like sensitivity to ITDs of SAM tones are frequently excited contralaterally, but inhibited ipsilaterally when tested with pure tones, unlike neurons of the MSO itself, which are mostly excited by stimulation of either ear. It appears that a transformation has occurred from the superior olivary complex to the inferior colliculus, but what can the purpose of this transformation be?

Neurons that are excited by stimulation of one ear but inhibited by stimulation of the other are thought to encode the azimuth of a sound using interaural intensity differences as a cue. Perhaps neurons of the inferior colliculus encode the azimuth of a sound using *both* interaural intensity and interaural temporal differences. Thus, if a sound were located off the midline, and were a relatively pure tone, these neurons would use the interaural intensity cue, but if the sound had a rapidly fluctuating envelope, then they would use the interaural temporal cue.

Such conjoint coding could arise in the inferior colliculus from the convergence of direct and indirect inputs from the MSO and LSO, or, for that matter, from interaction of these inputs with direct inputs from the

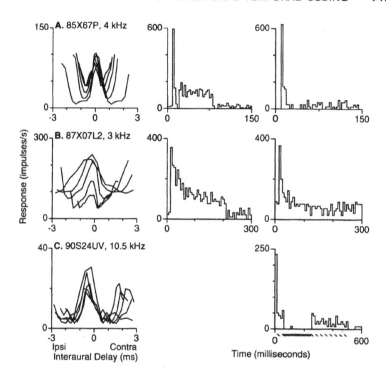

FIG. 9.4. Three neurons in the inferior colliculus with MSO-like sensitivity to ITDs. Each row depicts the response of a different neuron at its best frequency. Left column: Responses to ITDs of SAM tones. Intensity levels (contra/ipsi dB SPL): A – 39/63 dB; B – 44/43 dB; C – 56/55 dB. Modulation depth was 80% in all cases. Middle column: Responses to contralateral stimulation with pure tones, shown as PST histograms. Frequency and intensity level were the same as for stimulation with SAM tones. Stimulus duration: A – 75 ms; B – 200 ms. Right column: Responses to binaural stimulation. Frequencies and contralateral intensity levels were the same as before. Stimulus duration in A and B same as for middle column. In C, hatched bar marks contralateral stimulation alone, solid bar marks binaural stimulation. Ipsilateral intensity levels: A – 53 dB; B – 63 dB; C – 75 dB.

cochlear nucleus. The inferior colliculus receives direct input from the ipsilateral MSO and from both the ipsilateral and contralateral LSO (e.g., Brunso-Bechtold et al., 1981; Roth et al., 1978; Stotler, 1953). The uncrossed pathway actually comprises two projections: one of which is glycinergic and most likely inhibitory, the other of which is neither glycinergic nor GABAergic, and is most likely excitatory (Glendenning et al. 1992; Saint Marie, Ostapoff, Morest, & Wenthold, 1989). There are also indirect pathways from the LSO and MSO that arrive at the inferior colliculus by way of the dorsal nucleus of the lateral lemniscus of both sides and direct projections from both cochlear nuclei (reviewed by Oliver &

Shneiderman, 1991). Many of these inputs form terminal bands in the neuropil, which may or may not overlap. However, nonoverlapping inputs may still be connected by the extensive internal circuitry of the inferior colliculus (Oliver, Kuwada, Yin, Haberly, & Henkel, 1991). The complexity of the afferents to the inferior colliculus and the neural circuitry within it provide several ways in which the responses we observed could arise.

ACKNOWLEDGMENTS

This research was supported by the National Institute of Neurological Disorders and Stroke Grant NS-18027 to S. Kuwada, in whose laboratory this work was performed.

REFERENCES

Batra, R., Kuwada, S., & Standford, T. R. (1989). Temporal coding of envelopes and their interaural delays in the inferior colliculus of the unanesthetized rabbit. *Journal of Neurophysiology, 61* 257–268.

Bernstein, L. R., & Trahiotis, C. (1985). Lateralization of low-frequency, complex waveforms: The use of envelope-based temporal disparities. *Journal of the Acoustical Society of America, 77,* 1868–1880.

Boudreau, J. C., & Tsuchitani, C. (1968). Binaural interaction in the cat superior olive S segment. *Journal of Neurophysiology, 31,* 442–454.

Brunso-Bechtold, J. K., Thompson, G. C., & Masterton, R. B. (1981). HRP study of the organization of auditory afferents ascending to central nucleus of inferior colliculus in cat. *Journal of Comparative Neurology, 197,* 705–722.

Caird, D., & Klinke, R. (1983). Processing of binaural stimuli by cat superior olivary complex neurons. *Experimental Brain Research, 52,* 385–399.

Covey, E., Vater, M., & Casseday, J. H. (1991). Binaural properties of single units in the superior olivary complex of the mustached bat. *Journal of Neurophysiology, 66,* 1080–1094.

David, E. E. J., Guttman, N., & van Bergeijk, W. A. (1959). Binaural interaction of high-frequency complex stimuli. *Journal of the Acoustical Society of America, 31,* 774–782.

Finlayson, P. G., & Caspary, D. M. (1991). Low-frequency neurons in the lateral superior olive exhibit phase-sensitive binaural inhibition. *Journal of Neurophysiology, 65,* 598–605.

Frisina, R. D., Smith, R. L., & Chamberlain, S. C. (1985). Differential encoding of rapid changes in sound amplitude by second-order auditory neurons. *Experimental Brain Research, 60,* 417–422.

Glendenning, K. K., Baker, B. N., Hutson, K. A., & Masterton, R. B. (1992). Acoustic chiasm V: Inhibition and excitation in the ipsilateral and contralateral projections of LSO. *Journal of Comparative Neurology, 319,* 100–122.

Goldberg, J. M., & Brown, P. B. (1968). Functional organization of the dog superior olivary complex: An anatomical and electrophysiological study. *Journal of Neurophysiology, 31,* 639–656.

Guinan, J. J., Jr., Norris, B. E., & Guinan, S. S. (1972). Single auditory units in the superior olivary complex. II: Locations of unit categories and tonotopic organization. *International Journal of Neuroscience, 4,* 147–166.

PROCESSING OF AM BY THE AUDITORY NERVE

At low- and moderate-intensity levels, auditory nerve fibers give significant synchronous responses to AM tones. If AM frequency is varied, auditory nerve fibers act as lowpass filters for the encoding of tones and wideband noise whose envelopes are modulated (Frisina, Smith, & Chamberlain, 1985; Javel, 1980; Møller, 1976a). The frequency response starts to fall off at AM frequencies above 500 Hz, with some positive relationship observed between best frequency (BF) and the high cutoff for AM coding (Palmer, 1982). Local maxima in the AM frequency-response functions are sometimes seen at much higher AM frequencies for low-BF fibers. This effect may be due to complex interactions between the carrier and modulation frequencies which occur when low carrier frequencies are used.

Auditory nerve fiber phase locking to AM rapidly declines as the intensity of the stimulus is raised (Brachman, 1980; Evans & Palmer, 1980; Frisina, 1983; Møller, 1976a; Smith & Brachman, 1977, 1980a). In most cases, an auditory nerve fiber can only give a significant synchronous response to AM over a 30- to 40-dB range of average intensities. The decline at high AM frequencies is sometimes less than at low AM frequencies, because the synchronous response starts at a lower level at high AM frequencies. These findings apply to the typical, low-threshold, high spontaneous-activity auditory nerve fiber. High-threshold, low spontaneous-activiy auditory nerve fibers are similar except that they can have extended dynamic ranges for the steady-state encoding of AM (Joris & Yin, 1992).

NEURAL MECHANISM FOR AUDITORY NERVE AM ENCODING

What neural events govern and constrain the ability of auditory nerve fibers to encode AM? Why is the AM operating range so limited for a typical auditory nerve fiber relative to the overall perceptual operating range of hearing? The best theoretical model put forth to explain this situation comes from the work of Smith and Brachman (1980b). They observed that at frequencies between 150–300 Hz, the frequencies at which auditory nerve fibers give maximal responses to AM, if the rise time of a pure-tone burst is appropriate, the *onset* rate-intensity function of a fiber is a good, quantitative predictor of how phase locking to AM varies with the average intensity of sound. The onset function is a measure of the firing rate of the fiber during the initial, peak 1 ms of the response. We subsequently demonstrated that the rising and falling phases of the AM are encoded differentially, consistent with adaptational processes in the auditory nerve (Smith, Brachman, & Frisina, 1985).

Harnischfeger, G., Neuweiler, G., & Schlegel, P. (1985). Interaural time and intensity coding in superior olivary complex and inferior colliculus of the echolocating bat, *Molussus ater*. *Journal of Neurophysiology, 53*, 89–109.

Henning, G. B. (1974). Detectability of interaural delay in high-frequency complex waveforms. *Journal of the Acoustical Society of America, 55*, 84–90.

Javel, E. (1980). Coding of AM tones in the chinchilla auditory nerve: Implications for the pitch of complex tones. *Journal of the Acoustical Society of America, 68*, 133–146.

Joris, P. X., & Yin, T. C. T. (1990). Time sensitivity of cells in the lateral superior olive (LSO) to monaural and binaural amplitude-modulated complexes. *Association for Research in Otolaryngology Abstracts, 13*, 267–268.

Joris, P. X., & Yin, T. C. T. (1992). Responses to amplitude-modulated tones in the auditory nerve of the cat. *Journal of the Acoustical Society of America, 91*, 215–232.

Kim, D. O. (1990). Responses of DCN-PVCN neurons and auditory nerve fibers in unanesthetized decerebrate cats to AM and pure tones: Analysis with autocorrelation/power-spectrum. *Hearing Research, 45*, 95–113.

Kuwada, S., & Batra, R. (1991). Sensitivity to interaural time differences (ITDs) of neurons in the superior olivary complex (SOC) of the unanesthetized rabbit. *Society for Neuroscience Abstracts, 17*, 450.

Kuwada, S., Batra, R., & Stanford, T. R. (1989). Monaural and binaural response properties of neurons in the inferior colliculus of the rabbit: effects of sodium pentobarbital. *Journal or Neurophysiolgy, 61*, 269–282.

Kuwada, S., Batra, R., & Stanford, T. R., (1987). Interaural phase senistive units in the inferior colliculus of the unanesthetized rabbit. Effects of changing frequency. *Journal of Neurophsiology, 57*, 1338–1360.

Langford, T. L. (1984). Responses elicited from medial superior olivary neurons by stimuli associated with binaural masking and unmasking. *Hearing Research, 15*, 39–50.

Leakey, D. M., Sayers, B. M. A., & Cherry, C. (1958). Binaural fusion of low- and high-frequency sounds. *Journal of the Acoustical Society of America, 30*, 222.

McFadden, D., & Pasanen, E. G. (1976). Lateralization at high-frequencies based on interaural time differences. *Journal of the Acoustical Society of America, 59*, 634–639.

Møller, A. R. (1976). Dynamic properties of primary auditory fibers compared with cells in the cochlear nucleus. *Acta Physiologica Scandinavia, 98*, 157–167.

Moore, M. J., & Caspary, D. M. (1983). Strychnine blocks binaural inhibition in lateral superior olivary neurons. *Journal of Neuroscience, 3*, 237–242.

Neutzel, J. M., & Hafter, E. R. (1976). Lateralization of complex waveforms: Effects of fine structure, amplitude, and duration. *Journal of the Acoustical Society of America, 60*, 1339–1346.

Oliver, D. L., Kuwada, S., Yin, T. C. T., Haberly, L. B., & Henkel, C. K. (1991). Dendritic and axonal morphology of HRP-injected neurons in the inferior colliculus of the cat. *Journal of Comparative Neurology, 303*, 75–100.

Oliver, D. L., & Shneiderman, A. (1991). The anatomy of the inferior colliculus: A cellular basis for integration of monaural and binaural information. In: R. A. Altschuler, R. P. Bobbin, B. M. Clopton, & D. W. Hoffman (Eds.), *Neurobiology of hearing: The central auditory system* (pp. 195–222). New York: Raven Press.

Palmer, A. R. (1982). Encoding of rapid amplitude fluctuations by cochlear-nerve fibres in the guinea-pig. *Archives of Oto-Rhino-Laryngology, 236*, 197–202.

Roth, G. L., Aitkin, L. M., Andersen, R. A., & Merzenich, M. M. (1978). Some features of the spatial organization of the central nucleus of the inferior colliculus of the cat. *Journal of Comparative Neurology, 182*, 661–680.

Saint Marie, R. L., Ostapoff, E. - M., Morest, D. K., & Wenthold,R. J. (1989). Glycine-immunoreactive projection of the cat superior olive: Possible role in midbrain ear dominance. *Journal of Comparative Neurology, 279*, 382–396.

Smith, R. L., & Brachman, M. L. (1980). Response modulation of auditory-nerve fibers by AM stimuli: Effects of average intensity. *Hearing Research, 2,* 123–133.

Stotler, W. A. (1953). An experimental study of the cells and connections of the superior olivary complex of the cat. *Journal of Comparative Neurology, 98,* 401–431.

Tsuchitani, C. (1977). Functional organization of lateral cell groups of cat superior olivary complex. *Journal of Neurophysiology, 40,* 296–318.

Wu, S. H., & Kelly, J. B. (1991). Physiological properties of neurons in the mouse superior olive: Membrane characteristics and postsynaptic responses studied in vitro. *Journal of Neurophysiology, 65,* 230–246.

Yin, T. C. T., & Chan, J. C. K. (1990). Interaural time sensitivity in medial superior olive of cat. *Journal of Neurophysiology, 64,* 465–488.

10 Differential Abilities to Extrac Sound-Envelope Information by Auditory Nerve and Cochlear Nucleus Neurons

Robert D. Frisina
Joseph P. Walton
Kenneth J. Karcich
University of Rochester School of Medicine & Dentistry

INTRODUCTION

Investigating responses of auditory neurons to critical features of important sounds is one approach to understanding the neural basis of complex sound encoding by the auditory nervous system. Key features of speech and other biologically relevant sounds include rapid changes in sound amplitude — amplitude modulation (AM). Single-neuron studies of AM coding are timely, because interest in temporal-processing mechanisms of the peripheral and central auditory systems is currently a favored topic of many auditory and sensory neuroscientists.

Reviewing what we know about how single neurons of the auditory nerve and cochlear nucleus encode amplitude modulation is a major goal of this chapter. All of these studies have been conducted by presenting AM sounds in a *quiet* acoustic environment. It will be evident that we have learned much from these previous efforts about how the cochlear nucleus abstracts important information about rapid sound-amplitude changes. However, it remains uncertain, for example, how the remarkable abilities of some cochlear nucleus neurons to give an amplified response to AM over a wide range of average intensities would be effected by a more realistic auditory setting containing background noise. We will present some initial data directed at answering this question toward the end of this chapter.

Insights can be gained from previous articles into the nature of how the auditory system responds to complex sound features such as AM. Representative, key studies will be described that have set the stage for the new findings put forth later.

Because a quantitative relation exists between auditory nerve AM encoding and the onset rate-intensity function, and the properties of the rate-intensity function are determined by adaptational properties at the hair cell/auditory nerve fiber synapse, it was hypothesized and subsequently demonstrated that the adaptational properties of the hair cell/auditory nerve synaptic transmitter kinetics can quantitatively predict AM processing capabilities of auditory nerve fibers (Brachman, 1980; Hewitt & Meddis, 1991; Schwid & Geisler, 1982; Westerman & Smith, 1988).

EFFECTS OF BACKGROUND NOISE ON AUDITORY NERVE CODING OF SIMPLE SOUNDS

Several studies have measured the effects of background noise on the operating ranges of auditory nerve fibers in regard to their abilities to encode tones and other temporally and spectrally simple sounds (Costalupes, Young, & Gibson, 1984; Geisler & Sinex, 1980; Gibson, Young, & Costalupes, 1985). The majority of evidence from these reports indicates that the operating range of most auditory nerve fibers, as measured in steady-state rate-intensity functions for tones, shifts to higher average intensities in the presence of wideband noise. Because the operating range per se (the sloping portion of the rate-intensity function) is shifted to higher levels but does not change much in magnitude, sound-intensity coding diminishes at low levels and can improve at certain higher levels.

COCHLEAR NUCLEUS PROCESSING OF AMPLITUDE MODULATION

Ground-breaking studies of AM responses in the cochlear nucleus of the rat were done by Møller (1972, 1973, 1974a, 1974b, 1975a, 1975b, 1976a, 1976b, 1976c). A key goal was to perform a linear systems analysis of single-unit responses to determine the fidelity with which AM is encoded. He discovered that, except at very high-stimulus modulation depths, most cochlear nucleus units encode AM with high fidelity. Some units were tuned to different AM frequencies (80–500 Hz), and their tuning properties were relatively resilient to alterations in stimulus parameters such as the depth of modulation, the duration of the stimulus, and whether repetitive bursts or continuous tones were used as stimuli. Single-unit AM tuning properties remained stable for hours and were found to be independent of the several procedures used to measure them. For example, in some instances tones or noise amplitude modulated with sinusoids were used, and the depth of modulation of the response obtained from period histograms phase locked to the stimulus envelope. In other cases, continuous tones or noise modulated with pseudorandom noise (random noise that is periodically repeated) were used and the cross-correlation functions obtained, allowing the computation of AM tuning properties using Fourier transforms.

Møller also found that cochlear nucleus units can amplify the depth of modulation in the stimulus at intensities up to 60 dB above threshold. He found, in contrast, that auditory nerve fibers show this amplification over only a 30-dB range. Lastly, he pointed out that the dynamic range for AM encoding can exceed that of the average rate-intensity function for some cochlear nucleus units.

As is true of noteworthy pioneering work, Møller's investigations raised many novel, interesting questions. For instance: Do all cochlear nucleus units encode AM equally well? If not, is there a relation between a unit's responses to simple sounds and its ability to encode dynamic features of complex sounds such as AM? Where are the units located that preferentially encode AM relative to auditory nerve fibers? What are the possible cellular or network mechanisms by which enhanced responses to AM are generated in the cochlear nucleus? What features of AM signals do cochlear nucleus units select for?

Insights into answers to some of these questions come from recent reports from Kim and coworkers (Arle & Kim, 1991; Kim, Sirianni, & Chang, 1990). For example, they have shown in decerebrate cat that pauser/ buildup, Type IV units in the dorsal cochlear nucleus (DCN) show amplified responses to AM. The frequency selectivity of this AM encoding is predictable from the unit's autocorrelation function. In addition, regularity analyses of pauser/buildup units in the DCN, as well as units of the ventral cochlear nucleus (VCN), indicate that a strong correlation exists between a unit's regularity of discharge to simple sounds and its ability to effectively encode AM. Their modeling efforts, and those of Banks and Sachs (1991) and Hewitt, Meddis, and Shackleton (1992), have suggested that part of a cochlear nucleus unit's ability to preferentially encode sinusoidally modulated tones comes from the dendritic filtering properties of stellate and fusiform extensive dendritic arbors.

We, too, have made progress in obtaining answers to the previously asked questions. Aside from advancing knowledge about how the auditory system encodes complex sounds, our efforts have provided insights into how the auditory system as a whole is able to neurally process acoustic information to operate over a range of intensities that greatly exceeds the dynamic range of individual auditory nerve fibers. One discovery is that certain cochlear nucleus units can maintain or even enhance their encoding of AM at high sound levels in the presence of a fairly intense wideband background noise. In addition, clarification of the significance of the pure-tone classification for cochlear nucleus neurons has been obtained (Frisina, Chamberlain, Brachman, & Smith, 1982).

NEURAL PROCESSING OF AM IN THE VENTRAL COCHLEAR NUCLEUS

A portion of our results to date help merge two lines of classical research of the cochlear nucleus: (a) cochlear nucleus responses to simple sounds, and (b) cochlear nucleus responses to dynamic sounds such as AM (Frisina, 1983; Frisina et al., 1985; Frisina, Smith, & Chamberlain, 1990a). To accomplish this, single-unit responses were recorded in intermediate regions of the VCN for pure-tone and sinusoidally AM stimuli. Four major VCN unit types were encountered: onset, chopper, primary-like with notch, and primary-like. The responses of these unit types were compared with responses of auditory nerve fibers of the same species to identical stimuli. It was found that all four unit types, as well as auditory nerve fibers, show strong synchronous responses or phase locking to 150-Hz AM at low intensities. However, neurons differ greatly in their abilities to encode AM at high intensities. Onset units tend to show the strongest phase locking to AM, followed by chopper, primary-like-with-notch, and primary-like, respectively. Auditory nerve fibers respond similarly to primary-like units, qualitatively.

A HIERARCHY OF ENHANCEMENT IN VCN FOR AM ENCODING

The 150-Hz findings do not necessarily reflect a neuron's overall ability to encode AM, because some cochlear nucleus neurons are tuned to different AM frequencies. To get a comprehensive understanding of each unit type's ability to encode AM, we varied the AM frequency and intensity of stimulation. To quantitatively measure phase locking, Fourier analyses were performed on steady-state portions of the peri-stimulus-time (PST) histograms generated in response to AM, which yields measures of the first-harmonic and average responses. The percent modulation of the response is defined as the ratio of the first-harmonic response to the average response. A neuron's synchronous response was reported in terms of the gain scale:

$$\text{response gain in dB} = 20 \times \log_{10}\left(\frac{\text{percent modulation of response}}{\text{percent modulation of stimulus}}\right) \quad (1)$$

Note that for a gain of 0 dB, the percent modulation of the response equals that of the stimulus. The results were plotted as three-dimensional surfaces displaying response gain versus AM frequency and sound level. It was found that throughout their AM response areas, all four VCN unit types show stronger phase locking than auditory nerve fibers. The distances between the response surfaces of VCN neurons and auditory nerve fibers are measures of the amount of *enhancement* or amplification performed by VCN neurons relative to their ascending input. The distances are greatest for onset units, followed in order by chopper, primary-like-with-notch, and primary-like units. The greatest amount of enhancement occurs at *high* intensities.

AM RESPONSE AREAS BECOME BANDPASS AT HIGH INTENSITIES IN VCN

It was also found (Frisina et al., 1985, 1990a) that at low intensities the shapes of the response surfaces are similar for each of the VCN unit types and auditory nerve fibers. The surfaces are lowpass in nature, that is, low AM frequencies evoke strong synchronous responses, and this response diminishes as the AM frequency increases. At high intensities, in contrast, the response surfaces tend to be tuned or bandpass in nature with peaks occurring at AM frequencies between 80 and 700 Hz. The response surfaces of onset and chopper units usually show a single, easily identified AM frequency at which there is a maximal response. However, the response surfaces of primary-like-with-notch units, and to a greater extent, primary-like units and auditory nerve fibers are fairly flat with several, shallow local maxima. A quantitative measure of the amount of enhancement of AM encoding of a VCN unit relative to auditory nerve fibers was calculated by subtracting the mean response gain of our sample of auditory nerve fibers from the mean response gain of each of the four groups of VCN units. This quantitative analysis substantiated the hierarchy of enhancement as described above, with onset units being the best encoders of AM in the VCN, followed by choppers, primary-like-with-notch, and primary-like units respectively.

SUMMARY OF VCN AM ENCODING IN QUIET

These findings demonstrate that a relation exists between the pure-tone classification scheme and the encoding of a complex-sound feature: AM. Specifically, the further a neuron's pure-tone responses deviate from a primary-like pattern, the greater its ability to produce strong, synchronous responses to AM. These results, aside from advancing knowledge of the functional organization of the VCN, also provide new clues about the neural correlates of the wide dynamic range of the auditory system. For instance, previous investigations of the auditory nerve reviewed earlier, which we have built on and extended, show that most single fibers encode AM over only about a 30- to 40-dB intensity range. We found that some onset and chopper units show significant temporal processing of AM over a *90-dB* range of average intensities. This is a remarkable operating range for a second-order sensory neuron. If a 25-dB spread of absolute thresholds exists within an animal for these unit types in a particular BF region (Bourk, 1976; Frisina, 1983), a population of these units could encode rapid sound-amplitude changes over the auditory system's entire operating range.

NEURAL MECHANISMS FOR AM PROCESSING IN VCN

Our progress to date has elucidated some of the mechanisms by which VCN neurons enhance their responses to rapid changes in sound amplitude relative to their ascending inputs. As previously mentioned, for auditory nerve fibers, the onset rate-intensity function is a good qualitative and quantitative predictor of a fiber's ability to encode AM. This implies that similar dynamic response characteristics of a neuron are responsible for onset responses to pure tones and encoding of AM. Logically, because onset and chopper units in the VCN have relatively precisely timed onset responses, it seemed worthwhile to examine the relationship between their onset rate-intensity functions and their AM encoding abilities as a function of average sound intensity. We investigated this situation for VCN units (Frisina, Smith, & Chamberlain, 1990b). We found that the onset and steady-state rate-intensity functions of all VCN units have very limited dynamic ranges of 20–30 dB (with the exception of On-C unit steady-state rate-intensity functions which had extended operating ranges). Thus, the tight relationship found in the auditory nerve was *not* present in the VCN, because VCN units continue to give strong synchronous responses to AM at intensities above the saturation points of their rate-intensity functions.

As presented earlier (Frisina et al., 1985, 1990a), AM gain surfaces of VCN units consist of two main features: a lowpass characteristics which dominates at low intensities, and a bandpass characteristic that is preeminent at high sound levels. The lowpass characteristic is similar to that seen in the responses of auditory nerve fibers. However, the bandpass characteristics asserts itself in varying degrees in the four main VCN unit types. A path of inquiry that we pursued was aimed at trying to explain how this bandpass characteristic arises.

BF AND OFF-BF EXCITATORY INPUTS

One possibility for producing the extended AM operating range for sinusoidally modulated tones in quiet is that VCN units get inputs not only from auditory nerve fibers with the same BF, but also from ascending inputs with higher or lower BFs. Thus, a subset of fibers that provide input to a VCN neuron could always be near threshold as stimulus intensity increases. This type of mechanism implies that the rate-intensity function of the cochlear nucleus cell should have the same operating range as that for the encoding of AM. As just mentioned, we found that except for On-C unit steady-state rate-intensity functions, the VCN onset and steady-state input–output functions for tones saturate 20–30 dB above threshold, whereas the operating range for AM encoding is up to 90 dB for some VCN units. Also, an off-BF excitatory input hypothesis requires that the excitatory response area would be larger than the excitatory response area of a typical auditory nerve fiber. The abundance of evidence from our lab and others refutes this notion in that VCN On-L, chopper, primary-like-with-notch, and primary-like units, although some variability exists, have excitatory response areas that are as sharp or as narrowly tuned as auditory nerve fibers. Lastly, we have found that if a wideband noise is used as a carrier, instead of a BF tone, VCN units can encode AM over a large a dynamic range as for BF tones (Frisina et al., 1990b). Therefore, AM responsiveness occurs at high intensities despite the probable saturation of off-BF inputs. (This criticism applies to the next possible neural mechanism for VCN AM encoding.) In light of all this evidence, it is quite *unlikely* that off-BF excitatory inputs are responsible for the bandpass characteristic of VCN AM encoding at high sound levels. The exception to this conclusion is that On-C units, which have extended steady-state rate-intensity functions and broad excitatory response areas for tones, may receive help from off-BF excitatory inputs to explain their superior AM encoding abilities, but as explained later other neural processes also probably contribute to their enhanced AM processing capabilities.

BF EXCITATORY INPUTS AND OFF-BF INHIBITORY INPUTS

The extended AM operating range for VCN units could also be due to off-BF inhibitory inputs from primary fibers via interneurons or a lateral inhibitory network. If this were the case for VCN units, a 180° phase shift (or at least a phase discontinuity) of the fundamental-frequency response to AM would occur at the intensity level in which the phase-locked BF excitatory inputs become weaker than the phase locking to the off-BF inhibitory inputs. We investigated this hypothesis by measuring the phase-intensity functions for chopper units in regard to AM encoding (Frisina et al., 1990b). These functions are quite smooth, lacking any phase shifts or discontinuities at suprathreshold intensity levels. Also, an off-BF inhibitory mechanism for increased AM synchrony requires that, to supply a strong phase-locked input, off-BF auditory nerve fibers must be within their AM operating range (within 30 dB above threshold). Because we have shown that auditory nerve fiber AM gain surfaces are lowpass in nature at low sound levels (Frisina et al., 1985, 1990a), it is not clear where the differentially tuned bandpass characteristics of the VCN cells would originate from with this type of mechanism. (This criticism also applies to the first possible mechanism discussed earlier.) Therefore, it is *not* likely that the increased fundamental-frequency response of VCN units comes from off-BF or lateral inhibitory inputs, however, these inputs could play a role in lowering the average response of a VCN unit for AM. The latter hypothesis is consistent with the presence of lateral inhibitory sidebands in the response areas of VCN chopper units (Martin & Dickson, 1983; Young, 1984). We pursued this hypothesis as follows.

As defined earlier in Equation 1, the synchronous response to AM (response gain) is proportional to the percent modulation of the response. Therefore, the response gain can be increased by either *increasing the first-harmonic response* or *decreasing the average response*. As just argued, it is unlikely that off-BF inhibitory inputs act to increase the first-harmonic response. To investigate the notion that off-BF inhibitory inputs could decrease the average response, we measured the first-harmonic and average response firing rates to AM quantitatively for the four VCN unit types and for auditory nerve fibers (Frisina et al., 1990b). We found that all four VCN unit types had reduced average responses to AM relative to their inputs, whereas only onset and chopper units achieved their increased AM response gains by significant increases in the first-harmonic response. Another finding supports the notion that *separate mechanisms* are responsible for the increase in first-harmonic response on the one hand and decrease in the average response on the other. Responses of chopper units to AM stimuli with non-BF carriers show that gain increases over BF AM responses are obtained, likewise, by lowering the average response without affecting the fundamental-frequency response (Frisina et al., 1990b).

These analyses support the notion that two mechanisms may be responsible for the amplification of eighth nerve inputs by VCN cells. One mechanism, which results in a *lowering of the average response* to AM may involve off-BF, lateral inhibitory inputs, or efferent inhibitory inputs originating from other brainstem auditory centers. The other mechanism, which is primarily present in onset and chopper units, causes an *increase in the first-harmonic response*. Our next step is to probe into the origins of this latter mechanism.

BF EXCITATORY DRIVE FROM TWO TYPES OF
AUDITORY NERVE INPUTS

The extent of spread of absolute thresholds for mammalian auditory nerve fibers was a controversial topic (Katsuki, Suga, & Khanno, 1962; Kiang, 1968; Schmiedt, 1977). The current evidence substantiates that there are at least two populations of auditory nerve fibers that are distinguishable on the basis of threshold and spontaneous activity rates (Liberman, 1978, 1982; Salvi, Perry, Hamernik, & Henderson, 1982). One population has low thresholds and high rates, and the other high thresholds and low spontaneous rates. The latter comprises about 10% of auditory nerve fibers and has thresholds 20–80 dB higher than the main population. The encoding of AM in high-threshold fibers is as good or better than low-threshold fibers (Joris & Yin, 1992). Therefore, the high-threshold population is capable of providing a strong synchronous input to VCN units with the same BF at high intensities.

One implication of this dual-input type of mechanism is that the VCN BF rate-intensity might have an operating range similar to that for the encoding of AM. As presented previously, we found this not to be the case. However, this would not necessarily be true if the increase in average response at high intensities caused by the high-threshold primary fiber inputs were counterbalanced by inhibitory inputs which simultaneously decrease the average response due to spread of excitation. If this mechanism is correct, the first-harmonic response at high intensities would be strong and the average response kept low so as to optimize the signal-to-noise ratio available to the next level of the auditory system. Lastly, the tuning of VCN neurons to different AM frequencies could be due to variations in properties of high-threshold fibers providing inputs or perhaps to differences in the electronic properties of VCN postsynaptic cells (Manis & Marx, 1991; Oertel, 1983; Oertel, Wu, Garb, & Dizack, 1990).

SPATIALLY DISTRIBUTED BF EXCITATORY INPUTS

The dendritic and somatic morphology of a neuron as well as the degree to which its ascending inputs are distributed onto these structures has been implicated as an important factor in determining the temporal response properties of cochlear nucleus units (Banks & Sachs, 1991; Colombo, Frisina, & Karcich, 1992; Colombo, Frisina, Karcich, & Swartz, 1991; Fernald & Gerstein, 1971; Molnar & Pfeiffer, 1968; Young, Robert, & Shofner, 1988). More specifically, evidence to date suggests that in the anterior and posterior AVCN bushy cells of Golgi impregnated material correspond to primary-like and primary-like-with-notch or On-G units, respectively (Bourk, 1976; Kiang, 1975; Morest, 1975; Pfeiffer, 1966a, 1966b; Rhode, Oertel, & Smith, 1983b). Spherical cells of Nissl preparations are associated with primary-like units and globular cells with primary-like-with-notch or On-G units. Chopper and On-L units may correspond to the stellate cells of Golgi preps (Cant, 1981; Rhode et al., 1983b). Stellate cells are equivalent to the multipolar cells of Nissl material. Bushy cells receive inputs from one or more primary fibers via the large, axosomatic end-bulbs of Held (Cant & Morest, 1979; Tolbert & Morest, 1982). Thus, the units that show *amplified first-harmonic responses* (chopper, onset) *receive distributed inputs* from many auditory nerve fibers, and the units that show very little change of the first-harmonic response relative to the auditory nerve (primary-like, primary-like-with-notch) receive fewer, larger endings from a smaller number of primary fibers. The distributed inputs of chopper and onset neurons onto their dendrites, combined with the lowpass filtering effect of the dendrites, may be the mechanism by which the small amount of first-harmonic response modulation at high intensities in the auditory nerve is amplified by stellate cells. In sum, our analyses suggest that an anatomical hierarchy of distributed inputs is correlated with the physiological hierarchy of the degree of amplification of AM responses and temporal precision of the onset response. Hence, an appropriate analytical model of AM encoding for VCN cells has to explain how differences in AM tuning could result from slightly different dendritic innervation patterns or from different postsynaptic cell membrane properties.

A current major goal of our laboratory is to pursue an interrelated series of experiments geared toward multiple hypothesis testing concerning the nature of the two independent mechanisms we have proposed for cochlear nucleus encoding of temporal fluctuations of complex sound envelopes.

AMPLIFIED ENCODING OF AM IN THE DORSAL COCHLEAR NUCLEUS

As mentioned before, it was recently discovered that pauser/buildup units give very strong synchronous responses to AM tones. The prevailing evidence suggests that the pauser/buildup unit type of the DCN corresponds to the Type IV unit of the Evans and Nelson (1973) pure-tone classification scheme, and both are highly correlated with the fusiform cell anatomical variety (Rhode, Smith, & Oertel, 1983a). Our findings indicate that the AM encoding abilities of pauser units can be as impressive as the best AM encoders in the VCN (Frisina & Walton, 1991; Frisina, Walton, Karcich, & Colombo, 1992). One study, utilizing procedures similar to our previous publications, included extracellular recordings from 104 single neurons of the cochlear nucleus. Recordings were made in adult chinchillas anesthetized with an initial dose of Nembutal with maintained anesthesia provided by urethane. Using a lateral surgical approach that does not require the removal of any brain tissue, stable recordings from single units were made from periods of a few minutes to a couple hours, thus allowing extensive parametric studies of many units. Stimuli consisted of pure-tone bursts and sinusoidally AM tone bursts with carrier frequencies at a unit's BF or at 1 kHz. Stimulus tone bursts had durations of 100 or 125 ms, rise/decay times of 2.5 ms, repetition rates of 2.5 per sec, and AM bursts had fixed AM frequencies that varied from 10 to 500 Hz across sets of 75 repetitions. Stimulus recording sites in a particular division of the cochlear nucleus were localized by a focal, extracellular injection of HRP utilizing procedures similar to our previous publications (e.g., Frisina, O'Neill, & Zettel, 1989).

An example of a pauser unit's BF pure-tone response pattern is shown in Fig. 10.1 at 50 dB above this unit's threshold (which was 41 dB SPL, BF = 13.2 kHz). The thickening of the abscissa starting at 5 ms marks the time that the stimulus-tone burst was on. The post-stimulus-time (PST) histogram displays a classic pauser response pattern. Specifically, a significant onset response occurs shortly after the start of the stimulus, followed by a period of low activity which for this unit extends from about 15–27 ms, and then a slow buildup of the response after 28 ms.

An example of this same unit's AM response is given in Fig. 10.2 for an AM stimulus with carrier frequency at the unit's BF, at 50 dB above threshold (91 dB SPL). Notice the very prominent synchronous response to

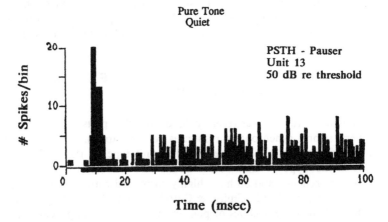

FIG. 10.1.   Best-frequency pure-tone response of a representative pauser unit in quiet, in PSTH format. These responses were recorded at a high intensity level (50 dB re threshold = 91 dB SPL). Unit 13, BF = 13.2 kHz, Threshold = 41 dB SPL, Bin width = 667 μs; the thickening of the abscissa starting at 5 ms indicates when the stimulus tone burst was present. Note: the actual peak onset firing level was 63 spikes/bin, which was truncated to allow better presentation of the steady-state response.

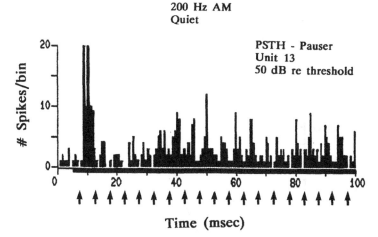

FIG. 10.2. Best-frequency AM response of a pauser unit in quiet, at the same high intensity level as the data of Fig. 10.1. Notice the significant degree of synchronous firing to each cycle of the AM stimulus. Unit 13, PSTH format same as Fig. 10.1. Each arrowhead below the abscissa represents the time of occurrence of 1 cycle of the AM stimulus. Note: the actual peak onset firing level was 61 spikes/bin, which was truncated to allow better presentation of the steady-state response.

the 200 Hz AM, that is, there is an increase in firing rate for each cycle of the AM sound (each period of the AM stimulus is indicated by one of the arrowheads below the PST histogram). This vigorous AM encoding at a high sound level can be particularly appreciated by comparing the synchronous AM firing of Fig. 10.2 with the pure-tone PST histogram of Fig. 10.1. One should also be aware that this synchronous response by pauser units at high sound levels is at an intensity level at which about 90% of auditory nerve fibers show very little synchronous response to AM because of their limited dynamic ranges.

Unlike units of the VCN, pauser/buildup units of the DCN have nonmonotonic pure-tone rate-intensity functions. A BF rate-intensity function for the unit whose data were presented in Figs. 10.1 and 10.2 is displayed in Fig. 10.3. The overall firing rate of the unit increases from the spontaneous rate of 38 sp/sec (S) to 354 sp/sec at about 20 dB above threshold, then declines with further increases in the average stimulus intensity. This decline in responsivity at high sound levels results from inhibitory inputs to pauser/buildup units. The point on the input/output function that the data of Figs. 10.1 and 10.2 were collected at is indicated by the straight arrow of Fig. 10.3 (91 dB SPL).

Responses of another representative pauser/buildup unit are shown in Fig. 10.4 for a BF stimulus at 46 dB above threshold (threshold = 29 dB SPL, BF = 355 Hz). The pauser response to a 125 msec pure-tone burst at BF is evident. This unit's response to an AM stimulus at the same intensity

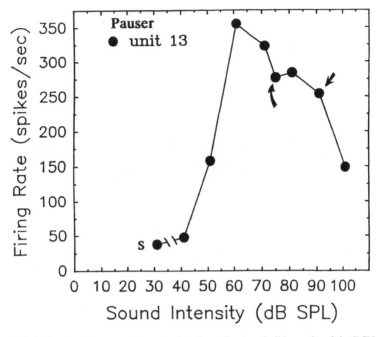

FIG. 10.3. Steady-state rate-intensity functions of pauser/buildup units of the DCN are nonmonotonic in shape. Each data point represents the average firing rate for the total number of spikes in response to a BF tone burst of 100-ms duration. Unit 13, S denotes the spontaneous firing rate as measured during the time before the start of the stimulus. Straight arrow = denotes the intensity level for the data of Figs. 10.1, 10.2, and 10.6. Curved arrow = indicates the intensity level of the data of Figs. 10.8 to 10.9.

level as the data of Fig. 10.4 (46 dB re threshold = 75 dB SPL) are presented in Fig. 10.5. Notice the very strong synchronous response of the pauser to 80 Hz AM, at an intensity level at which the vast majority of auditory nerve fibers are saturated (75 dB SPL). It is also interesting to note, as also can be seen for the unit of Fig. 10.2, the synchronous response to AM does not show signs of adapting or fatiguing for the 100–125 msec stimuli, that is, the response peaks to AM do not systematically decline during stimulation.

PAUSER/BUILDUP MODULATION TRANSFER FUNCTIONS

Given the finding that pauser/buildup units tend to give very strong synchronous responses to AM, we set out to explore how this AM encoding ability would change with AM frequency, particularly at high intensities at which the biggest enhancement of auditory nerve AM encoding occurs. To do this we measured the AM response of DCN units quantitatively utilizing

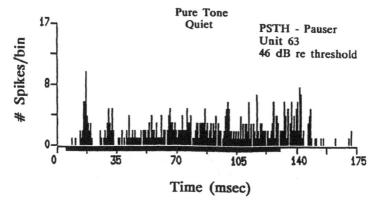

FIG. 10.4.   Best-frequency pure-tone response of another representative pauser unit in quiet at a high intensity level (46 dB re threshold = 75 dB SPL). Unit 63, PSTH format same as Fig. 10.1.

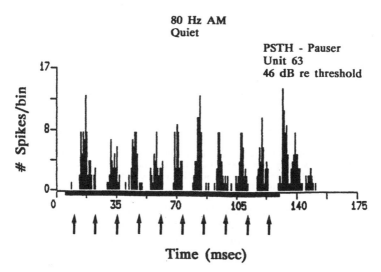

FIG. 10.5.   Amplitude-modulated response of the pauser unit of Fig. 10.4 at the same high intensity level. Notice, comparing these data with the previous figure, there is a dramatic synchronous response to each cycle of the AM stimulus. Unit 63, PSTH format same as Fig. 10.2.

the analysis paradigm of Equation 1. A modulation transfer function (MTF) is displayed in Fig. 10.6, for the same unit whose data were presented in Figs. 10.1–10.3, for an intensity 50 dB above threshold (91 dB SPL), as marked by the straight arrow of Fig. 10.3. The function shows the AM response gain during the last 50 ms of a 100-ms AM stimulus (adapted response). This

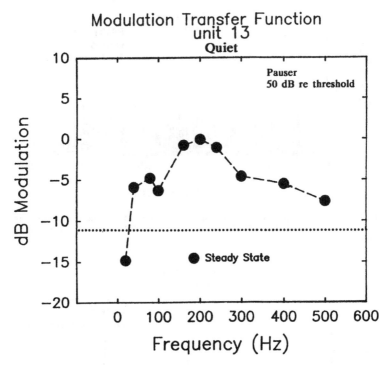

FIG. 10.6.   Bandpass MTF for a representative pauser unit at a high intensity level (50 dB re threshold, 91 dB SPL). The dotted line at -11 dB modulation response gain shows the low level of AM coding that the typical auditory nerve fiber would display at the same intensity under comparable stimulus conditions (from Frisina et al., 1990a). At all AM frequencies except the lowest (20 Hz), the pauser dB-modulation response (ordinate, as defined in Equation 1) significantly exceeds the response of a typical auditory nerve fiber. Unit 13.

steady-state measure is comparable to the AM response measure used in our previous work and reports by others. The flat, dotted line at-12-dB response modulation is the level at which the typical auditory nerve fiber would be giving its AM response under comparable stimulus conditions. It is important to realize that the steady-state AM encoding by the pauser unit is significantly above that of its ascending inputs. Second, pauser units have the bandpass characteristic of their AM transfer functions reminiscent of onset and chopper units of the VCN at high-average intensity levels.

EFFECTS OF SOUND LEVEL ON PAUSER/BUILDUP AM ENCODING

In the VCN we previously systematically investigated the effects of average intensity level on a unit's ability to process AM as a function of the modulation frequency, that is, the effect of sound level on the shape of the MTF (Frisina et al., 1985, 1990a). We found that the vast majority of VCN units had MTFs that were lowpass in nature at low sound levels. At high sound levels, primary-like units displayed flat MTFs with modest amounts of modulation gain, and onset and chopper units showed bandpass MTFs with higher modulation response gains. In our current study, we are finding that pauser/buildup units, like onset and chopper units of the VCN, show bandpass MTFs at high intensities (Fig. 10.6) and lowpass MTFs at low sound levels (Fig. 10.7). The data in Fig. 10.7 are for the same unit of Fig. 10.6, but were collected at a lower intensity of 14 dB above threshold (55 dB SPL).

EFFECTS OF BACKGROUND NOISE ON DCN AM PROCESSING

We investigated the effects of a continuous, wideband background noise on AM encoding in pauser/buildup units utilizing a stimulus control paradigm

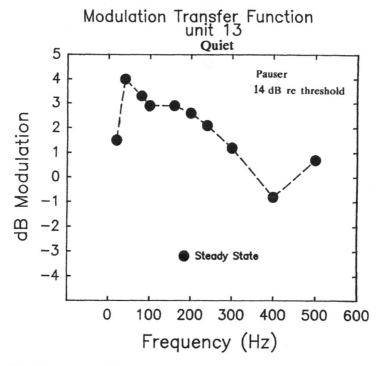

FIG. 10.7. Lowpass MTF for the pauser unit of the previous figure, these data were collected at a lower intensity level (14 dB re threshold = 55 dB SPL). MTF format same as Fig. 10.6 except that the ordinate has been autoscaled to cover a different range. Unit 13.

similar to Gibson et al. (1985). Differences in this case were that we used 100–125-ms test tones and utilized AM test tones at BF, as well as pure tones (Frisina & Walton, 1991; Frisina et al., 1992). Some representative findings for the same unit presented in Figs. 10.1–10.3 and 10.6–10.7 are displayed in Fig. 10.8 (intensity level: 75 dB SPL, steady-state measure of AM encoding). The solid data points show the steady-state AM response in quiet (similar to the data of Fig. 10.6, but at a slightly lower intensity level, as indicated by the curved arrow of Fig. 10.3). Open points of Fig. 10.8 show the AM transfer function for this unit, under identical stimulus conditions, except that a continuous wideband background noise at 75 dB SPL (0 dB signal/noise—S/N) was turned on 1 min before the AM transfer function data were collected. As one might predict, for a fairly intense noise, at many AM frequencies (in this case 160–300 Hz) there is a *decline* in AM reponsivity in the vicinity of the peak of the AM transfer function in quiet.

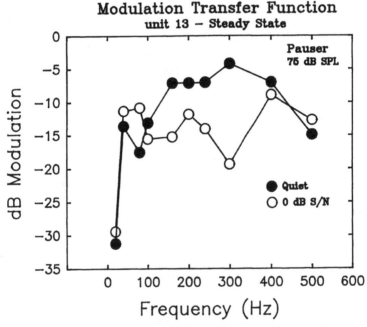

FIG. 10.8.   Bandpass MTFs for the pauser unit of the previous figure, at a high sound level (34 dB re threshold = 75 dB SPL). Filled data points give the synchronous response to BF AM tone bursts presented in quiet. The MTF is similar to that shown in Fig. 10.6. The open data points give the response of this unit under identical stimulus conditions, except that the AM tone bursts were delivered in the presence of a wideband background noise at 75 dB SPL (0 dB S/N). For the middle AM frequencies the noise *decreases* the synchronous response to AM. However, at low and high AM frequencies, the temporal coding of AM is relatively *unaffected* by the loud noise. Unit 13.

However, it is also noteworthy that at certain AM frequencies (20–100 Hz, 400–500 Hz), the AM processing of this pauser unit is relatively unaffected by the intense background noise. Thus, at some AM frequencies, preservation of AM processing takes place in pauser/buildup units, despite the presence of acoustic clutter from a fairly intense wideband background noise.

To gain more insights into this interesting behavior we varied the level of the background stimulation, therefore altering the S/N. The results of lowering the background noise level by 5 dB relative to that of Fig. 10.8, and otherwise keeping all other stimulus parameters the same, are shown in Fig. 10.9. The solid data points are the same as the solid points of Fig. 10.8. The open points show the MTF with the noise at 70 dB SPL (+5 dB S/N). As was discovered for the 0 dB S/N condition, near the peak of the AM transfer function in quiet (200–300 Hz), the noise has a deleterious effect on AM processing. However, at the low and high AM frequencies (20–160 Hz,

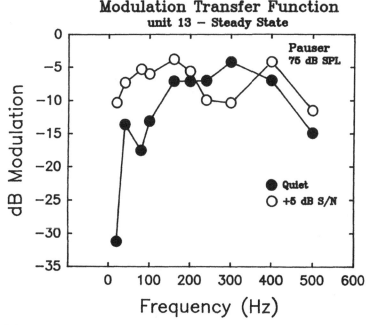

FIG. 10.9. Reducing the level of the background noise allows for better temporal coding of AM for the pauser unit of Fig. 10.8. The filled data points are replotted from the previous figure. The open data points give the response of this unit to AM in the presence of a 70 dB SPL wideband noise (+5 dB S/N). Although the noise is still relatively loud, there are low and high AM frequencies at which the AM coding of this unit is *improved* compared to quiet. At the middle AM frequencies, the AM temporal responsiveness of the unit is diminished. Unit 13.

400–500 Hz), not only is AM encoding preserved in the presence of the noise, but it is actually *enhanced*.

In contrast to the findings of beneficial effects of background noise on AM processing in DCN pauser/buildup units, under some conditions, background noise can be quite devastating to encoding of sound-envelope fluctuations. For instance, the effects of background noise on AM processing for the unit whose AM response in quiet is shown in Fig. 10.5 are presented in Fig. 10.10 for the same stimulus configuration, except that a continuous wideband noise at +6 dB S/N was simultaneously present. In this case, the evoked activity in response to the AM stimulus is virtually obliterated (compare Fig. 10.5 synchronous activity with the lack of response in Fig. 10.10).

To start to understand whether the obliteration of the evoked response was somehow unique to AM, we compared the effects of noise on the AM stimulus with its effects on a pure tone at the same sound level and carrier frequency. These effects of noise on the pure-tone response are shown in Fig. 10.11. Comparison of Fig. 10.4, 10.5, 10.10, and 10.11 show that for this pauser unit the background noise seems to inhibit the unit's evoked response, regardless of whether the evoking tone is modulated or unmodulated.

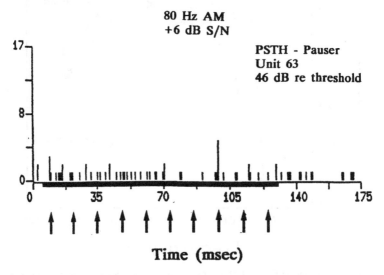

FIG. 10.10.   The AM processing of some pauser units is obliterated by the presence of a wideband background noise. Here, responses to the same AM stimulus presented in Fig. 10.5 are shown when the AM tone burst was delivered in the presence of a continuous background noise (70 dB SPL, +5 dB S/N). Unit 63, PSTH format same as Fig. 10.5.

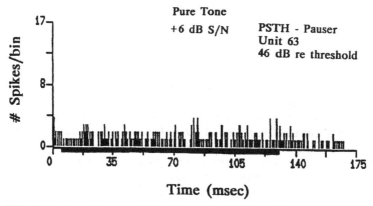

FIG. 10.11. The obliteration of the AM response by background noise for this unit is not a response unique to modulated stimuli. Here it can be seen that the response to a pure tone is also tremendously decreased under stimulus conditions comparable to those of the previous figure. Unit 63, PSTH format same as Fig. 10.5.

BIOMEDICAL AND BIOENGINEERING RELEVANCE

Because a major approach in the design of auditory prosthetic devices, designed to restore hearing in deaf patients, is to mimic the natural responses to complex sounds made by the normal auditory nervous system, findings concerning the normal coding of complex sound elements will be critical and directly applicable for developing and testing protheses. These protheses include both cochlear implants and the newer cochlear nucleus implants that directly stimulate cochlear nucleus neurons (Anderson et al., 1989; Shannon, 1989). The latter are particularly exciting, because in cases of deafness due to cochlear pathology, more cochlear nucleus cells generally survive than auditory nerve fibers (Kiang, 1975; Morest & Bohne, 1983), making direct stimulation of a brainstem nucleus potentially quite valuable. Our results will also be essential to speech scientists who are trying to build real-time speech decoders, and in some cases, the information will be directly applicable to device design (e.g., Rhody, Houde, Parkins, & Dianat, 1986). Lastly, if we can continue to describe which subdivisions and pathways of the auditory system are more specialized for encoding rapid changes in sound frequency or amplitude and other complex sound features, and how these features subserve auditory functions such as arousal, localization, or loudness coding, neurologists, otolaryngologists, and neurosurgeons will be greatly assisted in their diagnoses of the functional implications of CNS lesions, cerebrovascular malformations, and accidents such as stroke and trauma due to head injury.

CONCLUSION

Many units of the dorsal and ventral cochlear nuclei, especially those with inhibitory inputs, have the ability to amplify information about temporal aspects of sound envelopes, over a very wide range of sound levels relative to their auditory nerve inputs. Our ongoing studies indicate that many units with good AM processing capabilities are able to maintain, or in some specific cases even *enhance*, their AM coding in the presence of significant levels of a wideband background noise. Other cochlear nucleus units are quite adversely affected in terms of their AM processing capabilities in the presence of noise. One of our present goals is to systematically study enough units of a particular type to discover under what conditions its AM processing is preserved or enhanced, and how this is due to shifts in auditory nerve AM operating ranges, and how much is due to unique neuronal circuitry of the cochlear nucleus.

ACKNOWLEDGMENTS

We especially thank Dr. William O'Neill, Dr. D. Robert Frisina, Joseph Colombo, Todd Tracey and Daniel Sullivan for assistance in carrying out this research. This research was supported by a grant DC 00408 from the National Institute for Deafness & Other Communication Disorders, National Institute of Health, U.S. Department of Health and Human Services, and the International Center for Hearing & Speech Research—RICHS, Rochester, NY.

REFERENCES

Anderson, D. J., Najafi, K., Tanghe, S. J., Evans, D. A., Levy, K. L., Hetke, J. F., Xue, X., Jappia, J. J., & Wise, D. K. (1989). Batch-fabricated thin-film electrodes for stimulation of the central auditory system. *IEEE Transactions on Biomedical Engineering, 36*, 693–704.

Arle, J. E., & Kim, D. O. (1991). Neural modeling of intrinsic and spike-discharge properties of cochlear nucleus neurons. *Biological Cybernetics, 64*, 273–283.

Banks, M. I., & Sachs, M. B., (1991). Regularity analysis in a compartmental model of chopper units in the anteroventral cochlear nucleus. *Journal of Neurophysiology, 65*, 606–629.

Bourk, T. R. (1976). *Electrical responses of neural units in the anteroventral cochlear nucleus of the cat.* Unpublished doctoral dissertation, MIT, Cambridge, MA.

Brachman, M. L. (1980). *Dynamic response characteristics of single auditory nerve fibers.* Unpublished doctoral dissertation and Special Rep. ISR-S-19. Institute for Sensory Research, Syracuse, NY.

Cant, N. B. (1981). The fine structure of two types of stellate cells in the anterior division of the anteroventral cochlear nucleus. *Neuroscience, 6*, 2643–2655.

Cant, N. B., & Morest, D. K. (1979). The bushy cells in the anteroventral cochlear nucleus of the cat. A study with the electron microscope. *Neuroscience, 4*, 1925–1945.

Colombo, J., Frisina, R. D., & Karcich, K. J. (1992). Quantitative models of ventral cochlear nucleus neurons: Pure tone response predictions. *Association for Research in Otolaryngology, Abstracts, 15*, 27.

Colombo, J., Frisina, R. D., Karcich, K. J., & Swartz, K. P. (1991). Computational models of ventral cochlear nucleus neurons. *International Brain Research Organization — World Congress Abstracts, 3*, 250.

Costalupes, J. A., Young, E. D., & Gibson, D. J. (1984). Effects of continuous noise backgrounds on rate response of auditory-nerve fibers in cat. *Journal of Neurophysiology, 51*, 1326–1344.

Evans, E. F., & Nelson, P. G. (1973). The responses of single neurones in the cochlear nucleus of the cat as a function of their location and the anesthetic state. *Experimental Brain Research, 17*, 402–427.

Evans, E. F., & Palmer, A. R. (1980). Dynamic range of cochlear nerve fibers to amplitude modulated tones. *Journal of Physiology, 298*, 33–34.

Fernald, R. D., & Gerstein, G. L. (1971). A model of cochlear-nucleus neurons responding to complex stimuli. In M. B. Sachs (Ed.), *Physiology of the auditory system* (pp. 189–196). Baltimore: Educational Association.

Frisina, R. D. (1983). *Enhancement of responses to amplitude modulation in the gerbil cochlear nucleus: Single-unit recordings using an improved surgical approach.* Unpublished doctoral dissertation and Special Rep. ISR-S-23. Institute for Sensory Research, Syracuse, NY.

Frisina, R. D., Chamberlain, S. C., Brachman, M. L., & Smith, R. L. (1982). Anatomy and physiology of the gerbil cochlear nucleus: An improved surgical approach for microelectrode studies. *Hearing Research, 6*, 259–275.

Frisina, R. D., O'Neill, W. E., & Zettel, M. L. (1989). Functional organization of mustached bat inferior colliculus. II. Connections of the FM$_2$ region. *Journal of Comparative Neurology, 284*, 85–107.

Frisina, R. D., Smith, R. L., & Chamberlain, S. C. (1985). Differential encoding of rapid changes in sound amplitude by second-order auditory neurons. *Experimental Brain Research, 60*, 417–422.

Frisina, R. D., Smith, R. L., & Chamberlain, S. C. (1990a). Encoding of amplitude modulation in the gerbil cochlear nucleus: I. A hierarchy of enhancement. *Hearing Research, 44*, 99–122.

Frisina, R. D., Smith, R. L., & Chamberlain, S. C. (1990b). Encoding of amplitude modulation in the gerbil cochlear nucleus: II. Possible neural mechanisms. *Hearing Research, 44*, 123–141.

Frisina, R. D., & Walton, J. P. (1991). Processing of rapid changes in sound amplitude in the cochlear nucleus in quiet and in the presence of noise. *International Brain Research, Organization — World Congress Abstract, 3*, 250.

Frisina, R. D., Walton, J. P., Karcich, K. J., & Colombo, J. (1992). Effects of background noise on the processing of amplitude modulation in the cochlear nucleus. *Association for Research in Otolaryngology, Abstracts, 15*, 78.

Geisler, C. D., & Sinex, D. G. (1980). Responses of primary auditory fibers to combined noise and tonal stimuli. *Hearing Research, 3*, 317–334.

Gibson, D. J., Young, E. D., & Costalupes, J. A., (1985). Similarity of dynamic range adjustment in auditory nerve and cochlear nuclei. *Journal of Neurophysiology, 53*, 940–958.

Hewitt, M. J., & Meddis, R. (1991). An evaluation of eight computer models of mammalian inner hair cell function. *Journal of the Acoustical Society of America, 90*, 904–917.

Hewitt, M. J., & Meddis, R., & Shackleton, T. M. (1992). A computer model of a cochlear nucleus cell: Responses to pure-tone and amplitude-modulated stimuli. *Journal Acoustical Society of America, 91*, 2096–2109.

Javel, E. (1980). Coding of AM tones in the chinchilla auditory nerve: Implications for the pitch of complex tones. *Journal of the Acoustical Society America, 68*, 133–146.

Joris, P. X., & Yin, T. C. T. (1992). Responses to amplitude-modulated tones in the auditory nerve of the cat. *Journal of the Acoustical Society of America, 91*, 215–232.

Katsuki, Y., Suga, N., & Khanno, Y. (1962). Neural mechanisms of the peripheral and central auditory system in monkeys. *Journal of the Acoustical Society of America, 34*, 1396–1410.

Kiang, N. Y. S. (1968). Survey of recent developments in the study of auditory physiology. *Annals of Otology, Rhinology and Laryngology, 77*, 656–676.

Kiang, N. Y. S. (1975). Stimulus representation in the discharge patterns of auditory neurons. In D. B. Tower (Ed.), *The nervous system* (pp. 81–96). New York: Raven Press.

Kim, D. O., Sirianni, J. G., & Chang, S. O. (1990). Responses of DCN-PVCN neurons and auditory nerve fibers in unanesthetized decerebrate cats to AM and pure tones: Analysis with autocorrelation/power-spectrum. *Hearing Research, 45*, 95–113.

Liberman, M. C. (1978). Auditory-nerve response from cats raised in a low-noise chamber. *Journal of the Acoustical Society of America, 63*, 442–455.

Liberman, M. C. (1982). The cochlear frequency map for the cat: Labeling auditory-nerve fibers of known characteristic frequency. *Journal of the Acoustical Society of America, 72*, 1441–1449.

Manis, P. B., & Marx, S. O. (1991). Outward currents in isolated ventral cochlear nucleus neurons. *Journal of Neuroscience, 11*, 2865–2880.

Martin, M. R., & Dickson, J. W. (1983). Lateral inhibition in the anteroventral cochlear nucleus of the cat: A microiontophoretic study. *Hearing Research, 9*, 35–42.

Møller, A. R. (1972). Coding of amplitude and frequency modulated sounds in the cochlear nucleus of the rat. *Acta Physiologica Scandinavica, 86*, 223–238.

Møller, A. R. (1973). Statistical evaluation of the dynamic properties of cochlear nucleus units using stimuli modulated with pseudorandom noise. *Brain Research, 57*, 443–456.

Møller, A. R. (1974a). Coding of amplitude and frequency modulated sounds in the cochlear nucleus. *Acustica, 31*, 202–299.

Møller, A. R. (1974b). Responses of units in the cochlear nucleus to sinusoidally amplitude-modulated tones. *Experimental Neurology, 45*, 104–117.

Møller, A. R. (1975a). Dynamic properties of excitation and inhibition in the cochlear nucleus. *Acta Physiologica Scandinavica, 93*, 442–454.

Møller, A. R. (1975b). Latency of unit responses in cochlear nucleus determined in two different ways. *Journal of Neurophysiology, 38*, 812–821.

Møller, A. R. (1976a). Dynamic properties of primary auditory fibers compared with cells in the cochlear nucleus. *Acta Physiologica Scandinavica, 98*, 157–167.

Møller, A. R. (1976b). Dynamic properties of excitation and 2-tone inhibition in the cochlear nucleus studied using amplitude modulated tones. *Experimental Brain Research, 25*, 307–321.

Møller, A. R. (1976c). Dynamic properties of the responses of single neurones in the cochlear nucleus of the rat. *Journal of Physiology, 259*, 63–82.

Molnar, C. E., & Pfeiffer, R. R. (1968). Interpretation of spontaneous spike discharge patterns in the cochlear nucleus. *Proceedings of the IEEE, 56*, 993–1004.

Morest, D. K. (1975). The structural organization of the auditory pathways. In D. B. Tower (Ed.), *The nervous system* (pp. 19–29). New York: Raven Press.

Morest, D. K., & Bohne, B. A. (1983). Noise-induced degeneration in the brain and representation of inner and outer hair cells. *Hearing Research, 9*, 145–151.

Oertel, D. (1983). Synaptic responses and electrical properties of cells in brain slices of the mouse anteroventral cochlear nucleus. *Journal of Neuroscience, 3*, 2043–2053.

Oertel, D., Wu, S. H., Garb, M. W., & Dizack, C. (1990). Morphology and physiology of cells in slice preparations of the posteroventral cochlear nucleus of mice. *Journal of Comparative Neurology, 295*, 136–154.

Palmer, A. R. (1982). Encoding of rapid amplitude fluctuations by cochlear-nerve fibers in the guinea pig. *Archives of Otology, Rhinology & Laryngology, 236*, 197–202.

Pfeiffer, R. R. (1966a). Anteroventral cochlear nucleus: Waveforms of extracellularly recorded spike potentials. *Science, 154*, 667–668.

Pfeiffer, R. R. (1966b). Classification of response pattern of spike discharges for units in the cochlear nucleus: Tone burst stimulation. *Experimental Brain Research, 1*, 220–235.

Rhode, W. S., Smith, P. H., & Oertel, D. (1983a). Physiological response properties of cells labeled intracellularly with horseradish peroxidase in cat dorsal cochlear nucleus. *Journal of Comparative Neurology, 213*, 426–447.

Rhode, W. S., Oertel, D., & Smith, P. H. (1983b). Physiological response properties of cells labeled intracellularly with horseradish peroxidase in cat ventral cochlear nucleus. *Journal of Comparative Neurology, 213*, 448–463.

Rhody, H. E., Houde, R. A., Parkins, C. W., & Dianat, S. (1986). *Speech analysis based on a model of the auditory system* (RADC-TR-85-265 Final Tech. Rep.). Rome, NY: Air Development Center.

Salvi, R. J., Perry, J., Hamernik, R. P., & Henderson, D. (1982). Relationships between cochlear pathologies and auditory and behavioral responses following acoustic trauma. In R. P. Hamernik, D. Henderson, & R. Salvi (Eds.), *New perspectives on noise-induced hearing loss* (pp. 165–188). New York: Raven Press.

Schmiedt, R. A. (1977). *Single and two-tone effects in normal and abnormal cochleas: A study of cochlear microphonics and auditory-nerve units.* Unpublished doctoral dissertation and Special Rep. ISR-S-16. Syracuse, NY: Institute for Sensory Research.

Schwid, H. A., & Geisler, C. D. (1982). Multiple reservoir model of neurotransmitter release by cochlear inner hair cells. *Journal of the Acoustical Society of America, 72*, 1435–1440.

Shannon, R. V. (1989). Threshold functions for electrical stimulation of the human cochlear nucleus. *Hearing Research, 40*, 173–178.

Smith, R. L., & Brachman, M. L. (1977). Responses of auditory-nerve fibers to sinusoidal amplitude modulation. *Journal of the Acoustical Society of America, 62*, S46(A).

Smith, R. L., & Brachman, M. L. (1980a). Response modulation of auditory-nerve fibers by AM stimuli: Effects of average intensity. *Hearing Research, 2*, 123–144.

Smith, R. L., & Brachman, M. L. (1980b). Operating range and maximum response of single auditory-nerve fibers. *Brain Research, 184*, 499–505.

Smith, R. L., Brachman, M. L., & Frisina, R. D. (1985). Sensitivity of auditory-nerve fibers to changes in intensity: A dichotomy between decrements & increments. *Journal of the Acoustical Society of America, 78*, 1310–1316.

Tolbert, L. P. & Morest, D. K. (1982). The neuronal architecture of the anteroventral cochlear nucleus of the cat in the region of the cochlear nerve root: Electron microscopy. *Neuroscience, 7*, 3053–3067.

Westerman, L., & Smith, R. L. (1988). A diffusion model of the transient response of the cochlear inner hair cell synapse. *Journal of Acoustical Society of America, 83*, 2266–2276.

Young, E. D. (1984). Response characteristics of neurons of the cochlear nuclei. In C. I. Berlin (Ed.), *Hearing science, recent advances* (pp. 423–460). San Diego: College Hill Press.

Young, E. D., Robert, J. -M., & Shofner, W. P. (1988). Regularity and latency of units in ventral cochlear nucleus: Implications for unit classification and generation of response properties. *Journal of Neurophysiology, 60*, 1–29.

11 Representing the Surface Texture of Grooved Plates Using Single-Channel, Electrocutaneous Stimulation

Clayton L. Van Doren
Lisa L. Menia
Case Western Reserve University

A dive to a vent site in a submersible is at once thrilling and frustrating. With about five hours of ocean-bottom time on a dive—much of which is spent navigating to a vent field—there is little enough time for operations with a cumbersome and insensitive manipulator. Tunnicliffe (1992, p.349)

INTRODUCTION

Artificial Sensory Feedback

People are often in situations in which they must grasp and manipulate objects with hands that have no sensation. In some cases the insensate hands are their own, such as when diabetes mellitus or Hansen's disease has severely damaged the peripheral nerves; or the insensate hands may be mechanical, such as a motorized prosthetic gripper. It was, in fact, the development of the myoelectrically controlled prosthetic hand shortly after World War II (Reiter, 1948, cited in Körner, 1978) that brought the problem of manipulation without sensation into focus (Wiener, 1951; see also Sueda & Tamura, 1969). Prior to that time, upper-extremity prostheses were controlled by a cable connected to a shoulder harness at one end and connected to the prosthetic hand (typically a Dorrance hook) at the other. The user pulled on the cable by shrugging the shoulders, opening or closing the hand. Some sense of grip force was provided by the tension developed in the cable. In the myoelectric hand, in contrast, a user generates an electrical signal (EMG) by contracting one or more muscles. The EMG is amplified and used to control a motor that opens or closes the artificial hand. In this case, there is very little sensory feedback from the prosthesis. Some users report that they can feel vibrations when the mechanical clutch shifts from one gear to another, or they can hear the motor noise, but the information is quite limited. There also may be some sense of effort provided by the muscles that are contracting to produce the EMG. In most cases, though, users report that such feedback is inadequate to control the hand as they would like.

Artificial sensory feedback, that is, presentation of missing sensory information through an alternate sensory channel, can improve the dexterous control of an otherwise insensate prosthetic hand. Meek, Jacobsen, and Goulding (1989) found that grasp-force feedback via a mechanical indenter on the upper arm improved the success rate for normal subjects using a modified myoelectric prosthesis to lift a heavy object without breaking it. Similarly, Kawamura and Sueda (1968) reported that electrocutaneous feedback of grasp force and finger span in a myoelectric hand increased the success rate for picking up quail's eggs from 60% to 100%. Patterson and Katz (1992) found that feedback via a pressure cuff allowed subjects to match grasp forces more accurately, and Mann and Reimers (1970) showed that a vibrotactile code for elbow angle improved the accuracy of elbow flexion with the Boston arm.

Sensory feedback also has received considerable recent attention in the field of telerobotics. In this case, an operator moves a controller, often an exoskeleton mounted on his hand and arm, so that his movements are mimicked by a robot. Through this linkage, the user can make the robot pick up objects, but unless there is some form of sensory feedback, the user has to rely on open-loop control or visual information to monitor the amount of force applied to the object and the movements of the device. A few companies have been developing force reflection to assist in controlling robots. For example, Kraft Telerobotics (Kansas City, MO) has developed an excavator that can be operated remotely, and reflects a fraction of the force that is being applied by the shovel at the end of the excavator's arm to the end of the control arm that is manipulated by the operator. If the excavator is digging through soft soil, the operator does not feel much resistance; but if the excavator suddenly hits a rock, the operator feels a sudden increase in force.

A recent study (Hannaford & Wood, 1992) has shown that force reflection can improve the performance of a teleoperator performing everyday tasks. Subjects controlled a robotic arm to perform a variety of tasks, with and without force reflection. They exchanged the position of two blocks attached to a board with velcro, inserted pegs into holes with different diameters and chamfers, and connected and disconnected three standard electrical connectors. The sensory feedback reduced the time of completion, the number of errors, and the amount of force that was used by the operators in manipulating the objects. In other words, force reflection allowed the operators to use more appropriate forces for the task, which resulted in less risk of damaging the objects and a more economic use of energy.

The control difficulties imposed by the lack of sensory information from mechanical devices such as prostheses and telerobots are shared by upper extremity neuroprostheses. In these devices electrodes are placed on the paralyzed muscles in the forearm which control the fingers through tendons that cross the wrist (for a review, see Gorman & Peckham, 1991). The electrodes are used to deliver stimuli in controlled patterns so that a paralyzed individual with an injury at the C5 or C6 spinal level can open and close their hand to grasp objects used for activities of daily living (Wijman et al., 1990). The neuroprosthesis developed at Case Western Reserve University and the Cleveland Veterans Administration Medical Center is controlled with an angle transducer mounted on either the wrist or the shoulder, so that flexion and extension of the joint causes the hand to open or close (Smith, Peckham, Keith, & Roscoe, 1987).

The spinal injury abolishes not only the motor function of the hand, but eliminates the sensory information coming back from the hand as well. Proprioceptive information about the force of hand grasp and the position of the finger joints, tactile information from cutaneous mechanoreceptors, temperature information from thermal receptors, and pain from nociceptors is all lost. Artificial sensory feedback can restore some of the missing information and enhance performance just as it has in prostheses and teleoperators. Riso, Ignagni, and Keith (1991) implemented an electrocutaneous code which mapped the force exerted by the neuroprosthesis into the frequency of stimulation at a surface electrode placed on the user's skin (at a location where sensation was preserved). The authors found that objects were grasped and lifted with less force when the feedback was available than when the feedback was absent. The reduced force resulted in an economy of grasp that could reduce muscle fatigue during object manipulation. Milchus and Van Doren (1990) have also shown that sensory feedback can improve the accuracy of shoulder movements used to generate grasp force. In that experiment, an electrocutaneous code was used to represent shoulder position. Subjects tried to repeat shoulder positions in a target-matching task, and feedback improved the accuracy of the matching responses and reduced the variability over multiple trials.

It is important to note that proprioceptive feedback was implemented in all of the examples cited above. Indeed, proprioception has received nearly all of the attention in feedback research for the last four decades—the use of tactile or cutaneous information has largely been ignored. Minsky, Ouh-young, Steele, Brooks, and Behensky (1990) describe one of the few implementations of a form of tactile feedback. These investigators provide feedback to a normal hand through a joystick so that users can perceive the roughness and texture of a virtual surface while they are tactually exploring a virtual environment. Users push the joystick in the direction that they want to explore the surface, and the joystick handle reacts with a force that is proportional to the gradient of the surface at that point. The handle of the joystick pushes against the hand and pulls the hand as the point of exploration moves up and down the gradients of the surface. Subjects are able to order surfaces by perceived roughness using this feedback system.

The experiments described in this chapter represent the first step in developing a feedback system that can represent the texture of real surfaces, rather than virtual surfaces, for users of the hand neuroprostheses, conventional and myoelectric prostheses, and telerobotics. For this preliminary study we chose to represent the texture of especially simple surfaces — grooved plates (flat metal or plastic plates with parallel grooves cut or etched in the surface) — because (a) they vary in only one dimension, (b) they can be characterized by one or two parameters, (c) they are easy to fabricate, and (d) there is a large body of physiological and psychophysical data on the tactile responses to such surfaces. The extant data provide us with important clues that can guide our development of a texture feedback system.

PHYSIOLOGY AND PSYCHOPHYSICS OF TEXTURE PERCEPTION

The earliest studies of surface texture, and roughness in particular, were only descriptive (Meenes & Zigler, 1923; Katz, 1925, 1989). Stevens and Harris (1962) were the first to characterize texture perception quantitatively using magnitude estimates of the roughness of 12 different grades of emery cloth. The perceived roughness was a power function of the grit number with an exponent of 1.5 (when no modulus was used). Grit size, unfortunately, provides an inexact description of surface texture. Lederman and her colleagues (e.g., Lederman, Loomis, & Williams, 1982; Lederman & Taylor, 1972; Taylor & Lederman, 1975) recognized this limitation of emery cloth and other "natural" surfaces and were the first investigators to use grooved plates or "gratings." The plates had groove widths G from 0.125 to 1.00 mm cut at varying separations into their surface. The sum of the groove width and the ridge width R (i.e., the raised area between the grooves) is the spatial period of the grating. Lederman consistently found that the perceived roughness increased as the groove width or contact force increased. Increasing the ridge width or finger speed either had little effect or slightly reduced the perceived roughness.

These psychophysical results were replicated by Goodwin and colleagues (Goodwin & John, 1990; Sathian, Goodwin, John, & Darian-Smith, 1989). These investigators also recorded the activity from peripheral mechanoreceptors in monkey fingertips that were passively stroked with the same gratings in order to identify potential neural codes for perceived roughness (Goodwin, John, Sathian, & Darian-Smith, 1989; Goodwin & Morley, 1987). The principal criterion for such a code would be an increase in neural activity with increased groove width, but little change or perhaps a slight decrease with increased ridge width. All three types of cutaneous mechanoreceptors found in monkey skin—RA (rapidly adapting), SA (slowly adapting) and PC (Pacinian)—responded with one to a few impulses every time a groove passed over the receptive field. That is, the output of a receptor was phase-locked to the grating spatial cycle. The mean cyclic response (i.e., the average discharge rate over one sinusoidal stroke of the grating) increased with groove width for all three receptor types, but decreased with ridge width only for the PCs. The average number of impulses evoked by each grating period consisting of a groove and a ridge also increased with groove width for all receptors, but increased with ridge width as well. In summation, temporal neural codes such as the mean cyclic response or the number of impulses evoked by each grating period accounted for the psychophysical effect of groove width, but did not account well for ridge width.

Connor, Hsiao, Phillips, and Johnson (1990) likewise found that neural codes based on average firing rates are inadequate to represent the perceived roughness of tetragonal patterns of embossed dots. Magnitude estimates of roughness for the dot patterns were nonmonotonic—at first increasing with increased dot spacing and then decreasing for separations greater than 3 mm. Roughness also increases as the dot size decreases from 1.2 to 0.5 mm. The mean firing rate was poorly correlated with perceived roughness for all afferent types and produces too large a response at small dot spacings and too small a response at moderate to large spacings. Measures of firing-rate variation (mean absolute deviation, standard deviation, and variance), however, were all well correlated with the roughness judgments. The correlation was highest for the SAs, somewhat lower for the RAs, and only modest for the PCs.

In addition to measures based on the average activity of individual receptors at a single time, Connor et al. (1990) derived two measures based on the average absolute differences in activity between firing rates at times separated by an interval dt, and firing rates at locations separated by a distance d. For both, the correlation between the SA response and the roughness judgments was excellent. The optimal value of dt decreased as the scanning velocity v increased, which suggests that the critical parameter is spatial separation ($v \times dt$ = constant) rather than temporal separation.

The product of the scanning velocity and the optimal delay was 2.2 mm for a scan velocity of 50 mm per sec, and 2.6 mm for a velocity of 20 mm per sec. The optimal separation for the mean absolute difference calculated over space, rather than time, was also 2.2 mm for the SA responses. It is important to note that a neural code based on spatial differences in activity would be independent of the velocity, consistent with the observed invariance of perceived roughness (Lederman, 1974). It appears, then, that the best neural code for roughness is based on the instantaneous difference in firing rate for receptors separated by about 2 mm (about twice the size of the receptive field for SA units), averaged over the population of receptors.

ELECTROCUTANEOUS CODE FOR TEXTURE

If we want to develop an electrocutaneous stimulus to represent surface texture, we would like ideally to replicate the neural responses evoked by the natural stimuli. If the neural code is the average spatial variation in firing rate, as suggested by the results of Connor et al. (1990), we will need an array of stimulators that can produce differences in the level of activation over space with a resolution of about 2 mm. Unfortunately, arrays of electrodes are difficult to produce, and it is unlikely that they will be suitable for prosthetic applications. The current version of the hand neuroprosthesis has only 8 stimulation channels, 7 of which are devoted to muscle stimulation (Keith et al., 1989; Smith et al., 1987). The energy costs of supporting even a modest array of electrodes for sensory feedback would be too high for a battery-powered device.

We chose, instead, to use a more economical alternative—a single electrode. But how can we adequately represent texture with just one electrode? One approach would be to have an array of sensors that measures the surface profile, a processor that calculates what the mean difference in firing rate should be based on a model of receptor response, and a stimulator that delivers a stimulus equivalent to the neural code described by Connor et al. (1990). The output of this system, however, would be related only to the roughness of the surface—all other textural qualities would be discarded by the processing.

A more general approach could use a spatial-to-temporal transformation, in which the spatial texture of a surface is transformed into the temporal texture of the feedback stimulus. Katz (1925, 1989) observed that the texture of a surface could be appreciated by stroking a pencil or stylus across it. As the stylus moves across the surface, it produces vibrations that are transmitted to the receptors in the fingertips. The spatial surface texture is then inferred from the temporal variations of the vibrations. In contrast to normal texture perception in which the receptors in the skin fire at all different phases of the surface simultaneously, the receptors in the finger-tips are stimulated synchronously by the stylus vibrations. The overall spatial variation in activity across the population is small, but the temporal variations are distinct.

As a stylus moves over a grating (perpendicular to the grooves), it will oscillate with a temporal period T equal to the spatial period P of the grating (where $P = G + R$), divided by the scan velocity V. Furthermore, it is plausible that the stylus will protrude further into wider grooves and produce stronger vibrations. As the groove width increases, then, we would expect that the roughness of the surface as perceived through the stylus will increase, because the size of the vibrations produced by the stylus increases and the frequency decreases.

We attempted to represent the surface texture of grooved plates by using an electrocutaneous stimulus that mimicked "feeling with a stylus." The stimulus consisted of bursts of pulses, and the burst period and the burst amplitude (i.e., the current in the pulses) were variable. The major features of the grooved surface were represented by these two stimulus parameters. Subjects performed a matching experiment in which they stroked gratings with different groove widths and adjusted the intensity and temporal period of the electrocutaneous stimulus in order to make a subjective match between the texture of the surface and the texture of the stimulus.

METHODS

Six subjects, ages 21 to 33 years, performed the matching experiments.

The gratings were made from a commercial photosensitive plastic (Anderson-Vreeland, Bryan, OH). Although we made gratings with a range of groove and ridge widths, we used only four gratings in this experiment with groove widths of 0.25, 0.75, 1.25, and 1.75 mm. The ridge width was constant at 1.5 mm. This range of grating parameters is commensurate with the stimuli used by previous investigators (Goodwin & John, 1990; Sathian et al., 1989). The gratings were 2.5 cm wide (i.e., parallel to the grooves) and 5.0 cm long.

The electrocutaneous stimuli consisted of bursts of balanced, biphasic pulses, as shown in Fig. 11.1, generated by an isolated, constant-current stimulator. Each pulse consisted of a cathodic phase, an interphase interval, and an anodic phase (in that order), all with durations of 30 μsec. The currents in the cathodic and anodic phases were equal so that no net charge (current X duration) was delivered by the pulse. In order to maximize the available range of perceived intensity without evoking painful sensations (Kaczmarek, Webster, & Radwin, 1992), the pulses were delivered in bursts of 10 pulses each at a pulse frequency of 1 KHz. All stimuli were 1 sec in

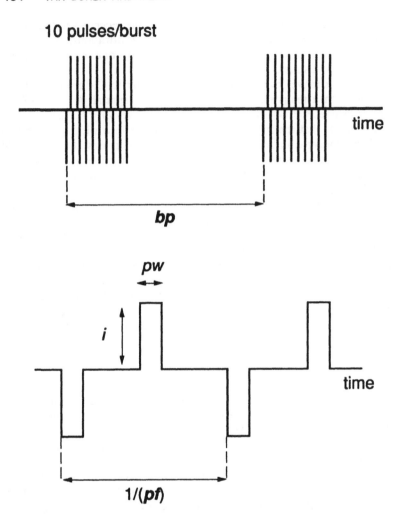

FIG. 11.1.   Electrocutaneous stimulus used to represent the texture of grooved plates. The balanced, biphasic, constant-current pulses are presented in bursts of 10. The pulse frequency pf is 1 kHz; the burst frequency bf is adjustable by the subject. The subject can also adjust the current i, typically within the range of 2 to 20 mA. The pulse widths pw of the cathodic (first) and anodic (second) phases were 30 μs. The charge per phase of each pulse is the product of the current and the pulse width. Stimuli were delivered to the skin on the lateral surface of the upper arm via a concentric surface electrode.

duration. At the beginning of the stimulus, the number of pulses increased from 2 pulses to 10 pulses over a period of 250 msec to avoid a sudden onset transient. The stimulus current and the burst period were adjusted by the subject during the matching experiment.

The stimuli were delivered through a surface electrode strapped or taped to the lateral surface of the subject's upper-right arm. The diameter of the electrode's central, circular cathode was 0.64 cm. The cathode was separated by an insulator from an annular anode, 2.5 cm in diameter with a wall thickness of 0.32 cm. Prior to placing the electrode on the skin, the skin was washed with alcohol and then moistened with tap water (Kaczmarek, Webster, Bach-y-Rita, & Tompkins, 1991; Saunders, 1974). Before the electrode was strapped or taped, the stimulus was set at a moderate intensity, and the subject was allowed to move the electrode over the upper arm in order to find a comfortable location. The site was chosen so that the stimulation did not produce any stinging, indicative of the recruitment of small nociceptive afferents. After the site was chosen, the subjects received a 5-minute "warm-up" period in which the stimulus was applied intermittently (1 sec on, 1 sec off) at a moderate intensity level in order to stabilize the skin impedance (Kaczmarek et al., 1991). Threshold was measured using the method of limits after the warm-up period and was remeasured in the middle and at the end of each session.

The subjects used the tip of the index finger of their right hand to stroke one of the four gratings in each trial. The subjects adjusted the stimulus parameters (burst period and current) with their left hand using rotary encoders equipped with large, unmarked knobs. During the experiment, the stimulus was delivered to the subject for 1 sec every other sec. Subjects were instructed to stroke the gratings in the intervals in which the stimulus was absent. In other words, the subject would experience the sensation from the fingertip for a second, followed by one second of electrocutaneous stimulation. Subjects were given as much time as they liked in each trial, making as many adjustments as necessary to match the electrocutaneous stimulus to the texture of the grating. The four different gratings were presented in blocks, with the order randomized within each block. Each session included five blocks. The entire session lasted for approximately 1 to $1\frac{1}{2}$ hours.

RESULTS

The matching results are plotted in Fig. 11.2, in which the coordinates of each point are the charge per phase q (in dB SL) and the burst period bp selected to match a particular grating in one trial. The four different groove widths are represented by the different symbols. Although the subjects reported that the electrocutaneous textures were indeed similar subjectively to the cutaneous textures, they did find it difficult to make matches — as evidenced by the scatter in the data.

The most important question, then, is whether there is any systematic effect of groove width on charge and burst period. Most subjects showed a tendency to match coarser gratings using higher charges and longer burst periods, as indicated by the average data plotted in Fig. 11.3.

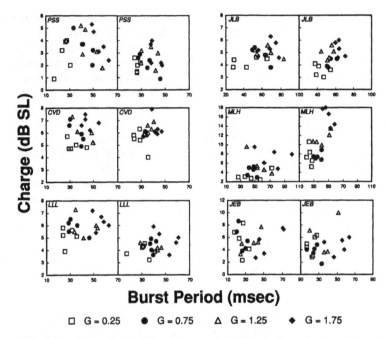

Burst Period (msec)

□ G = 0.25   ● G = 0.75   △ G = 1.25   ◆ G = 1.75

FIG. 11.2.   Charges (in dB SL) and burst periods (in ms) chosen by the subjects to optimize the perceptual match between the sensations evoked by the electrocutaneous stimulus and the sensations evoked by stroking a particular grating with the index fingertip. Each point represents one match, and the different symbols represent the four different gratings with groove widths of 0.25 mm (□), 0.75 mm (●), 1.25 mm (△), and 1.75 mm (◆). The ridge width was 1.5 m in all cases. Each grating was matched five times in two sessions.

The results from a MANOVA for each subject are given in Table 11.1 (univariate tests) and Table 11.2 (multivariate tests), which list the significance of the effects of groove width, session (first or second), and their interaction on the matched values of q and bp. Groove width had a significant univariate effect on burst period for all subjects, but produced a significant effect on charge in only four subjects (JLB, CVD, LLL, and MLH). A fifth subject, PSS, also showed a trend towards increasing charge with increasing groove width, but the effect was not statistically significant ($p = 0.22$) due to the wide range of charges used with each grating. Univariate session effects were mixed, producing the most dramatic differences in subject LLL, who had a pronounced change in the charges used in the two sessions, and subject MLH, who used markedly different charges and burst periods. The latter subject also had a clear change in the slope of the matching function, as indicated by the significant interaction of session and groove width effects. The multivariate effect of groove width on burst

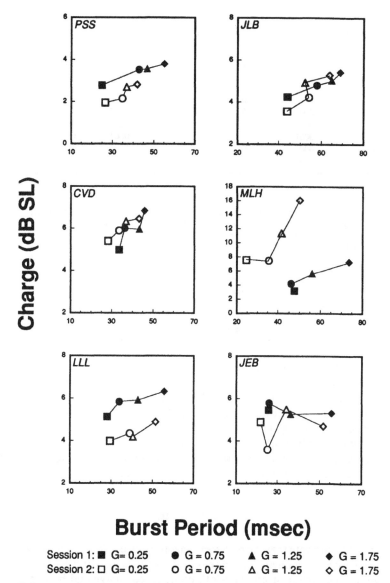

Burst Period (msec)

Session 1: ■ G= 0.25   ● G = 0.75   ▲ G = 1.25   ◆ G = 1.75
Session 2: □ G= 0.25   ○ G = 0.75   △ G = 1.25   ◇ G = 1.75

FIG. 11.3. Matched charges and burst periods for each subject, averaged across five trials in both the first (closed symbols) and second (open symbols) sessions. The different symbols represent the four gratings with groove widths of 0.25 mm (□), 0.75 mm (○), 1.25 mm (△), and 1.75 mm (◇).

TABLE 11.1

Significance (p values) of univariate effects of groove width (G) and session (S) on matched burst period and charge. Cells with $p > 0.05$ are left blank for clarity.

SUBJECT	BURST PERIOD			CHARGE		
	G	*S*	*G × S*	*G*	*S*	*G × S*
PSS	.0001	.0005			.005	
CVD	.0001	.05		.0005		
LLL	.0001			.05	.0001	
JLB	.0001			.0001	.05	
MLH	.0001	.0001		.0001	.0001	.005
JEB	.0001					

TABLE 11.2

Significance (p values) of multivariate effects of groove width (G) and session(s). Cells with $p > 0.05$ are left blank for clarity.

SUBJECT	*G*	*S*	*G × S*
PSS	.0001	.0005	
CVD	.0001	.05	
LLL	.0001		
JLB	.0001	.02	
MLH	.0001	.0001	
JEB	.0001		

period and charge simultaneously was significant for all subjects; the effect of session was significant for all subjects except JEB; and the interaction of groove width and session was significant only for subject MLH.

The general trend towards higher q and bp with larger groove widths is more apparent in Fig. 11.4, in which the data have been averaged across all trials and all subjects. A MANOVA again showed that the multivariate effects of groove width and session on q and bp were highly significant ($p < 0.0001$), but their interaction was not ($p = 0.63$).

DISCUSSION

Our results indicate that the electrocutaneous code can be used to reproduce at least some components of the sensation of surface texture evoked by the gratings. The effect of groove width on matched charge and burst period, as shown in Fig. 11.4, was anticipated based on the physiological and psychophysical studies described earlier. First, the afferent discharge from any single receptor, and from the overall population of receptors, will increase with the groove width (Goodwin & John, 1990; Sathian et al.,

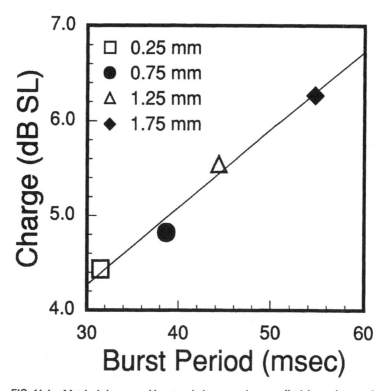

FIG. 11.4. Matched charges and burst periods averaged across all trials, sessions, and subjects for each of the four gratings.

1989). A similar effect will be produced by increasing the charge of the electrocutaneous stimulus. Second, the temporal burst period of the afferent discharge from any receptor is proportional to the spatial period of the grating. If subjects can perceive this temporal period and try to match it, the period of the electrocutaneous stimulus should also increase with the spatial period of the grating. The average burst period used to match each grating is plotted as a function of the spatial period in Fig. 11.5. The function is nearly linear with a slope of 1/(6.6 cm/sec). If the subjects did match the temporal period of the electrocutaneous stimulus to that of the afferent discharge, then this slope is the reciprocal of the average scanning velocity, that is, $v = 6.6$ cm/sec—a reasonable value.

The average results shown in Figs. 11.4 and 11.5 suggest that subjects adjusted the electrocutaneous stimulus to reproduce some basic features of the afferent response to the gratings. The average effects, however, were nearly obscured by the intertrial variation. Such variation could limit the usefulness of the feedback code in a prosthetic device, so it is important to

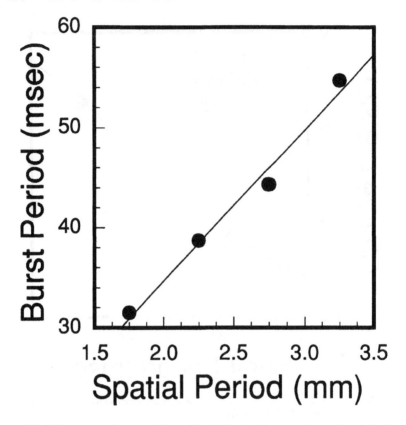

FIG. 11.5.   Average burst periods (see Fig. 11.4) plotted versus the spatial period of the gratings. The spatial period is the sum of the groove width and ridge width (1.5 mm). The line represents a least-squares linear fit with a slope of 1/(6.6 cm/s), which is the reciprocal of the average scanning velocity if subjects matched the burst period of the electrocutaneous stimulus to the temporal period of the afferent response to the gratings.

try to identify its source. One such source is adaptation. That is, if the electrocutaneous stimulus adapts, then the subjects will tend to use higher charges to achieve the same subjective intensity as the session progresses. The charges matched to all of the stimuli are plotted as a function of trial number for three subjects in Fig. 11.6 (the trial numbers were inadvertently discarded during data processing for the other three subjects).

Charge did not increase systematically for subject JLB, with the possible exception of the 1.75-mm grating (filled diamonds) in the first session. In contrast, all of the charges matched by PSS increased progressively throughout the session. In fact, the variation with trial number was more pronounced than the variation with groove width. Subject MLH had mixed

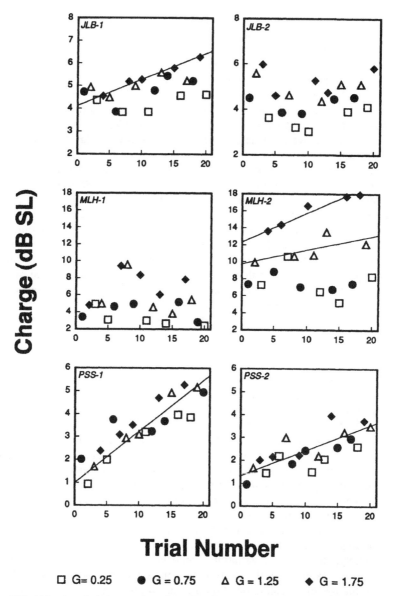

Trial Number

□ G= 0.25   ● G = 0.75   △ G = 1.25   ◆ G = 1.75

FIG. 11.6. Matched charges plotted as a function of trial number for three subjects for whom data were available. Increasing charge with trial number may indicate increasing adaptation, as in the case of subject PSS. The other two subjects showed little effect except for the larger groove widths (JLB: 1.75 mm, session 1; MLH: 1.75 and 1.25 mm, session 2). The lines were drawn by hand to indicate possible trends.

results. The charges matched to the wider grooves (1.25 and 1.75 mm) tended to increase with time in the second session, but there was little change in the first session.

The threshold data also provide a measure of adaptation. The thresholds measured at the beginning, middle, and end of each session are plotted in Fig. 11.7. The trends varied among subjects, and subject PSS showed the most pronounced elevation in threshold over time, consistent with the observed effect of trial number for this subject. The overall effect of time on threshold, averaged across subjects as shown in Fig. 11.8, was not significant.

The effects of time on both the threshold charge and suprathreshold charges used to match the gratings suggest that subject PSS was affected by adaptation, and that the other subjects were not. Adaptation, then, appears to be an infrequent problem at worst — and may not occur at all. That is, the observed threshold variations do not necessarily represent the amount of adaptation experienced at suprathreshold levels, and the effect of time on threshold or matched charge may not be due to adaptation per se. Such changes could be the result of fatigue or changes in the impedance of the skin-electrode interface (Kaczmarek et al., 1990). Other experiments are required to assess the effects of adaptation more directly.

Variation could also be introduced by an interaction between the perceived intensity and perceived burst frequency (pitch) of the electrocutaneous stimulus. The data in Fig. 11.9 for subjects JLB and PSS are replotted from Fig. 11.1.

Note that the matches for subject JLB are uniformly clustered, whereas the matches for PSS seem to follow an inverse relationship (dotted lines) between charge and burst period for each of the three largest groove widths. That is, for a fixed groove width, PSS chose high charges and short burst periods or low charges and long burst periods. Perhaps there is a perceptual tradeoff between the perceived pitch of the electrocutaneous stimulus and its perceived loudness (Szeto, 1985), analogous to similar effects in audition (e.g., Rossing & Houtsma, 1986; Stevens, 1935; Terhardt, 1974). The apparent interaction is strongest for subject PSS, but is also evident in matches made to some gratings by the other subjects. The interaction does not appear to be a particularly robust effect, but could confound the choice of unique stimulus parameters for any given grating.

Finally, the observed variations could be due to changes in the tactile sensations, rather than the electrocutaneous sensations. Kinematic and kinetic changes in the palpation of the gratings would change the temporal and intensive components of the tactile sensations, resulting in concomitant adjustments of the electrocutaneous parameters. The subjects were instructed to stroke the grating with their fingertip using a comfortable but consistent force, and to do so only during the 1-sec intervals between suc-

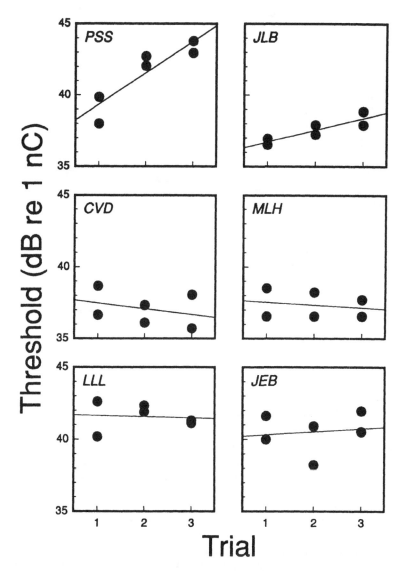

FIG. 11.7. Threshold charges (in dB re 1 nC) measured at the beginning (Trial 1), middle (Trial 2), and end (Trial 3) of each session. As in Fig. 11.6, increasing threshold over the duration of the experiment may indicate adaptation. Again, subject PSS shows the strongest effect.

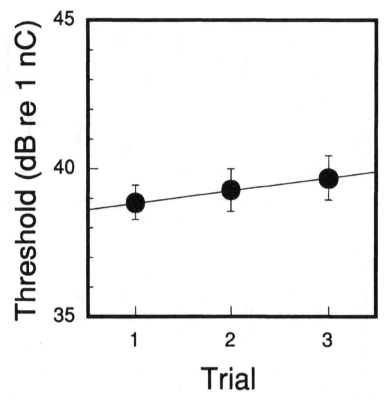

FIG. 11.8.   Threshold charges (in dB re 1 nC) averaged across both sessions and all subjects at the three measurement times. Error bars represent ± 1 standard error. Overall, the effect of time was not significant.

cessive stimuli. There were no further controls or constraints on contact force or finger speed. If the subjects pressed harder in a particular trial, they would be expected to match the grating with a higher charge. Likewise, if they moved their finger faster, the burst period would be lower. Some subjects, in fact, remarked that they had a tendency to change their finger speed in order to match the tactile perception to the electrocutaneous stimulus once the match was reasonably close to the optimum. Ideally, speed and force should be controlled using a mechanical apparatus such as a rotating drum or moving plate (Goodwin, Morley, Clarke, Lumaskana, & Darian-Smith, 1985), or the parameters of unrestricted movements should be measured.

CONCLUSIONS

Our initial attempt to represent surface texture using electrocutaneous stimulation was successful. The average matching results showed that

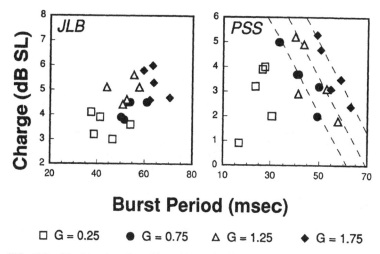

Burst Period (msec)

☐ G = 0.25   ● G = 0.75   △ G = 1.25   ◆ G = 1.75

FIG. 11.9. Matching data for subjects JLB and PSS replotted from Fig. 11.1. Note that the matches for any particular grating appear to be randomly scattered for JLB. In contrast, the matches for PSS tend to fall on the dashed lines, at least for the three largest groove widths, suggesting that there is a systematic tradeoff between charge and burst period for equally perceived textures.

coarser gratings were best matched by electrocutaneous stimuli with higher currents and longer burst periods—consistent with our expectations based on previous psychophysical and physiological studies. The main effect, however, was nearly obscured by substantial intra- and intersubject variations in the matches made to each grating. The variations may have been caused by adaptation, which seemed particularly strong in one subject, by a perceptual interaction between burst period and charge, or by changes in finger speed and contact force. Control or measurement of the movement parameters, measurement of adaptation effects, and characterization of potential perceptual interactions between the temporal and intensive dimensions of electrocutaneous stimuli will provide important data for further development of electrocutaneous codes of surface texture for prosthetic, neuroprosthetic, and robotic applications.

REFERENCES

Connor, C. E., Hsiao, S. S., Phillips, J. R., & Johnson, K. O. (1990). Tactile roughness: Neural codes that account for psychophysical magnitude estimates. *Journal of Neuroscience, 10,* 3823–3836.

Goodwin, A. W., & John, K. T. (1990). Tactile perception of texture: Peripheral neural correlates., In M. Rowe & L. Aitkin (Eds.), *Information processing in mammalian auditory and tactile systems* (pp. 7–18). New York: Wiley-Liss.

Goodwin, A. W., John, K. T., Sathian, K., & Darian-Smith, I. (1989). Spatial and temporal factors determining afferent fiber responses to a grating moving sinusoidally over the monkey's fingerpad. *Journal of Neuroscience, 9*, 1280-1293.

Goodwin, A. W., & Morley, J. W. (1987). Sinusoidal movement of a grating across the monkey's fingerpad: Representation of grating and movement features in afferent responses. *Journal of Neuroscience, 7*, 2168-2180.

Goodwin, A. W., Morley, J. W., Clarke, C., Lumaskana, B., & Darian-Smith, I. (1985). A stimulator for moving textured surfaces sinusoidally across the skin. *Journal of Neuroscience Methods, 14*, 121-125.

Gorman, P. H., & Peckham, P. H. (1991). Upper extremity functional neuromuscular stimulation. *Journal of Neurologic Rehabilitation, 5*, 5-12.

Hannaford, B., & Wood, L. (1992). *Evaluation of performance of a telerobot* (Jet Propulsion Laboratory New Tech. Rep. NPO 17924/7419). Pasadena: California Institute of Technology.

Kaczmarek, K. A., Webster, J. G., Bach-y-Rita, P., & Tompkins, W. J. (1991). Electrotactile and vibrotactile displays for sensory substitution systems. *IEEE Transactions on Biomedical Engineering, 38*, 1-16.

Kaczmarek, K. A., Webster, J. G., & Radwin, R. G. (1990, November). Periodic variations in the electrotactile sensation threshold. *Proceedings of the 12th Annual International Conference of the IEEE Engineering in Medicine & Biology Society*. Philadelphia, PA.

Kaczmarek, K. A., Webster, J. G., & Radwin, R. G. (1992). Maximal dynamic range of electrotactile stimulation waveforms. *IEEE Transactions on Biomedical Engineering, 39*, 701-715.

Katz, D. (1989). *The world of touch* (L. Krueger & L. Erlbaum, Eds. & Trans.). Hillsdale, NJ: Lawrence Erlbaum Associates. (Original work published 1925).

Kawamura, Z., & Sueda, O. (1968). Sensory feedback device for the artifical arm. *4th Pan Pacific Rehabilitation Conference, Hong Kong*.

Keith, M. W., Peckham, P. H., Thrope, G. B., Stroh. K. C., Smith, B., Buckett, J. R., Kilgore, K. L., & Jatich, J. W. (1989). Implantable functional neuromuscular stimulation in the tetraplegic hand. *Journal of Hand Surgery, 14A*, 524-530.

Körner, L. (1978). Afferent electrical nerve stimulation for sensory feedback in hand prostheses: Clinical and physiological aspects. *Acta Orthopaedica Scandinavica*, (Supplement 178), 1-52.

Lederman, S. J. (1974). Tactile roughness of grooved surfaces: The touching process and effects of macro- and microsurface structure. *Perception & Psychophysics, 16*, 385-395.

Lederman, S. J., Loomis, J. M., & Williams, D. A. (1982). The role of vibration in the tactual perception of roughness. *Perception & Psychophysics, 32*, 109-116.

Lederman, S. J., & Taylor, M. M. (1972). Fingertip force, surface geometry, and perception of roughness by active touch. *Perception & Psychophysics, 12*, 401-408.

Mann, R. W., & Reimers, S. D. (1970). Kinesthetic sensing for the EMG controlled "Boston arm." *IEEE Transactions, Man Machine Systems, 11*, 110-115.

Meek, S. G., Jacobsen, S. C., & Goulding, P. P. (1989). Extended physiologic taction: Design and evaluation of a proportional force feedback system. *Journal of Rehabilitation Research & Development, 26*, 53-62.

Meenes, M., & Zigler, M. J. (1923). An experimental study of the perceptions of roughness and smoothness. *American Journal of Psychology, 34*, 542-549.

Milchus, K. L., & Van Doren, C. L. (1990, November) Psychophysical parameterization of synthetic grasp force feedback. *Proceedings of the 12th Annual International Conference IEEE Engineering in Medicine and Biology Society*, Philadelphia, PA.

Minsky, M., Ouh-young, M., Steele, O., Brooks, F. P. Jr., & Behensky, M. (1990). Feeling and seeing: Issues in force display. *Computer Graphics, 24*(2), 235-243.

Patterson, P. E., & Katz, J. A. (1992). Design and evaluation of a sensory feedback system that provides grasping pressure in a myoelectric hand. *Journal of Rehabilitation Research & Development, 29*, 1-8.

Riso, R. R., Ignagni, A. R., & Keith, M. W. (1991). Cognitive feedback for use with FES upper extremity neuroprostheses. *IEEE Transactions on Biomedical Engineering, 38*, 29-38.

Rossing, T. D., & Houtsma, A. J. M. (1986). Effects of signal envelope on the pitch of short sinusoidal tones. *Journal of the Acoustical Society of America, 79*, 1926-1933.

Sathian, K., Goodwin, A. W., John, K. T., & Darian-Smith, I. (1989). Perceived roughness of a grating: Correlation with responses of mechanoreceptive afferents innervating the monkey fingerpad. *Journal of Neuroscience, 9*, 1273-1279.

Saunders, F. A. (1974). Electrocutaneous displays. In F. A. Geldard (Ed.), *Cutaneous communication systems and devices* (pp. 20-26). Austin, TX: Psychonomic Society.

Smith, B., Peckham, P. H., Keith, M. W., & Roscoe, D. D. (1987). An externally-powered, multichannel, implantable stimulator for versatile control of paralyzed muscle. *IEEE Transactions on Biomedical Engineering, 34*, 499-508.

Stevens, S. S. (1935). The relation of pitch to intensity. *Journal of the Acoustical Society of America, 6*, 150-154.

Stevens, S. S., & Harris, J. R. (1962). The scaling of subjective roughness and smoothness. *Journal of Experimental Psychology, 64*, 489-494.

Sueda, O., & Tamura, H. (1969, July). Sensory device for the artificial arm. *Proceedings of the Eighth International Conference on Medical and Biological Engineering*, Chicago, IL.

Szeto, A. Y. J. (1985). Relationship between pulse rate and pulse width for a constant-intensity level of electrocutaneous stimulation. *Annals of Biomedical Engineering, 13*, 373-383.

Taylor, M. M., & Lederman, S. J. (1975). Tactile roughness of grooved surfaces: A model and the effect of friction. *Perception & Psychophysics, 17*, 23-36.

Terhardt, E. (1974). Pitch of pure tones: Its relation to intensity. In E. Zwicker & E. Terhardt (Eds.), *Facts and models in hearing* (pp. 353-360). New York: Springer-Verlag.

Tunnicliffe, V. (1992). Hydrothermal-vent communities. *American Scientist, 80*, 336-349.

Wiener, N. (1951). Problems of sensory prostheses. *Bulletin of the American Mathematical Society, 56*, 27-35.

Wijman, C. A. C., Stroh, K. C., VanDoren, C. L., Thrope, G. B., Peckham, P. H., & Keith, M. W. (1990). Functional evaluation of quadriplegic patients using a hand neuroprosthesis. *Archives of Physical Medicine & Rehabilitation, 71*, 1053-1057.

12 Loudness Evaluation by Subjects and by a Loudness Meter

Hugo Fastl
Technische Universität München, Germany

INTRODUCTION

Loudness represents a hearing sensation which attracts much attention not only in the field of psychoacoustics, but also in noise control. Because psychoacoustic experiments are very time-consuming, it is a long-standing endeavor of engineers to simulate the relation between sound stimuli measured by physical means and the correlated loudness of the psychoacoustic hearing sensation. It is anticipated that algorithms can be proposed and implemented which give a correspondence between physical magnitude in line length and the loudness sensation. Instruments which produce an indication that is directly proportional to loudness perception are called *loudness meters*. A well-known example for this family of instruments is Zwicker's loudness meter for time-varying sounds (Zwicker & Fastl, 1983), which is successfully applied in noise evaluation and noise control.

The performance of a loudness meter has to be tested on the basis of psychoacoustic results on loudness evaluation. For physically well-defined stimuli, the perceived loudness is measured by different psychophysical procedures. A huge amount of psychoacoustic data have been compiled which serve among other things as an input to test and to improve the accuracy of loudness meters.

In the 1950s, seminal work on loudness evaluation was done in the Psychoacoustics Lab of S. S. Stevens at Harvard University. Since the 1960s, loudness evaluation is extensively studied in Zwislocki's laboratory as well as in other places in the United States and in Europe, especially in Germany. The effects of different methods and procedures on the results of loudness experiments have received much attention at the Institute for Sensory Research at Syracuse University since its founding in 1957. A special conference in Syracuse on the scaling of psychological magnitudes recently assembled specialists on that topic from all over the world. The proceedings (Bolanowski & Gescheider, 1991) not only display the state of the art on scaling of psychological magnitudes, but also give guidelines for future research.

Along these lines, three main issues are discussed in this chapter. First, it shows how excellent the results of two eminent scientists in psychoacoustics agree: Psychoacoustic loudness data from Zwislocki are compared to data from Zwicker's loudness meter. Second, the influence of different methods on loudness evaluation is shown, not for synthetic sounds like pure-tones or broadband noise, but for actual environmental sounds produced by different types of aircraft during takeoff. Again, the subjective evaluations are compared to data from the loudness meter. Noise *emissions* of single take-off sounds as well as noise *immissions* of several take-off sounds within 15 min were studied. (Immission is a product of energy and time, usually used to designate the emissions of sound over an extended period of time.) For noise immissions of aircraft sounds, the effects of different procedures to indicate the instantaneous loudness on the evaluation of the global overall loudness are tested. Third, the practical implications of phasing out loud aircraft on the "noise climate" around airports are assessed in terms of subjective and physical loudness evaluations.

EXPERIMENTS

Eight subjects with normal hearing, 26 to 32 years old (median = 27 yrs.) participated in the experiments. Sounds were presented diotically via electrodynamic earphones (Beyer DT 48) with freefield equalizer (Zwicker & Fastl, 1990) in a soundproof booth.

Sounds produced by different types of jet-aircraft during takeoff were recorded on DAT tape at the end of the runway of an airport. From the original recordings, sounds of 20-sec duration were edited. For the experiments on noise immissions, within a 15-min time period, four or eight take-off sounds were combined with a soft background of road traffic noise (see Fastl, 1990a, 1991a). Single take-off sounds (noise emissions) were subjectively measured by three different procedures:

1. Magnitude estimation with a reference or anchor sound (see, e.g., Hellman & Zwislocki, 1961; Stevens, 1955; Zwislocki & Goodman, 1980).
2. Absolute magnitude estimation (see, e.g., Zwislocki, 1983).
3. Matching of line length to loudness (see, e.g., Stevens & Guirao, 1963).

The third method was implemented as follows: By means of cursor keys, the subject could vary the length of a horizontal line displayed on the monitor of a PC up to a maximum length of 22 cm. The subjects were instructed to vary the length of the line in such a way that at any instant of time, the line length represented the actual perceived loudness (see Fastl, Zwicker, Kuwano, & Namba, 1989). The line length indicated by the subject was sampled every 100 ms and stored in the PC. For each take-off sound, the maximum line length was taken as a measure of the loudness corresponding to the noise emission. Each subject scaled each take-off sound presented in random order four times. Thus, for each of the three procedures and each take-off sound, 32 data points were obtained from which medians and interquartiles were calculated.

For the measurement of noise immissions, the following procedure was used: During the 15-min presentation of sounds, the subjects scaled the actual loudness by varying the length of a line displayed on a PC monitor as described above. After 15 min they were presented with a questionnaire on which they scaled the global average loudness of the preceeding 15 min by absolute-magnitude estimation and by marking the length of a line on a horizontal line with 15-cm total length (see Fastl, 1991b; Fastl et al., 1989; Kuwano & Fastl, 1989).

With four experienced subjects out of the group of eight, three additional experiments were performed to study possible interactions of instantaneous loudness scaling and global overall loudness scaling. In the first experiment, instantaneous loudness was scaled by line length displayed on a PC monitor as described above. In the second experiment, instantaneous loudness was indicated by the position of a slider from a mixing console (see Fastl, 1991b). In the third experiment, the subjects did *not* scale instantaneous loudness, but just listened to the sounds. After each of the three experiments, the subjects filled in the questionnaire and scaled overall loudness by absolute-magnitude estimation and by line length as described above.

All sounds presented to the subjects were analyzed by a loudness meter (Zwicker & Fastl, 1983) with a statistics analyzer. The loudness values N in Figs. 12.1 and 12.2 represent maximum values, loudness values N_5 in Figs. 12.4, 12.6, and 12.7 indicate the percentile loudness N_5 that is, the loudness value that is reached or exceeded in 5% of the measurement time.

RESULTS AND DISCUSSION

The results plotted in Fig. 12.1 enable a comparison of loudness evaluation for 1-kHz tones by subjects and loudness measurements of the same tones by a loudness meter. The subjective data (crosses) from Hellman and Zwislocki (1963, Fig. 12) are given as loudness in associated numbers n as

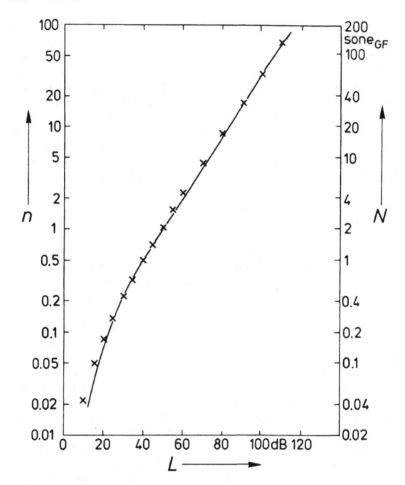

FIG. 12.1.   Loudness in assigned numbers *(n)* of a 1-kHz tone as a function of sound-pressure level *(L)* in dB. Crosses: Numbers associated to loudness (Hellman & Zwislocki, 1963). Curve: Loudness *(N)* measured by a loudness meter (Zwicker & Fastl, 1983).

a function of sound-pressure level L. The corresponding loudness N in some$_{GF}$ (curve) was measured by Zwicker's loudness meter (Zwicker, 1960; Zwicker & Fastl, 1983).

There is an excellent agreement between subjective and physical loudness evaluations of 1-kHz tones within a large dynamic range of more than 80 dB. The numbers n associated to loudness by the subjects of Hellman and Zwislocki (1963) and the numerical values of the loudness N measured by Zwicker's loudness meter differ by a factor of 2. This is primarily due to the fact that the loudness meter indicates values based on the sone scale in which, by definition, a 1-kHz tone at 40 dB produces a loudness of 1 sone.

In the 1960s the loudness of short sound impulses was studied extensively in several labs around the world, in particular in the United States and in Germany. In his classic paper "Temporal Summation of Loudness: An Analysis," Zwislocki (1969) compiled the data available at that time and developed his quantitative psychophysical theory of loudness summation. His results concerning the dependence of loudness on stimulus duration were confirmed in the 1970s in an international Round Robin Test (Pedersen, 1976) in which about 20 laboratories and more than 300 subjects participated.

In Fig. 12.2 temporal summation of loudness as proposed by Zwislocki is compared to data measured by Zwicker's loudness meter. The curve shows the dependence of relative loudness N/N_{ref} as a function of sound duration T_i (Zwislocki, 1969, Fig. 7). The circles indicate the loudness N in $sone_{GF}$ of impulses with a duration T_j, cut out of a continuous 2-kHz tone at 57 dB, as measured by the loudness meter (Zwicker & Fastl, 1983). There is good agreement between the data measured by Zwicker's loudness meter and the values predicted by Zwislocki's theory, which in turn is in line with subjective loudness evaluations.

Another interesting temporal effect with implications for the temporal structure of specific loudness N' (Zwicker & Feldtkeller, 1967) will be only briefly mentioned here, because it is described in detail elsewhere (Fastl, 1988): The decay of psychoacoustic excitation as seen in forward masking depends on stimulus duration (Zwicker, 1984; Zwicker & Fastl, 1972; Zwislocki, Pirodda, & Rubin, 1959). This nonlinear time effect represents an important feature of real-time loudness meters suitable for loudness measurements of signals with a strong temporal structure such as speech (Fastl, 1990b) or impulsive technical noises (Fastl, 1988).

In summary, it can be stated that several features of Zwicker's loudness meter can be regarded as technical simulation of loudness data obtained in

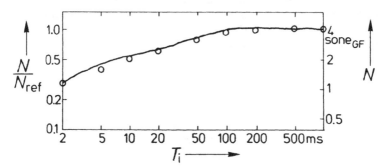

FIG. 12.2. Loudness as a function of stimulus duration. Curve: Normalized loudness values ($N/Nref$) in line with many compiled subjective data (Zwislocki, 1969). Circles: Loudness (N) of a 2-kHz tone impulse with duration T_i at 57 dB measured with a loudness meter (Zwicker & Fastl, 1983).

Zwislocki's laboratory in Syracuse. After all, this should not be too astonishing because during Fall 1961 and Spring 1962 Zwicker himself was a member of that laboratory.

Classic research on loudness scaling usually was performed with synthetic sounds like pure tones or broadband noise (see, e.g., Zwicker & Feldtkeller, 1967). In recent years, in addition to synthetic sounds, recorded environmental sounds are used in loudness experiments (e.g., Fastl, 1988; Namba, Kuwano, & Fastl, 1987). So far, methodological questions of loudness evaluation are studied mostly with synthetic sounds (for data and references see Bolanowski & Gescheider, 1991; Hellman & Zwislocki, 1961). However, in the following section some influences of different scaling procedures on loudness evaluation are studied with technical sounds, such as the noise produced by jet aircraft during takeoff.

Figure 12.3 shows the loudness time functions of the take-off sounds for aircraft A–I as measured with a loudness meter (Zwicker & Fastl, 1983). The sounds were produced by different types of commercial aircraft. Aircraft B and C have about the same seating capacity of 135 seats. Aircraft B developed in the 1960s produces about twice the loudness compared to aircraft C developed in the 1980s, despite the fact that the payload of C is about three times *higher* than that of B. This means that old stage-2 aircraft are considerably louder than modern stage-3 aircraft.

Figure 12.4 shows the loudness evaluation of the take-off sounds obtained by different psychoacoustic methods in comparison to values measured by the loudness meter. Circles show the numbers n_r associated with loudness when sound E is taken as reference sound (anchor) and its loudness is assigned the number 100. Squares represent data from absolute-magnitude estimation. The numbers n assigned to the respective loudnesses are arranged on the second-left ordinate in such a way that for sound E the medians indicated by circles and squares coincide. The triangles show loudness data obtained by line-length matching. The ordinate scale of line length 1 in mm again was chosen to get a coincidence of medians at sound E. The crosses in Fig. 12.4 represent values of physically measured percentile loudness N_5 arranged along the rightmost ordinate to fit the medians for sound E.

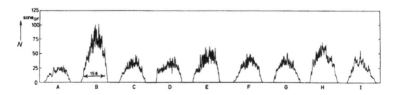

FIG. 12.3.   Loudness time functions produced by different aircraft A–I during take off.

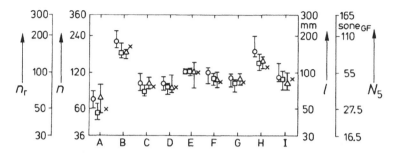

FIG. 12.4.   Loudness of aircraft sounds A through I. Circles: Magnitude estimation (n_r) with sound (E) as reference. Squares: Absolute magnitude estimation (n). Triangles: Matching sounds to line-length 1. Crosses: Percentile loudness (N_5) from loudness meter.

An analysis of the loudness data shown in Fig. 12.4 from an engineering point of view suggests that the three psychoacoustic methods produce very similar results (overlap of interquartiles), and that measurements by a loudness meter nicely simulate subjective loudness evaluation. Closer inspection shows that data obtained for magnitude estimation with an anchor (circles) are on the average somewhat higher than the other subjective estimates. For instance, if the loudness ratio is calculated for sound B versus sound C, we get as the median from 96 subjective ratios (8 subjects × 4 data × 3 methods) the factor 2.08 which is in good agreement with the ratio of 2.12 of physically measured loudness N_5.

Figure 12.5 shows the loudness time patterns of the sounds used for experiments on noise immissions. The loudness peaks produced by the take-off sounds and the relatively continuous road traffic background noise are easily identified. The loudness of the sounds displayed in Figs. 12.5a and 12.5b were scaled by four experienced subjects by three different methods as explained previously. Results are given in Fig. 12.6. The global overall loudness of the noise immissions was scaled by the subjects either by marking the length of a line (scale 1, unfilled symbols) or by absolute-magnitude estimation (assigned numbers n, filled symbols). The ordinate scales for line-length 1 and assigned numbers n were chosen to get equal maximum values for the situation 8 × B. During the 15-min sound presentation, subjects scaled the instantaneous loudness by line length (circles), or by slider potentiometer (squares) or just listened to the sounds without instantaneous loudness judgment (triangles). The crosses represent values of percentile loudness N_5 (right ordinate, adjusted to the maximum for 8 × B) measured with a loudness meter. The results shown in Fig. 12.6 suggest that for global average-loudness evaluation, line-length matching and absolute-magnitude estimation produce very similar results (unfilled vs. filled symbols).

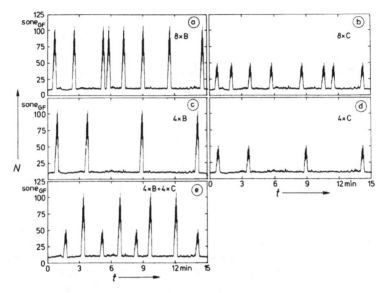

FIG. 12.5. Loudness time functions of noise emissions. Road-traffic background noise plus: a.eight take-off sounds of aircraft B; b.eight take-off sounds of aircraft C; c.four take-off sounds of aircraft B; d.four take-off sounds of aircraft C; e.eight take-off sounds, four from aircraft B and four from aircraft C.

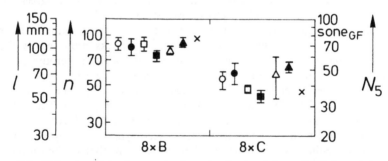

FIG. 12.6. Overall loudness evaluation of noise immissions. Unfilled symbols: Matching to line-length 1. Filled symbols: Absolute magnitude estimation (n). Scaling of instantaneous loudness by line length (circles), slide potentiometer (squares), no scaling (triangles). Crosses: Percentile loudness (N_5) from loudness meter.

For the noise immission with eight loud aircraft (8 × B), the global average loudness value depends very little on the method used for instantaneous loudness judgment. On the other hand, for the eight quieter aircraft (8 × C) global average loudness is scaled significantly lower when instantaneous loudness is indicated by movements of a slider (squares). This holds in particular for absolute-magnitude estimates of overall loudness. As described elsewhere (Fastl, 1991b) scaling of instantaneous loudness by a slider potentiometer can produce effects of clipping, and therefore other methods for scaling instantaneous loudness are preferred. If instantaneous loudness is not scaled (triangles), larger interindividual differences of the line length associated with overall loudness show up. The physical evaluation of overall loudness (crosses) frequently is in line with the subjective evaluation. However, for the noise immission produced by the softer aircraft (8 × C), larger differences to subjective evaluation show up for some methods used.

The results plotted in Fig. 12.7 can be regarded as indications for the variation in the "noise climate" around airports when loud old stage-2 aircraft (B) are replaced by more quiet aircraft (C). The circles represent medians of the line-length 1 associated by eight subjects to overall loudness when filling in the questionnaire. During the experiments, the subjects scaled instantaneous loudness by line length displayed on the monitor of a PC. The crosses in Fig. 12.7 represent the values of percentile loudness N_5 of the noise immissions as measured by the loudness meter. The corresponding scenarios are illustrated in Fig. 12.5.

If, for example, four old, loud aircraft are replaced by four modern quieter aircraft (Fig. 12.5c vs. Fig. 12.5d), according to the results plotted in Fig. 12.7 (4 × B vs. 4 × C), the loudness of the noise immission decreases by a factor of 2.03 which is in line with the decrease in noise emission by a factor of 2.08 as described earlier. Halving the number of operations (Fig. 12.5a vs. Fig. 12.5c and Fig.12.5b vs. Fig. 12.5d) leads approximately to half the overall loudness of the quieter aircraft (8 × C vs. 4 × C in Fig. 12.7), whereas for the loud aircraft (8 × B vs. 4 × B) the reduction in noise immission is much smaller than a factor of 2. Replacing only half of the loud old aircraft by more quiet modern aircraft (8 × B vs. 4 × B + 4 × C) leads to a loudness reduction by a factor of only 1.35, and

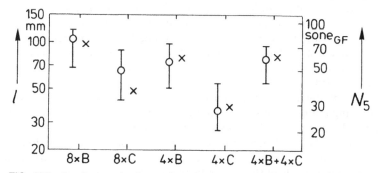

FIG. 12.7. Loudness evaluation of different scenarios of noise immissions around airports. Circles: Line-length 1 matched to overall loudness. Crosses: percentile loudness (N_5) from loudness meter.

replacing eight loud by eight quieter aircraft (8 × B vs. 8 × C) decreases the loudness of the noise immission by a factor of 1.56.

When calculating noise immissions according to the presently used standards based on L_{eq}, one single loud aircraft could be replaced by as many as 25 more quiet aircraft because of the level difference of 14 dB(A) of the take-off sounds. However, the data plotted in Fig. 12.7 suggest that the present calculation scheme for noise immissions is way off subjective evaluation: In terms of L_{eq}, take-off sounds of four loud aircraft (4 × B) should correspond to 100 takeoffs of quieter aircraft (100 × C), but according to Fig. 12.7, eight less loud aircraft (8 × C) produce almost the same overall loudness as four loud aircraft (4 × B). In contrast to the completely misleading concept of L_{eq}, the percentile loudness N_5 (crosses) simulates in good approximation the subjective evaluation of noise immissions by aircraft noise.

From a practical viewpoint, the results shown in Fig. 12.7 suggest that overall loudness of aircraft noise immissions is governed by the loud events. A similar result showing the large influence of loud events was also obtained for road traffic noise (see Fastl, 1991b).

CONCLUSION

From an engineering point of view, loudness evaluation by subjects can be simulated in good approximation by physical measurements with a loudness meter (Zwicker & Fastl, 1983). Subjective evaluation of the loudness produced by different aircraft during takeoff leads to similar results for the psychoacoustic methods of magnitude estimation and matching of loudness to line length. The subjective data are in line with physically measured percentile loudness N_5. When scaling the loudness ratio of noise immissions (eight take-off sounds of loud vs. quieter aircraft within 15 min), the global average- loudness evaluation may be somewhat influenced by the method used for scaling instantaneous loudness. While loudness matching to line length and just listening to the sounds lead to similar data, scaling of instantaneous loudness by slider potentiometer goes with a somewhat larger ratio in scaled overall loudness.

Different scenarios of the reduction in overall loudness around airports by phasing out old loud stage-2 aircraft suggest the following conclusions: Overall loudness crucially depends on the number of loud events. The presently used rule of thumb that for each reduction in noise emission by 3 dB the number of operations can be doubled is completely misleading! Instead, another rule of thumb can be proposed: A doubling of the number of operations is justified only if the loudness of the noise emission of aircraft is reduced by a factor of 2.

ACKNOWLEDGMENTS

The author gratefully acknowledges the assistence of Dipl.-Ing. U. Peschel who executed most of the experiments and Dr.-Ing. U. Widmann who gave valuable comments on the draft. This research is supported by Deutsche Forschungsgemeinschaft, SFB 204 Gehör München.

REFERENCES

Bolanowski, S. J., Jr., & Gescheider, G. A. (Eds.). (1991). *Ratio scaling of psychological magnitude.* Hillsdale, NJ: Lawrence Erlbaum Associates.

Fastl, H. (1988). Gehörbezogene Lärmmeßverfahren. *Fortschritte der Akustik, DAGA'88,* (pp. 111-124). Verl: DPG-GmbH, Bad Honnef.

Fastl, H. (1990a). Trading number of operations versus loudness of aircraft. *Proceedings Internoise '90, Vol. II, (pp. 1133-1136). Gothenburg, Sweden.*

Fastl, H. (1990b). Loudness of running speech measured by a loudness meter. *Acustica, 71,* 156-158.

Fastl, H. (1991a). Loudness versus level of aircraft noise. *Proceedings Inter-noise'91 Vol.* 1, pp. 33-36). Sydney, Australia. Poughkeepsie, NY: Noise Control Foundation.

Fastl, H. (1991b). Evaluation and measurement of perceived average loudness. In A. Schick, J. Hellbrück, & R. Weber (Eds.), *Contributions to psychological acoustics.*, Bibliotheks und Informationssystem der Universität Oldenburg. Poughkeepsie, NY: Noise Control Foundation.

Fastl, H., Zwicker, E., Kuwano, S., & Namba, S. (1989). Beschreibung von Lärmimmissionen anhand der Lautheit. *Fortschritte der Akustik, DAGA'89,* (pp. 751-754). Verl.: DPG-GmbH, Bad Honnef.

Hellman, R., & Zwislocki, J. (1961). Some factors affecting the estimation of loudness. *Journal of the Acoustical Society of America, 35,* 687-694.

Hellman, R., & Zwislocki, J. (1963). Monaural loudness function at 1000 cps and interaural summation. *Journal of the Acoustical Society of America, 35 ,* 856-865.

Kuwano, S., & Fastl, H. (1989). Loudness evaluation of various kinds of non-steady state sound using the method of continuous judgment by category. *Proceedings 13. ICA Belgrade, 1,* 365-368.

Namba, S., Kuwano, S., & Fastl, H. (1987). Cross-cultural study on the loudness, noisiness, and annoyance of various sounds. *Proceedings Inter-noise'87,* (Vol. II, pp. 1009-1012). Beijing, China, Poughkeepsie, NY: Noise Control Foundation.

Pedersen, O. J. (1976). Messung und Auswertung von impulsiven Geräuschen. *Fortschritte der Akustik, DAGA'76* (pp. 125-145). VDI-Verlag Düsseldorf.

Stevens, S. S. (1955). The measurement of loudness. *Journal of the Acoustical Society of America, 27,* 815-829.

Stevens, S. S., & Guirao, M. (1963). Subjective scaling of length and area and the matching of length to loudness and brightness. *Journal of Experimental Psychology, 66,* 177-186.

Zwicker, E. (1960). Ein Verfahren zur Berechnung der Lautstärke. *Acustica, 10,* 116-119.

Zwicker, E. (1984). Dependence of post-masking on masker duration and its relation to temporal effects in loudness. *Journal of the Acoustical Society of America, 75,* 219-223.

Zwicker, E., & Fastl, H. (1972). Zur Abhängigkeit der Nachverdeckung von der Störimpulsdauer. *Acustica, 26,* 78-82.

Zwicker, E., & Fastl, H. (1983). A portable loudness-meter based on ISO 532 B. *Proceedings 11. ICA Paris, 8,* 135-137.

Zwicker, E., Fastl, H. (1990). *Pscyhoacoustics—Facts and models.* Berlin/New York: Springer-Verlag.

Zwicker, E., & Feldtkeller, R. (1967). *Das Ohr als Nachrichtenempfänger, 2. erweiterte Auflage.* Stuttgart: Hirzel-Verlag.

Zwislocki, J. J. (1969). Temporal summation of loudness: An analysis. *Journal of the Acoustical Society of America, 46*, 431–441.

Zwislocki, J. J. (1983). Group and individual relations between sensation magnitudes and their numerical estimates. *Perception & Psychophysics, 33*, 460–468.

Zwislocki, J. J., & Goodman, D. A. (1980). Absolute scaling of sensory magnitudes: A validation. *Perception & Psychophysics, 28*, 28–38.

Zwislocki, J. J., Pirodda, E., & Rubin,, H. (1959). On some poststimulatory effects at the threshold of audibility. *Journal of the Acoustical Society of America, 31*, 9–14.

13 What is Absolute About Absolute Magnitude Estimation?

George A. Gescheider
Hamilton College and Syracuse University

INTRODUCTION

A fundamental problem in psychophysics is the measurement of the magnitude of sensations. There are no techniques for directly measuring the magnitudes of private sensations. The available methods are indirect, at best. The magnitude of a sensation must be inferred from the subject's responses to stimuli. To redefine sensation in terms of observable neural activity does not solve the problem, because to do so requires that we know the neural code for stimulus intensity, and presently no widespread agreement exists on this matter. The problem is further illustrated by the two-stage model of psychophysical scaling (e.g., Attneave, 1962; Curtis, Attneave, & Harrington, 1968; Shepard, 1981) in which sensation magnitude (φ) and its relation to stimulus intensity (ϕ), known as the psychophysical law [$\varphi = F_1 (\phi)$], must be inferred from the relationship between the stimulus and the observable response [$R = F_3 (\phi)$]. To do this, however, the relationship between the response and the sensation [$R = F_2 (\varphi)$] must be known. Unfortunately, the relationship between response and sensation is as inaccessible to direct observation and therefore is just as elusive as the relationship between stimulus and sensation. In spite of these difficulties, psychophysical scales of sensory magnitude have been constructed, and claims for their validity have been made.

In all psychophysical scales, the relationship between sensory magnitude and stimulus intensity must be inferred from the observable responses of subjects. The problem is that the subject's responses can easily be biased. Whatever the source of bias may be, there is wide agreement among sensory psychophysicists that the goal should be to develop and refine methods that minimize bias so that true sensory magnitude functions can be ascertained. One of many such efforts has been the development of the method of absolute magnitude estimation (Hellman & Zwislocki, 1961, 1963; Zwislocki, 1978; Zwislocki & Goodman, 1980) as a way of minimizing biases in magnitude-estimation experiments.

Absolute Magnitude Estimation

An important question recently asked is whether or not there is anything absolute about absolute magnitude estimation (Gescheider & Bolanowski, 1991). This issue has its origin in the problem of controlling bias in magnitude-estimation experiments (Hellman & Zwislocki, 1961). Absolute magnitude estimation (AME) requires subjects to match their subjective impression of the size of a number to their impression of the subjective magnitude of a stimulus, and to do so independently of prior matches. The method is based on the hypothesis that, at a particular time and in a particular setting, a subject has a strong tendency to assign a number to a stimulus in such a way that their psychological magnitudes match. Forcing the subject to use an arbitrary modulus associated with a particular standard stimulus can, by violating the natural tendency to match psychological magnitudes, cause bias. According to the AME hypothesis, subjects are capable of making unbiased numerical judgments of sensory magnitudes only when they are permitted to use their own natural units (Zwislocki & Goodman, 1980).

The first evidence that subjects tend to judge sensory magnitude on an absolute rather than on a ratio scale comes from experiments on the effect that the value of the standard stimulus and the associated modulus has on magnitude estimations. In accordance with the definition of a ratio scale in which the size of the unit of measurement is arbitrary (Stevens, 1951), a subject's numerical estimations of sensory magnitudes should be invariant to within a multiplicative transformation when the value of the modulus and/or standard stimulus is changed. Thus, it should be possible to make valid judgments of the sensation magnitudes of all stimuli in proportion to a modulus consisting of an arbitrary numerical value designated by the experimenter to represent the sensation magnitude of the standard stimulus. The work of Stevens (1956) and Hellman and Zwislocki (1961) on loudness scaling, in which the effects of using a standard stimulus with a particular modulus as a reference were investigated, casts serious doubt on the hypothesis that subjects, using an arbitrary unit, are capable of assigning numbers in proportion to the ratios of their sensations. Magnitude estimations of loudness when using a standard stimulus of 40 or 90 dB above threshold are seen in Fig. 13.1. Subjects were told to judge the loudness of

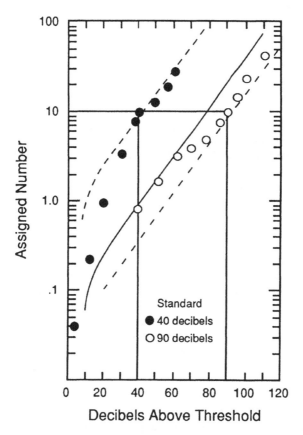

FIG. 13.1. Magnitude estimation of loudness as a function of sound intensity for standard stimuli of 40 and 90 dB SL. (Data from Hellman & Zwislocki, 1961.)

each tone relative to the loudness of 10 (the modulus) arbitrarily assigned to the standard stimulus. If the subjects had been able to make ratio judgments of loudness, the intensity of the standard stimulus would have had no effect on the form of the loudness scale, other than shifting all magnitude estimations by a constant ratio. Thus, ratio scaling would produce a vertical shift of the entire curve by a constant distance when magnitude estimations are plotted on a logarithmic axis. Under these conditions, the ratio of the magnitude-estimation values for various stimuli would remain constant, even though changing the standard stimulus would force the subject to assign higher or lower numbers.

It can be seen in Fig. 13.1 that when the standard stimulus was 40 and 90 dB above threshold, the resulting loudness scales were not parallel over the entire range of sound intensities. Only within a narrow range near the value of the standard stimulus are the curves approximately parallel. The solid curve is the binaural loudness scale derived from absolute magnitude estimation (Zwislocki & Goodman, 1980). The dashed curves are parallel to the absolute magnitude estimation curve. It is evident that when a standard stimulus is used, magnitude estimations of stimuli distant from the value of the standard tend to converge on the curve derived from absolute magnitude estimation. The finding that the loudness scales obtained with 40-and 90-dB standards are reasonably parallel within the intensity range of the standard stimulus suggests that, within this limited range, subjects are capable of making ratio judgments of sensation magnitude. On the other hand, outside this range, responses tend to drift toward what may be interpreted as a natural absolute scale.

The hypothesis that subjects tend to assign numbers to sensations on a natural absolute scale is also suggested by the work of Ward (1973), who had subjects make magnitude estimations of the loudnesses of 1000-Hz tones. At the start of an experimental session, the subject was presented with a standard stimulus of 56 dB above threshold and was told that this tone had a subjective value of 10. This and other stimuli were presented many times throughout the session, but no further statements were made by the experimenter on the subjective value of the standard stimulus. By the end of the session, the average value assigned to the standard by the subjects was not 10, but instead was 2.08. Zwislocki and Goodman (1980) have pointed out that 2.08 is almost exactly what subjects assign to this stimulus by absolute magnitude estimation. It appears that unless observers are repeatedly reminded of the arbitrary subjective value of a standard stimulus, they will eventually use their own natural numbers. It is this tendency of subjects to use their own natural numbers in judging psychological magnitudes and the inability of subjects to judge the ratios of their sensations in arbitrary units that best characterize what is absolute in absolute magnitude estimation.

The psychophysical scale resulting from AME is absolute in the sense that the unit of measurement employed by the subject in judging sensation magnitudes in a particular context has a fixed rather than arbitrary size. The value of the unit is determined by the size of the numbers that are natural for the subject to use in a particular context. Forcing the subject to change the unit produces bias. Thus, in accordance with the definition of an absolute scale, no transformation of the numbers is possible, because to do so induces bias in the subject's judgments which ultimately produces bias in the psychophysical scale. It should be made clear that the absolute in AME does *not* mean that all subjects will tend to make the same response to a particular stimulus nor does it mean that a particular subject will give the same number to a stimulus on all occasions or in differing stimulus contexts. Misunderstanding of this last point has given rise to false claims against the absolute magnitude estimation hypothesis (Foley, Cross, & O'Reilly, 1990; Mellers, 1983). Demonstrations that AME judgments can be influenced by the values of other stimuli presented in the session (Mellers, 1983) or on the values of stimuli presented in prior sessions (Foley et al., 1990) do not constitute evidence against the hypothesis. In his response to Mellers's paper, Zwislocki (1983b), one of the originators of AME, pointed out that a scale is called *absolute* not because it cannot be biased, but instead because it has the formal mathematical property of having a fixed unit. The absolute scale cannot be mathematically transformed without violating the properties of the scale, and therefore the scale consists of a special instance of a ratio scale in which the unit is fixed (e.g., numerosity). As well as having a fixed unit, the absolute scale in psychophysics is one that has the properties of transitivity and additivity characteristic of ratio scales. The fixed unit is implied by the results of Hellman and Zwislocki (1961), but the results of other experiments are pertinent to the issues of transitivity and additivity of AME scales. Let us consider the requirements of transitivity.

TRANSITIVITY OF AME JUDGEMENTS

Recent work on the prediction of cross-modality matches from AME judgments supports the hypothesis that valid absolute scales can be achieved in AME. If subjects assign numbers to their sensations on an absolute scale, then stimuli in two different modalities are equal in sensation magnitude when the stimuli are given the same number in magnitude estimation. It should, therefore, be possible to demonstrate the transitivity of scales by predicting the absolute values of cross-modality matches. The prediction is that stimuli from different modalities assigned the same number in magnitude estimation will be judged to be psychologically equal in cross-modality matching. Confirmation of this prediction would imply that the size of the numbers used in magnitude estimation are not arbitrary and thus result in psychophysical scales in which the unit of measurement is fixed. The prediction of cross-modality matches from absolute scales is based on the assumptions that (a) subjects are capable of making psychophysical matches between their impressions of the size of numbers and impressions of sensory stimuli, and (b) that subjects are capable of making psychophysical matches between their impressions of sensory stimuli.

Is it reasonable to assume that subjects have the ability to make matches of psychological magnitudes? The idea that matching is the fundamental operation underlying all physical and psychophysical measurement was recently expressed by Zwislocki (1991 p. 20) who stated that "measurement consists of matching common attributes of things and events" and "when a standard unit is involved, numbers come in to express the sum of the units required for a match." Zwislocki also pointed out that matching is natural, because it is something we all do every day in interacting with our environments. For example, the single act of picking up an object requires that a match be made between the impression of the object's mass and the impression of the needed effort to accomplish the task. That the matching operation is performed with a fairly high degree of accuracy is attested to by our survival. Moreover, we should, because of its simplicity, be very skilled at such a task. According to Zwislocki, the matching operation underlying measurement is performed on an ordinal scale, and this is true whether or not numbers are involved. The question in matching is simply which one of the items being matched is the greater, without a specification of how much. Thus, absolute magnitude estimation requires none of the complex judgments, such as ratio judgments or difference judgments, that other psychophysical scaling procedures depend on. Instead, in absolute magnitude estimation the subject is required, through ordinal judgments, to establish a match between the psychological magnitudes of numbers and of the stimuli.

Whether the subject is performing magnitude estimation or cross-modality matching, the task is essentially the same—to judge whether the psychological magnitude of a stimulus located on one stimulus continuum is less than, greater than, or equal to the psychological magnitude of a stimulus located on another stimulus continuum. It is assumed that the matches are made on a common abstract dimension of subjective magnitude (Zwislocki & Goodman, 1980). A match is made when the subjective magnitudes are judged to be equal. At this point, the two corresponding stimulus values are recorded by the experimenter. In AME, the two values that are recorded are the number selected by the subject and the physical value of the relevant dimension of the sensory stimulus (e.g., intensity, frequency, wavelength, etc.). In cross-modality matching, the physical values of the stimuli that are judged to be equal in sensory magnitude are recorded. Stevens (1975) also emphasized the fundamental nature of the matching operation in magnitude estimation and cross-modality matching.

Psychophysical matching by adults and children (age range 4–7 years) was investigated by Collins and Gescheider (1989) who had subjects match their impression of number size to their impressions of line length and to the loudness of 1000-Hz tones. In the second phase of the experiment, these same subjects matched their impressions of line length to the loudness of the tones. The results of one adult subject are seen in Fig. 13.2. The subjective line-length scale and the loudness scale were both power functions with exponents of .93 and .27, respectively. The solid line of the cross-modality matching function was predicted from the subjective line length and loudness functions. It is clear that, for this subject, the matches, as

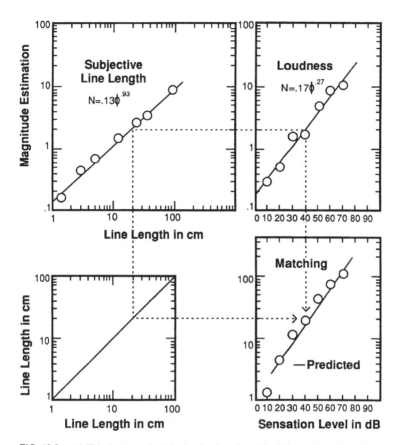

FIG. 13.2.   AME judgments of subjective line length and loudness as functions of line length in cm and the sensation level in dB of a 1000-Hz tone, respectively. The loudness exponent was determined over the range of 20–70dB SL. The predicted cross-modality matches of subjective line length to loudness (solid line) and the data for this task are shown in the lower part of the figure. The dashed lines illustrate the prediction of one cross-modality match when the AME value was 2.0 for both subjective line length and loudness. (Data for a single subject from Collins & Gescheider, 1989.)

indicated by the data points, are in reasonably close agreement with the predicted function. The dashed lines illustrate the prediction of a single point on the cross-modality matching function at which a magnitude estimation value of 2.0 corresponds to a line length of 20 cm and a tone of 40-dB sensation level.

The results of most of the other subjects also supported the hypothesis that, with proper instructions, both children and adults can judge sensory magnitude on an absolute scale. Specifically, for 9 out of 12 adults and 9 out of 11 children, lines and tones assigned the same number in absolute magnitude estimation were judged in cross-modality matching to be subjectively equal. Similar results have been obtained for AME judgments and cross-modality matches for brightness, loudness, the subjective magnitudes of vibration, and subjective line length (Bolanowski, Zwislocki, & Gescheider, 1991). In these experiments, the equality of assigned numbers in magnitude estimation fairly accurately predicted the results of cross-modality matches. This principle was also evident in a situation in which the response measure of applied pressure by the subject's fingertip was substituted for the AME response measure.

The transitivity of AME scales demonstrated in these cross-modality matching experiments has also been demonstrated in studies in which subjects made intramodality matches of the loudness of tones of different frequencies (Hellman, 1976), the loudness of tones presented in the presence of and in the absence of noise (Hellman & Zwislocki, 1964), and the subjective magnitude of vibrotactile stimuli of different frequencies (Verrillo, Fraioli, & Smith, 1969). In these studies, the values of intramodality matches of the psychological magnitude of qualitatively different stimuli were accurately predicted from AME judgments.

INDIVIDUAL DIFFERENCES AND RESPONSE TRANSFORMATION FUNCTIONS

An examination of exponents and the size of numbers used by individuals has revealed large individual differences. At the same time, an individual subject's responses show a high degree of stability over sessions, indicating that the subjects in AME experiments have individual ways of assigning numbers to sensations that tend to persist over time (Collins & Gescheider, 1989). Exponents for subjective line-length functions have been found to be highly correlated across sessions for both adults ($r = 0.97$) and children ($r = 0.87$) (Collins & Gescheider, 1989). In this study, loudness exponents were also found to be significantly correlated across sessions for both adults ($r = 0.86$) and children ($r = 0.82$). Teghtsoonian and Teghtsoonian (1983) favor the view that consistency in responding over sessions is due to memory of specific responses made in earlier sessions. It is doubtful that subjects would remember their judgments over the 5–14 days between sessions in the Collins and Gescheider study, or over 1 to 2 years, as in a study by Verrillo (1983) in which he found a high degree of reliability of responding in AME over these very long time intervals. Rather, it seems that subjects prefer to use certain numbers because of enduring modes of responding that are characteristically different for individual subjects.

Because the individual subject's responses tend to be stable over time, there is the possibility that the individual's response mode can be identified.

The stimulus transformation (psychophysical law) function cannot be determined from experimental data without knowing the response-transformation function describing the relationship between sensation magnitude and the subject's response. Zwislocki (1983b) has demonstrated that the AME exponent for subjective line length provides a direct measure of the exponent for the generalized response-transformation function that applies to all other sensory continuua. According to Zwislocki, given the correctness of the assumption that the perception of line length is veridical, any deviation of the exponent of the subjective line-length function from 1.0 is a reflection of bias (nonlinearity) in the response-transformation function. Assuming that this response bias generalizes across modalities, the response-transformation function obtained in judging subjective line length can be used to correct exponents obtained for other sensory dimensions. This is done simply by dividing the exponent in question by the subjective line-length exponent obtained from the same subject (see Collins & Gescheider, 1989, and Zwislocki, 1983a; for the formal logic).

What is the evidence that response-transformation functions generalize across modalities? In an experiment on loudness summation, Zwislocki (1983a) estimated the response-transformation function in two ways for the same subjects. In this study, the subjects made AME judgments of the overall loudness of two brief tones presented in rapid succession. The frequencies of the tones were in different critical bands, and therefore loudness summation was expected. Consistent with the hypothesis that loudness summates linearly in the nervous system and that subjects are capable of making valid judgments of loudness, AME judgments of the tone pair were equal to the sum of the AME judgments of the individual tones. Although this additivity was evident in the average data for the group of subjects, it was absent in the data of some of the individual subjects. In the cases in which subjects' responses were not additive, either loudness summation was nonlinear, the response transformation function in which loudness is transformed to magnitude-estimation responses was nonlinear, or both functions were nonlinear. If it is assumed that loudness summation is linear, it is possible to determine the nonlinear response transformations that are responsible for the lack of additivity of the magnitude estimations. Using this approach, Zwislocki determined the response transformation functions of individual subjects and found them to be power functions with exponents ranging from .83 to 1.33. It is clear that the data of individuals indicate that some subjects deviated somewhat from the ideal linear function with its exponent of 1.0. The second and independent estimation of the response-transformation functions of Zwislocki's subjects was obtained by having them estimate the subjective lengths of lines. Again the exponents were found to vary from individual to individual. Perhaps the most important finding of the study was the high correlation ($r = .95$) between the exponents for subjective line length and the theoretical response-transformation exponents calculated from the loudness summation data. Thus, similar estimates of the response-transformation function from line-length estimations and summation data indicate that systematic errors in assigning numbers to sensation magnitudes carry over from one modality to another.

The finding of Zwislocki that it is possible to determine a generalized response-transformation function from an individual subject's AME judgments of line length opens the possibility of using such estimations of the response-transformation function to obtain unbiased estimations of the stimulus transformation function (the psychophysical law). Collins and Gescheider (1989) used Zwislocki's correction procedure to correct loudness exponents of individual subjects and found that the intersubject variance of exponents for loudness was substantially reduced by dividing each individual loudness exponent by the line-length exponent of the same subject. The results are seen in Fig. 13.3. The line in Fig. 13.3a predicts the exponent for loudness from exponents of subjective line length under the assumptions that line-length exponents provide the exponents for the generalized re-

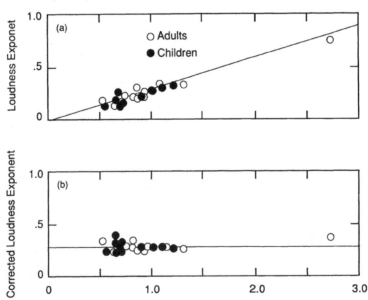

FIG. 13.3. Uncorrected (a) and corrected (b) loudness exponents for each individual as a function of his or her subjective line-length exponent. (From Collins & Gescheider, 1989. Reprinted with permission from the Journal of the Acoustical Society of America.)

sponse-transformation function and that the true loudness function exponent is 0.3 for every subject. Deviations of measured exponents from the prediction may reflect variability among the true loudness exponents of subjects. It is clear that the loudness exponents of individual subjects varied greatly and were highly correlated with their subjective line-length exponents. In Fig. 13.3b the corrected exponents for loudness are plotted as a function of the exponents for line length. The horizontal line represents the predicted function under the assumptions that the correction procedure works perfectly and that the true loudness exponent is 0.3 for every subject. One can see that, after correction, most of the loudness exponents clustered near the mean value of .3. This reduction in intersubject variability can be interpreted as an indication that the correction procedure has removed a source of variability in the loudness exponents attributable to differences in the response-transformation functions of individual subjects. Algom and Marks (1984), in a study of binaural summation, using conventional magnitude-estimation procedures, also attributed most of the individual differences in exponents to differences in the ways people assign numbers to sensations rather than to differences in sensory processes. It should be noted that the method of magnitude matching developed by Stevens and Marks (1980) has also been used to correct for idiosynchratic ways individual subjects use numbers in conventional magnitude estimation.

The substantial individual differences in response-transformation functions might lead one to distrust the results of studies in which this potential source of error was not eliminated. Fortunately,. average exponents for subjective line length are typically close to 1.0 (Collins & Gescheider, 1989; Stevens & Guirao, 1963; Teghtsoonian, 1965; Verrillo, 1981, 1983; Zwislocki, 1983a; Zwislocki & Goodman, 1980), indicating linearity of the average response-transformation function. Thus, given that the response-transformation function for line length is a generalized function applicable to other sensory continua, exponents for other sensory attributes, such as loudness, calculated from averaged magnitude-estimation data probably represent reasonably accurate estimations of the average exponents of the underlying stimulus transformation function. This conclusion is also suggested by group magnitude-estimation data in which the averaged responses indicate additivity of measurements (e.g., Bolanowski, 1987; Hellman & Zwislocki, 1963; Zwislocki, 1983a). In these experiments, the magnitude estimation of the overall sensation magnitude of two stimuli presented together was equal to the sum of the magnitude estimations obtained when the stimuli were presented separately. Analysis of individual differences in responding, however, demonstrates the importance of determining the response-transformation function of an individual subject. For example, the judgments of some of Zwislocki's (1983a) subjects were additive only after their nonlinear response-transformation functions were applied to the data. It is fundamental to recognize that without knowing the individual's response transformation function, the form of the underlying stimulus-transformation function for that subject is indeterminate from his or her magnitude estimations of the subjective magnitudes of stimuli.

THE EFFECTS OF STIMULUS CONTEXT

Do absolute magnitude estimations depend on stimulus context? Although there are those who interpret stimulus-context effects, in which AME judgments of a stimulus depend on the values of other stimuli presented in the session (e.g., Mellers, 1983), or on the values of stimuli presented in earlier session (Foley et al., 1990) as evidence against the AME hypothesis, there are others who have argued that the results of these experiments are irrelevant to this issue (Gescheider, 1988, Gescheider & Hughson, 1991, Zwislocki, 1983b). Nevertheless, if AME is to be useful as an experimental technique for measuring psychological magnitude, it is important to assess the degree to which results produced by the method are affected by stimulus context. Thus far, the findings on this issue are ambiguous with regard to the magnitude of context effects for AME. In the judgment of loudness, Zwislocki and Goodman (1980) found AME judgments to be fairly free from stimulus-context effects. Gescheider and Hughson (1991) also found context effects in AME judgments of loudness to be small for group data, as well as for the data of most of the individual subjects tested. Ellermeier, Westphal, and Heidenfelder (1991) found no significant effects of stimulus context on AME-type judgments or on verbally anchored category judgments of pain intensity. Ward (1987) reported context effects for several scaling methods, including AME, but they were smaller for AME and ratio magnitude estimation than for category rating. On the other hand, Mellers (1983) found substantial context effects in AME judgments. In her experiment, dot patterns of varied density were presented together, and subjects made AME judgments of their apparent densities. It was found that the judgment of a particular stimulus was substantially affected by the density values of other stimuli presented at the same time. It is not known, however, whether such context effects would have been found if these stimuli had been presented sequentially in the usual fashion rather than simultaneously.

The single-presentation mode of stimulus presentation was recently employed by Gescheider and Hughson (1991) in a study of stimulus-context effects in which it was determined whether AME judgments of the loudness of a tone are influenced by the intensities of other tones presented within the same session. In one experiment, a group of 18 subjects was tested in separate sessions in which judgments were made of the loudness of stimuli within either a low (10–60-dB SL) or high (40–90-dB SL) range of intensities. Examination of the results of individual subjects revealed that judgments of stimuli common to the two ranges (40-, 50-, and 60-dB SL) were, in most subjects, unaffected or only slightly affected by the position of the range. The data in Fig. 13.4 indicate that in the case of 10 subjects, subjects 1 through 5 and 9 through 13, there was very little tendency for AME values for the 40-, 50-, and 60-dB SL tones to be systematically influenced by the location of the range. In the case of the other six subjects, subjects 6 through 8 and 14 though 16, AME judgments of the loudness of the 40-, 50-, and 60-dB SL tones tended to be higher when these stimuli were presented in the context of the low range than when they were presented in the context of the high range. Of these six subjects whose judgments were

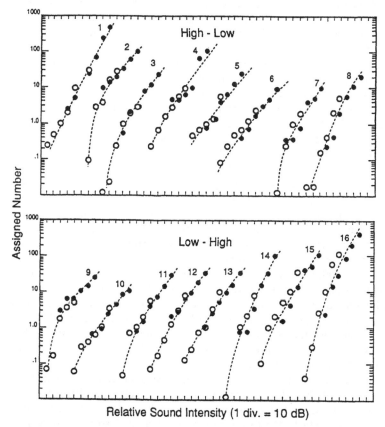

FIG. 13.4.   AME judgments of individual subjects as a function of relative sound intensity in dB. Subjects 1–8 received the high range first followed by the low range. Subjects 9–16 received the low range first followed by the high range. (From Gescheider & Hughson, 1992. Reprinted with permission from Perception & Psychophysics).

clearly affected by stimulus context, the loudness functions for the low and high range were separated on the intensity axis by no more than 5 to 10 dB. Thus, it seems that the results of the 16 subjects presented in Fig. 13.4 were predominately determined by a tendency of the subject to match impressions of number size to the subjective magnitude of the stimulus, with little, if any, influence of the subjective magnitudes of other stimuli presented in the same session. It appears that in most subjects, this tendency was so strong as to override any tendencies that might have existed to judge stimuli relative to one another. About one-third of the subjects in this study, however, did show some tendency to be influenced by context, but even in these cases, this tendency did not dominate the subject's judgments which were substantially more affected by changes in the intensity of the stimuli. Marks, Szczesiul, and Ohlott (1986), using instructions that were essentially the same as those used in AME, also found large individual differences in the degree to which context affected judgments. As in the Gescheider and Hughson study, some subjects were virtually unaffected by context, while others appeared to be greatly influenced.

It is possible that the effects of context are not due to relative judgments at all, but are instead the result of sensory contrast in which a tone is perceived as louder in the context of weaker than in the context of stronger tones. It is well established that such perceptual contrast effects occur in all sensory modalities, and the results of Gescheider and Hughson (1991) may be simply another example of the phenomenon. Results relevant to this hypothesis have been obtained by Ward (1982, 1985, 1986, 1990) who has argued that sequential dependencies in magnitude estimation are based on sensory processes when the subject's response contrasts with the value of the previous stimulus. In loudness judgments, for example, a tone is judged to be louder if heard after presentation of a weaker tone than after presentation of a stronger one. This contrast effect seems to be sensory as indicated by Ward's (1990) finding that the effect is not observed when subjects judge the loudness of tones of two different frequencies except when the frequencies fall within the same critical band. The hypothesis that context affects loudness is also supported by the work of Schneider and Parker (1990) whose procedures did not require subjects to make numerical judgments and by the work of Algom and Marks (1990) who found that context affects loudness summation, a process assumed to be purely sensory.

At the end of the second experimental session of the Gescheider and Hughson (1991) study, to ascertain whether subjects had followed the AME instructions, subjects were asked to write a brief description of how they performed the task. Most subjects reported that, as instructed, they tried to match their impression of number size to the loudness of the tone. A few reported assigning numbers proportionally so that small ones went with weak sounds and large ones went with loud sounds. The two subjects whose data are presented in Fig. 13.5, however, reported judging loudness in terms of categories. Subject 17 reported limiting the range of numbers to 1 through 30 with the exception that very weak sounds were given numbers less than 1.0. Subject 18 reported using a 0 through 10 scale with the exception that the loudest sound was given a value of 20. It is interesting that in these two cases in which the subject clearly failed to follow the AME instructions, very large biases occurred. The loudness functions obtained for the low- and high-stimulus ranges were separated by nearly 30 dB, indicating that nearly the same range of numbers were used for both stimulus ranges. This observation is a dramatic example of how failure of the subject to follow instructions in the AME experiment can result in unacceptable amounts of response bias.

The AME instructions, in which the subject is told to match impressions of number size to impressions of sensation magnitude independently for each stimulus, essentially tells the subject to produce an absolute scale (see Zwislocki, 1991). Thus, the question is whether or not the subjects can do what they are told to do. Only one number has exactly the same subjective magnitude as that of the stimulus. There should be nothing arbitrary about the subject's choice of the number. Compliance with instructions should produce judgments that form the basis of an absolute scale with its fixed unit.

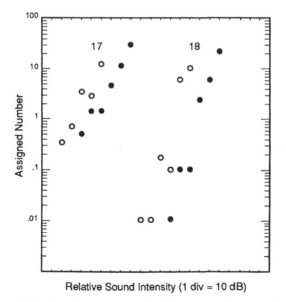

FIG. 13.5.   AME judgments as a function of relative sound intensity for two subjects who admitted using category scales in their judgments. (From Gescheider & Hughson, 1992. Reprinted with permission from Perception & Psychophysics.)

To determine the extent to which instructions in magnitude estimation influence the size of context effects, Gescheider and McDonnell (1991) compared results obtained using AME instructions with those obtained using more conventional magnitude-estimation (ME) instructions. In this study, the following ME instructions were given:

> Your task is to assign numbers to stand for the loudness of tones. Assign any number that you think is appropriate for the first tone you hear. Then, assign numbers to succeeding tones in proportion to your first judgment. You are free to use any positive numbers. You can use decimals or fractions if you feel they are appropriate.

These instructions can be contrasted with the AME instructions used by Gescheider and Hughson (1991, p. 46) which stated the following:

> You have impressions of quite, moderately loud and loud sounds. You also have impressions of what is a small, medium and large size number. When I present a tone, I would like you to assign a number to it so that your impression of the size of the number matches your impression of the loudness of the tone. Do not worry about comparing tones. Just listen to each tone and say a number that seems right for it. You can use any positive number that you want to. You can use decimals or fractions if you feel they are appropriate.

The procedures employed by Gescheider and McDonnell (1991) were virtually identical to those used by Gescheider and Hughson (1991) which even included having the same person give the instructions in both studies. The only difference was in the instructions given to the subjects. Shown in Fig. 13.6 are the geometric means of the data of the 16 subjects who followed the AME instructions and the data of 20 subjects who were given conventional magnitude-estimation instructions. In both AME and ME conditions, shifting from one stimulus range to another significantly affected the loudness judgement of the 40,- 50,- and 60-dB SL tones common to both ranges. The assigned numbers were always higher for these stimuli when presented in the context of the tones of lower than higher sensation levels. The magnitude of this context effect, however, was significantly greater for ME than for AME instructions. Furthermore, the data of only 3 of the 20 ME subjects exhibited insensitivity to context, whereas it should be recalled that the data of 10 of 16 AME subjects showed no context effects.

Why do stimulus-context effects in AME tend to be small or nonexistent but substantial for conventional magnitude estimation? The results of Gescheider and Hughson (1991) and Gescheider and McDonnell (1991) suggest that the answer is attributable to the difference in instructions used in the two methods. Although in both methods the subject is free to choose any numbers that seem appropriate, in conventional magnitude estimation

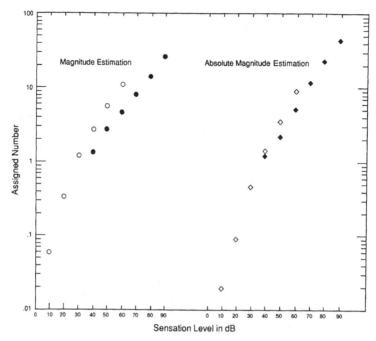

FIG. 13.6.   AME and ME judgments of loudness as a function of the sensation level of a 1000-Hz tone. Data are presented for a low (10–60-dB SL) and high (40–90-dB SL) stimulus range. (AME data from Gescheider & Hughson, 1992.)

there is no requirement that the subjective magnitudes of numbers and of the stimuli match. Instead, the subject is instructed to assign any number to the sensation magnitude of the first stimulus and to assign numbers proportional to this first judgment for the sensation magnitudes of all subsequently presented stimuli. If subjects interpret these instructions to mean that they can assign an arbitrary number to the first stimulus of the session, then they may have a tendency to work with the same set of numbers for different stimulus ranges. The consequence of this tendency would be to assign a new number to a stimulus when it is presented in the context of a new stimulus range.

The tendency for subjects in conventional magnitude estimation to work within the same number range independent of the position of the stimulus range does not always dominate the subject's judgments, as indicated by individual differences in the magnitude of context effects when the position of the stimulus range is varied. Finally, it must be said that the use of AME instructions does not always eliminate this tendency, as indicated by the existence of context effects in the AME judgments of some subjects. In extreme cases, such as subjects 17 and 18 in the Gescheider and Hughson (1991) study, the results may indicate a failure to follow instructions.

The effects of the width of the stimulus range was also examined by Gescheider and Hughson (1991) and Gescheider and McDonnell (1991). In the wide range, the sensation levels of the tones were 20, 30, 40, 50, 60, 70, and 80 dB, whereas the narrow range consisted of tones with sensation levels of 35, 40, 45, 50, 55, 60, and 65 dB. The center of both the 60-dB and the 30-dB range was the same 50-dB SL tone, and 7 stimuli were presented in both ranges. As in the experiments on the position of the stimulus range, the important question was whether the subject's judgments of the stimuli common to both the narrow and wide range (40,- 50,- and 60-dB SL) were significantly different, and whether prior experience with one range influenced judgments of the loudness of stimuli in the other. As seen in Fig. 13.7, Gescheider and Hughson found that AME judgments were not significantly affected by the size of the stimulus range. Furthermore, the mean power-function exponents of individual subjects fitted to overlapping portions of the two ranges were nearly identical for the narrow (mean exponent, = .359) and the wide (mean exponent = .357) range. In the case of nearly every subject, the exponents of the power functions fitted to the data were essentially the same for the two ranges.

This, however, was not the case in the study of Gescheider and McDonnell in which this experiment was repeated with conventional magnitude-estimation instructions. The judgments of many of the subjects in this experiment were affected by the size of the stimulus range, and these context effects are clearly manifested in the average data for the group of 20 subjects shown in Fig. 13.7. The mean exponents for the narrow and wide ranges were .352 and .241, respectively. This range effect, in which the slope of the sensation-magnitude function is inversely related to the width of the stimulus range, has also been reported in other studies using conventional magnitude-estimation instructions (e.g., Foley, Cross, Foley, & Reeder, 1983; Frederiksen, 1975; Montgomery, 1975; Teghtsoonian, 1973; Teghtsoonian & Teghtsoonian, 1978). The results shown in Fig. 13.7 indicate that there is no evidence that subjects, in performing AME, commit what Poulton (1979) has identified in magnitude estimation as the stimulus-range equalizing bias in which the subject uses much the same range of numbers, regardless of the size of the stimulus range. That some subjects in conventional magnitude estimation tend to use the same response range when the stimulus range is changed might result from how the task is interpreted. Many of the subjects tested by Gescheider and McDonnell (1991) reported that they choose a scale at the start of the experiment and spread their responses over the entire range. When such subjects decide on their response ranges before experiencing the stimuli, one would expect that their responses would be fairly insensitive to changes in the width of the stimulus range. One consequence of this strategy would be the observed

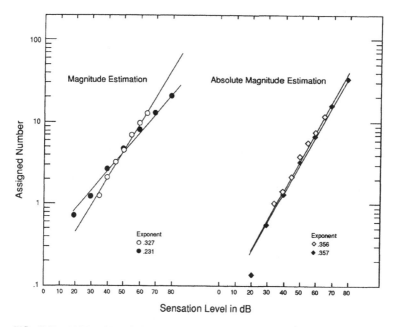

FIG. 13.7.   AME and ME judgments of loudness as a function of the sensation level of a 1000-Hz tone. Data are presented for a narrow (30-dB) and wide (60-dB) range. (AME data from Gescheider & Hughson, 1992.)

change in the slope of the sensation-magnitude function determined by ME when the width of the stimulus range is changed.

The results of Gescheider and McDonnell (1991) suggest that the response bias associated with subjects setting scales for themselves in advance of the presentation of the stimuli may frequently result from giving subjects ME rather than AME instructions. Thus, in experiments in which the width of the stimulus range could artifactually influence the results, it is highly recommended that appropriate means be taken to eliminate this source of bias in ME, or, alternatively, that relatively bias-free AME instructions be used.

ACKNOWLEDGMENTS

This work was supported in part by Grants PO 1 DC 00380 and RO 1 DC-00098 from the National Institutes of Health, U.S. Department of Health and Human Services.

REFERENCES

Algom, D., & Marks, L. E. (1984). Individual differences in loudness processing and loudness scales. *Journal of Experimental Psychology: General, 113*, 571–593.

Algom, D., & Marks, L. E. (1990). Range and regression, loudness scales, and loudness processing: Toward a context bound psychophysics. *Journal of Experimental Psychology: Human Perception & Performance, 16,* 706-727.

Attneave, F. (1962). Perception and related areas. In S. Koch (Ed.), *Psychology: A study of a science* (pp. 619-659). New York: McGraw-Hill.

Bolanowksi, S. J., Jr. (1987). Contourless stimuli produce binocular brightness summation. *Vision Research, 27,* 1943-1951.

Bolanowski, S. J., Jr., Zwislocki, J. J., & Gescheider, G. A. (1991). Intersensory generality and psychological units. In S. J. Bolanowski, Jr. & G. A. Gescheider (Eds.), Ratio scaling of psychological magnitude: A tribute to the memory of S. S. Stevens (pp. 277-293). Hillsdale, NJ: Lawrence Erlbaum Associates.

Collins, A. A., & Gescheider, G. A. (1989). The measurement of loudness in children and adults by absolute magnitude estimation and cross-modality matching. *Journal of the Acoustical Society of America, 85,* 2012-2021.

Curtis, D. W., Attneave, F., & Harrington, T. L. (1968). A test of a two-stage model of magnitude judgment. *Perception & Psychophysics, 3,* 25-31.

Ellermeier, W., Westphal, W., & Heidenfelder, M. (1991). On the "absoluteness" of category and magnitude scales of pain. *Perception & Psychophysics, 49,* 159-166.

Foley, H. J., Cross, D. V., Foley, M. A., & Reeder, R. (1983). Stimulus range, number of categories and the "virtual" exponent. *Perception & Psychophysics, 34,* 505-512.

Foley, H. J., Cross, D. V., & O'Reilly, J. A. (1990). Pervasiveness and magnitude of context effects: Evidence for the relativity of absolute magnitude estimation. *Perception & Psychophysics, 48,* 551-558.

Frederiksen, J. R. (1975). Two models for psychological judgment: Scale invariance with changes in stimulus range. *Perception & Psychophysics, 17,* 147-157.

Gescheider, G. A. (1988). Psychophysical Scaling. *Annual Review of Psychology, 39,* 169-200.

Gescheider, G. A., & Bolanowski, S. J., Jr. (1991). Final comments on ratio scaling of psychological magnitude. In S. J. Bolanowski, Jr. & G. A. Gescheider (Eds.), *Ratio scaling of psychological magnitude: A tribute to the memory of S. S. Stevens* (pp. 295-311). Hillsdale, NJ: Lawrence Erlbaum Associates.

Gescheider, G. A., & Hughson, B. A. (1991). Stimulus context and absolute magnitude estimation: A study of individual differences. *Perception & Psychophysics, 50,* 45-57.

Gescheider, G. A., & McDonnell, K. A. (1991) The effects of context on magnitude estimation and absolute magnitude estimation. In G. R. Lockhead (Ed.), *Proceedings of the seventh annual meeting of the international society for psychophysics* (pp. 109-113). Durham, NC: Duke University.

Hellman, R. P. (1976). Growth of loudness at 1000 and 3000 Hz. *Journal of the Acoustical Society of America, 60,* 672-679.

Hellman, R. P., & Zwislocki, J. J. (1961). Some factors affecting the estimation of loudness. *Journal of the Acoustical Society of America, 33,* 687-694.

Hellman, R. P., & Zwislocki, J. J. (1963). Monaural loudness function at 1000 cps and interaural summation. *Journal of the Acoustical Society of America, 35,* 856-865.

Hellman, R. P., & Zwislocki, J. J. (1964). Loudness function of a 1000 cps tone in the presence of a masking noise. *Journal of the Acoustical Society of America, 36,* 1618-1627.

Marks, L. E., Szczesiul, R., & Ohlott, P. (1986). On the cross-modality perception of intensity. *Journal of Experimental Psychology: Human Perception and Performance, 12,* 517-534.

Mellers, B. A. (1983). Evidence against "absolute" scaling. *Perception & Psychophysics, 33,* 523-526.

Montgomery, H. (1975). Direct estimation: Effect of methodological factors on scale type. *Scandinavian Journal of Psychology, 16,* 19-29.

Poulton, E. C. (1979). Models for biases in judging sensory magnitude. *Psychological Bulletin, 86,* 777-803.

Schneider, B., & Parker, S. (1990). Does stimulus context affect loudness or only loudness judgments? *Perception & Psychophysics, 48*, 409–418.

Shepard, R. N. (1981) . Psychological relations and psychophysical scales: On the status of "direct" psychophysical measurement. *Journal of Mathematical Psychology, 24*, 21–57.

Stevens, J. C., & Marks, L. E. (1980). Cross-modality-matching functions generated by magnitude estimation. Perception & Psychophysics, 27, 379–389.

Stevens, S. S. (1951). Mathematics, measurement and psychophysics. In S. S. Stevens (Ed.), *Handbook of experimental psychology* (pp. 1–49). New York: Wiley.

Stevens, S. S. (1956). The direct estimation of sensory magnitude: loudness. *American Journal of Psychology, 69*, 1-25.

Stevens, S. S. (1975). *Psychophysics: Introduction to its perceptual, neural, and social prospects.* New York: Wiley.

Stevens, S. S., & Guirao, M. (1963). Subjective scaling of length and area and the matching of length to loudness and brightness. *Journal of Experimental Psychology, 66*, 177–186.

Teghtsoonian, M. (1965). The judgment of size. *American Journal of Psychology, 78*, 392–402.

Teghtsoonian, M., & Teghtsoonian, R. (1983). Constancy of individual exponents in cross-modality matching. *Perception & Psychophysics, 33*, 203–214.

Teghtsoonian, R. (1973). Range effects in psychophysical scaling and a revision of Stevens' Law. *American Journal of Psychology, 86*, 3–27.

Teghtsoonian, R., & Teghtsoonian, M. (1978). Range and regression effects in magnitude scaling. *Perception & Psychophysics, 24*, 305–314.

Verrillo, R. T. (1981). Absolute estimation of line length in three age groups. *Journal of Gerontology, 36*, 625–627.

Verrillo, R. T. (1983). Stability of line-length estimates using the method of absolute magnitude estimation. *Perception & Psychophysics, 33*, 261–265.

Verrillo, R. T., Fraioli, A. J., & Smith, R. L. (1969). Sensory magnitude of vibrotactile stimuli. *Perception & Psychophysics, 6*, 366–372.

Ward, L. M. (1973). Repeated magnitude estimations with a variable standard: sequential effects and other properties. *Perception & Psychophysics, 13*, 193–200.

Ward, L. M. (1982). Mixed-modality psychophysical scaling: Sequential dependencies and other properties. *Perception & Psychophysics, 31*, 53–62.

Ward, L. M. (1985). Mixed-modality psychophysical scaling: Inter- and intramodality sequential dependencies as a function of lag. *Perception & Psychophysics, 38* 512–522.

Ward, L. M. (1986). Mixed-modality psychophysical scaling: Double cross-modality matching for "difficult" continua. *Perception & Psychophysics, 39*, 407–417.

Ward, L. M. (1987). Remembrance of sounds past: Memory and psychophysical scaling. *Journal of Experimental Psychology: Human Perception Performance, 13*, 216–227.

Ward, L. M. (1990). Critical bands and mixed-frequency scaling: Sequential dependencies, equal-loudness contours, and power function exponents. *Perception & Psychophysics, 47*, 551–562.

Zwislocki, J. J. (1978). Absolute scaling. *Journal of the Acoustical Society of America, 63*, 516.

Zwislocki, J. J. (1983a). Group and individual relations between sensation magnitudes and their numerical estimates. *Perception & Psychophysics, 33*, 460–468.

Zwislocki, J. J. (1983b). Absolute and other scales: Question of validity. *Perception & Psychophysics, 33*, 593–594.

Zwislocki, J. J. (1991). Natural measurement. In S. J. Bolanowski, Jr. & G. A. Gescheider (Eds.), *Ratio scaling of psychological magnitude: A tribute to the memory of S. S. Stevens (pp. 18–26). Hillsdale, NJ: Lawrence Erlbaum Associates.*

Zwislocki, J. J., & Goodman, D. A. (1980). Absolute scaling of sensory magnitude: A validation. *Perception & Psychophysics, 28*, 28–38.

14 Involvement of Different Isoforms of Actin in Outer Hair-Cell Motility

Joan E. Savage
Norma B. Slepecky
Syracuse University

INTRODUCTION

Previous studies have documented slow shape changes in outer hair cells, and it was suggested that this form of motility was caused by a calcium-activated actin and myosin system like that seen in muscle. Supporting evidence for a muscle-like mechanism involved in outer hair cell motility includes: the presence of actin filaments in the cytoplasm and lateral wall; the colocalization of calcium-binding and calcium-regulatory proteins (calsequestrin, calmodulin, and calbindin) with calcium; the activation of the response by second messengers; and sensitivity of outer hair cells to the neurotransmitter acetylcholine. However, more recent results from this lab argue against such a similarity. Unlike muscle cells, outer hair cells lack: an organized contractile apparatus; caldesmon, a major regulatory protein for smooth muscle; and muscle-type myosins in the cytoplasm, although myosin has been found in the cuticular plate and along the lateral wall.

Because actin plays such a prominent role in maintaining cell shape and causing cell motility, we have further investigated this protein in outer hair cells. It is well known that all actins are not alike. Six isoforms have been well characterized: two are specific for striated muscle fibers, two are specific for smooth muscle cells, and two cytoplasmic forms are predominant in nonmuscle cells. They differ only in about 10% of their amino acid sequences and can be distinguished by their differing isoelectric points as designated by the prefixes α, β, and γ. These six actin isoforms differ in their ability to interact with actin-binding and regulatory proteins, which is reflected in the differences in structural organization and mechanical properties of the actin monomers and filaments. Thus the mechanisms resulting in the shape changes seen in outer hair cells must depend in part on the isoforms that are present and their subcellular localization. The focus of this study is to determine if muscle isoforms of actin are present in the organ of Corti, and if their subcellular location could explain the different forms of slow shape changes that have been observed in outer hair cells.

METHODS

Control Tissues

At present, the six different isoforms of actin have been found to be enriched in different tissues throughout the body (Garrels & Gibson, 1976; Otey, Kalnoski, & Bulinski, 1987; Pinder & Gratzer, 1983; Rubenstein & Spudich, 1977; Vandekerckhove & Weber, 1981). Thus, control tissues were selected to determine the specificity of the antibodies available for the different isoforms. Striated muscle from leg was used for the α-skeletal isoform; the heart muscle was used for the α-cardiac isoform; the bladder was used for the α-smooth muscle isoform; the turkey gizzard was used for the γ-smooth muscle isoform; red blood cells were used for the β-cytoplasmic isoform; and the brain was used for the γ-cytoplasmic isoform.

Immunofluorescence

Control tissues and the inner ear from a guinea pig were immersion fixed in 2–4% paraformaldehyde in 0.1-M phosphate buffer pH 7.2 for 2 hours. They were washed in phosphate buffer, dehydrated in ethanol, and dissected into small pieces prior to embedding in Polyethylene glycol (Wolosewick & deMey, 1982). Sections ranging in thickness from 0.5 to 1 μm were cut, placed in a drop of water onto subbed slides, and processed through the following series at room temperature for immunocytochemical labeling: blocking serum, 10 min; specific antibody of interest, overnight; PBS wash, 30 min; blocking serum, 10 min; fluoresceine or rhodamine conjugated secondary antibody, 30 min; and PBS wash, 30 min. Details for labeling have previously been described in detail (Slepecky & Ulfendahl, 1992). Sections were mounted in a mixture of n-propyl gallate, glycerol, PBS, and observed with a Zeiss Axioskop equipped with a 40-X oil objective and a 100-watt UV light source. Photographs were taken with Kodak T-Max 400 film and developed in a T-Max developer according to directions.

Immunoblots

Control tissues and the organ of Corti from guinea pigs were homogenized into a 2X sample buffer containing tris/glycerol, β-mercaptoethanol, and the detergent sodium dodecyl sulfate (SDS) prior to subjecting them to electrophoresis (Laemmli, 1970) under denaturing conditions on polyacrylamide gels (PAGE). For slab gels of tissue homogenates, 100 to 1,000 μg wet weight of tissue corresponding to 10 to 100 μg total protein was dissolved in 100 μl sample buffer and loaded into a 7.4-cm well across the top surface of a BioRad vertical minigel. For the organ of Corti, cochleas were opened in L-15 tissue culture medium (Gibco, Garden City, NY), and each sensory epithelium containing hair cells and supporting cells was scraped off the basilar membrane. The samples from two inner ears were pooled, diluted to 20 μl in a 1X sample buffer, and half ear equivalents were loaded into 0.5-cm wells along the top surface of a gel. Gels composed of 7% acrylamide/bis (37.5:1) were cast 1-mm thick and were run at 200 volts for 0.34 hr in the BioRad minigel format using tris/glycine/SDS running buffer in the upper and lower buffer chambers.

Proteins were transferred from the SDS-PAGE gels onto BioRad nitrocellulose 0.45 μm on the BioRad electroblot unit. Gels were presoaked in transfer buffer composed of tris/glycine with 20% methanol. Transfers were carried out at 100V for 1 hr. The nitrocellulose sheet was rinsed in tris-buffered saline, air dried, and stored at room temperature until used for staining with antibody. Dry electroblots were cut into 0.5-cm strips and rewetted in tris-buffered saline with Tween for 15 min. They were then treated sequentially with blockers (avidin, wash, biotin, wash, bovine serum albumin and nondairy creamer, wash), primary specific antibodies of interest, wash, secondary antibody conjugated to biotin, wash, avidin conjugated to the enzyme alkaline phosphatase, wash. The enzyme alkaline phosphatase produces the final color indication of antibody binding when exposed to BCIP/NBT (Kirkgaard & Perry, Gaithersburg, MD). Similar results indicating binding of antibodies to actin were obtained when a streptavidin-alkaline phosphatase system was used without the avidin and biotin blockers, but numerous background lines indicating endogenous biotin or biotin-binding proteins were present. The nitrocellulose strips were stored in the dark until photographed using Kodak T-Max 100 film developed with T-Max developer according to directions.

Antibodies

Various antibodies were tested for specificity against the control tissues enriched for each of the different isoforms of actin. Each was tested for cross-reactivity with guinea pig tissue as well as for isoform specificity, regardless of manufacturer's claims. The antibodies were from commercial sources such as Amersham (Arlington Hts, IL), Sigma (St Louis, MO), ICN Immunobiologicals (Lisle, IL), and Biomedical Technologies (Stoughton, MA). Antibodies to the cytoplasmic isoforms of actin were gifts from Drs. Bulinski and Herman. Secondary antibodies were from Vector (Burlingame CA) or Accurate (Westbury, NY).

RESULTS

One method for detecting the presence of a protein of interest in cells is to use immunochemical techniques. These require having a purified protein of interest, injecting it into an animal to elicit production of antibodies to this protein, purifying the antibodies, and conjugating the antibodies to a detectable substance so that they may be visualized (colorimetrically, for example). At this point, the antibodies are applied to tissue sections or tissue homogenates. If a color can be detected, that indicates that the antibody binds and the protein of interest is present. Two typical applications of this technique—immunoblots and immunocytochemistry—have been used in our lab to address questions about actin in sensory hair cells.

Immunoblots are used to test the specificity of antibodies to proteins of interest. It is important to know that the antibody obtained after the immune challenge is specific for the protein injected and does not cross-react with a similar sequence of amino acids in another protein. To determine this, individual proteins must be isolated prior to reaction with the antibody. One way to do this is to denature the proteins and then separate them according to their size. Homogenized tissue samples are placed along the top edge of an acrylamide gel. When a voltage is applied, the proteins migrate through the gel at a rate that is inversely proportional to their molecular weight. Thus, small proteins move faster and reach the bottom of the gel, while large proteins remain near the top of the gel. If the electrophoresis is stopped before the proteins run off of the gel, it is possible to obtain a gradient of all proteins present in the sample in discrete bands arranged according to their molecular weight. Proteins of known molecular weight are also run to be used as standards against which the proteins in the tissue homogenate are compared. The banded proteins are transferred out of the gel onto a sheet of nitrocellulose.

When an antibody is applied to the sheet containing the proteins, if the antibody is specific, it should stain only one band. For actin, all antibodies to it should stain one band on the sheet at the position that corresponds to that of a protein with a molecular weight of 43 kDa. If more than one band is stained, then the antibody may be said to cross-react with other proteins and can not be used for specifically localizing the protein of interest. As seen in the immunoblots in Fig. 14.1, each of the antibodies used in this study stained at most one band on immunoblots of the control tissues surveyed.

In our studies of the inner ear, we are interested in the different isoforms of actin present. Our first step is to determine if the available antibodies for the detection of actin cross-react with the actin present in guinea pig and if

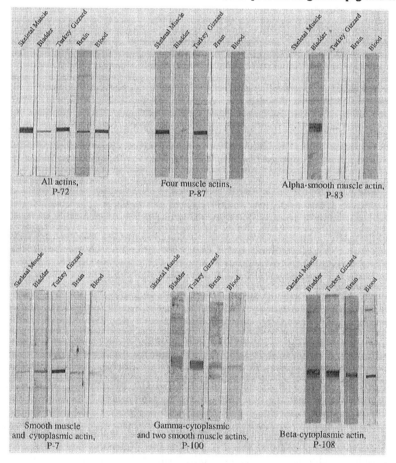

FIG. 14.1. Immunoblots of control tissues to determine isoform specificity. Homogenates of control tissues were subjected to SDS-PAGE. Proteins distribute throughout a polyacrylamide gel according to their molecular weight. The proteins have been transferred to nitrocellulose, and one strip from each sheet were incubated in a solution containing each of the antibodies used in the present study. All antibodies stained only one protein with an approximate size of 43 KDa. Each antibody displayed a pattern of staining and indicated the specificity of that antibody to the predominant actin isoform present in that tissue.

they are specific for the different isoforms. This was accomplished by performing immunoblots using several different tissues from the guinea pig known to be enriched in each of the isoforms in other species. If the antibodies worked as expected, a pattern of staining across the control tissues would emerge. Skeletal muscle was used as a marker for the α-skeletal muscle isoform; heart muscle was used as a marker for the α-cardiac isoform (data not shown); the bladder was used as a source of the α-smooth muscle isoform; and the gizzard from the turkey for γ-smooth muscle isoform. Cytoplasmic isoforms are present in all muscle cells, but can be found without muscle isoforms in nonmuscle tissue such as brain and red blood cells.

As can be seen in the immunoblots presented in Fig. 14.1, there is a pattern to antibody staining that shows isoform specificity of the various antibodies. It should be noted, however, that although the antibodies were stated to bind to specific isoforms (see the legend at the top of the figure) we did not always find the claims of the supplier to be valid. For example, P-72 which was supposed to stain "all" actins gave strong lines on all of the control tissues except the bladder, indicating that it did not have a high affinity for the α-smooth muscle isoform. P-87 which was supposed to stain all muscle actins also only weakly stained the bladder (α-smooth muscle isoform), while it stained the actin band in the other three muscle tissues strongly (skeletal and cardiac α-isoforms, and turkey gizzard γ-smooth isoform). P-83, an antibody specific only for the α-smooth muscle isoform, did stain the bladder strongly as expected, while leaving the actin from all the other control tissues unstained. P-7 which was supposed to stain smooth muscle and cytoplasmic actin showed a strong affinity for the smooth muscle actin in the turkey gizzard (γ-smooth muscle isoform) and weak affinity for bladder (α-smooth isoform).

Cytoplasmic actins are present in both nonmuscle and muscle cells. Thus the finding of positive staining lines on the control tissues of skeletal muscle (not shown) and smooth muscle of the bladder and gizzard would not be surprising. What can be said from the pattern of staining seen in the immunoblots is that the two antibodies that are specific for muscle actins, P-87 (α-skeletal, α-cardiac, and γ-smooth) and P-83 (α-smooth), do not stain the actin found in nonmuscle tissues such as neurons of the brain and red blood cells. From the staining pattern on the nonmuscle tissues, it is possible to characterize the antibodies which bind to the cytoplasmic isoforms. P-108 is specific for β-cytoplasmic (found alone in red blood cell ghosts and co-localized with α- and γ- smooth muscle isoforms in bladder and gizzard), and P-72 stains the β-cytoplasmic isoform in addition to binding to the muscle isoforms. P-100 is specific for the γ-cytoplasmic isoform in the brain (as well as binding to both smooth muscle isoforms), but does not stain the β-cytoplasmic isoform in red blood cells.

Because each of the antibodies stains the band of actin in the immuno-blots of control tissues with a different intensity, it is possible to identify each of the isoforms based on a staining pattern utilizing several of the antibodies. This pattern, which allows for the identification of the actin isoforms, is summarized in Table 14.1. For example, the presence of the α-striated and/or the α-cardiac isoforms of actin can be determined if there is staining with P-72 and P-87, but not with P-83 and P-7. The α-smooth muscle isoform can be identified if there is staining with P-83, but not with and P-87 and P-7. The γ- smooth isoform can be identified if there is staining with P-7 and P-87, but not with P-83. The cytoplasmic isoforms are more difficult to identify, because they colocalize with the muscle isoforms in muscle tissue. However, in nonmuscle tissues such as brain and red blood cells, if staining is negative for the two antibodies that are specific for the muscle isoforms (P-87 and P-83), then P-108 and P-100 can distinguish between the β- and γ-cytoplasmic isoforms respectively.

The antibodies thus characterized on the immunoblots have been further used to localize actin isoforms at the cellular level. For this, skeletal muscle and the small intestine can be used as control tissues, because they contain different subsets of 5 of the isoforms (the α-cardiac isoform is only present in heart muscle). In skeletal muscle the α-skeletal muscle isoform is found in sarcomeres of the striated muscle fibers, the α-smooth muscle isoform is found in the smooth muscle cells of the arterioles, and the cytoplasmic isoforms are found in the endothelial cells of the capillaries. Two different antibodies can be used to stain different isoforms in the same tissue section if each of the antibodies is labeled with a different color marker (Fig. 14.2). P-87 labeled with fluoresceine, which appears green in the microscope, binds to only muscle isoforms and stains only the actin in muscle fibers (Fig. 14.2a). P-100 labeled with rhodamine which appears red in the microscope stains the α-smooth muscle isoform of actin in the arterioles and the γ-cytoplasmic isoform in the endothelial cells of the capillaries (Fig. 14.2b).

On the small intestine (Fig. 14.3) antibodies which bind to the muscle

TABLE 14.1
Staining Pattern for Positive Identification of Each of the Different Isoforms of Actin

Actin Isoform	Antibodies					
	P-72	P-87	P-83	P-7	P100	P-108
α-skeletal		+	−	−		
α-cardiac		+	−	−		
α-smooth		−	+	−		
γ-smooth		+	−	+		
β-cytoplasmic		−	−		−	+
γ-cytoplasmic		−	−		+	−

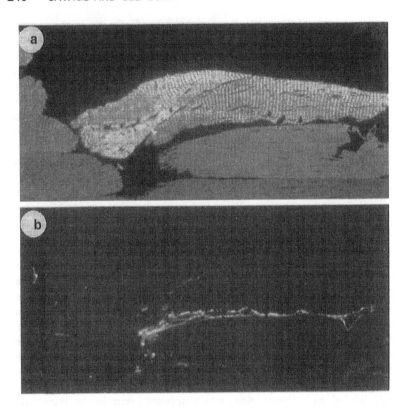

FIG. 14.2.   Tissue sections of control tissues that have been stained with antibodies to
the specific isoforms of actin. a. A section of skeletal muscle that has been labeled with
P-87, an antibody that labels α-skeletal muscle actin in the sarcomeres of the muscle
fibers. The same section of skeletal muscle that has been labeled with P-100, an
antibody that labels α-smooth muscle actin in the arterioles and γ-cytoplasmic actin in
the capillaries.

isoforms of actin can be seen localized in the smooth muscle cells running
through the villi (Fig. 14.3a). The antibodies that stain the cytoplasmic
isoforms of actin stain the epithelial cells of the brush border and the
lacteals (Fig. 14.3b).

   To investigate the isoforms of actin present in the organ of Corti, it is
necessary to isolate the organ from the rest of the cochlea, because there are
a variety of cell types within the cochlea which could contribute actin. For
histological investigations this is relatively easy to do after all staining is
completed, because the isolation can be accomplished visually at the
microscope. However, for immunoblots it is necessary to dissect the organ
of Corti away from all surrounding tissues. This is accomplished by opening
the cochlea, while the temporal bone is immersed in cold tissue culture

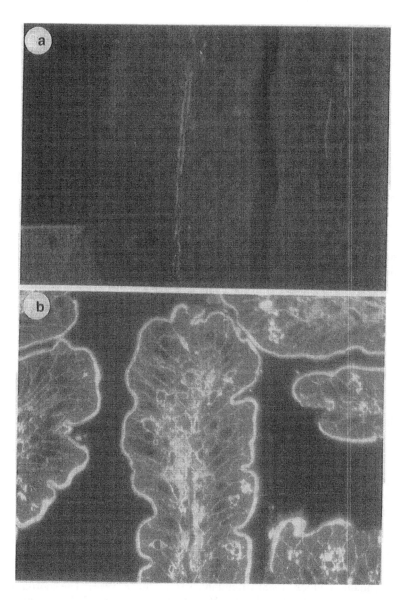

FIG. 14.3. Tissue sections of control tissues that have been stained with antibodies to the specific isoforms of actin. a. A section of small intestine that has been labeled with P-87, an antibody that labels smooth muscle isoforms in the smooth muscle cells in the villi. b. A section of small intestine that has been labeled with P-72, an antibody that labels β-cytoplasmic actin in the epithelial cells of the brush border and the lacteals.

medium. The thick bone at the back part of the cochlea is thinned by gentle shaving, then the thin bone surrounding the entire cochlea is picked off, leaving the spiral ligament exposed. This lateral wall soft tissue is then removed, leaving the sensory epithelium on the basilar membrane. With the tip of a scalpel, the organ of Corti is gently scraped off the basilar membrane and placed in the sample buffer described above for control tissue.

In tissue sections (Fig. 14.4) only cytoplasmic isoforms are labeled in the organ of Corti. There was no staining with any of the antibodies that were muscle specific (P-87 or P-83), while there was intense staining with all antibodies that bind cytoplasmic isoforms (P-72, P-7, P-100, and P-108). Supporting cells and sensory cells were stained with equal intensity, when they were stained positively. Similar results were seen in immunoblots (Fig. 14.5, in which each lane represents 3μ total protein (or one-half of one sensory epithelium from one cochlea). At the present level of sensitivity, no muscle isoforms can be detected. Based on this finding it can therefore be determined that both the β-cytoplasmic and γ-cytoplasmic isoforms are present in the organ of Corti.

DISCUSSION

Hearing depends critically on the structural and functional integrity of the outer hair cells in the inner ear. Changes in the shape of these cells provide active feedback which has been shown to contribute to normal hair cell sensitivity and frequency selectivity. Two types of movement have been describe *in vitro*: a slow response resulting either in a shortening or an elongation of the outer hair cell, and a fast response that follows the frequency of stimulus up to several thousand cycles per second. These types of motility have different rates and metabolic requirements suggesting different cellular mechanisms, and the changes in cell shape resulting from their activation are thought to affect the micromechanics of the cochlea differentially.

This laboratory has been involved in studying the slow form of motility, which is characterized by a sustained shortening or elongation, and has been observed to occur in isolated cells by chemical stimulation (Dulon, Zajic, & Schacht, 1990; Flock, Flock, & Ulfendahl, 1986; Slepecky, 1989; Slepecky, Ulfendahl, & Flock, 1988; Ulfendahl, 1987; Zenner, 1986). The shortening may also occur, coupled with the DC response of the hair cell during normal sinusoidal stimulation and superimposed on the fast motility displaying the frequency following AC response (Brownell, 1986; Evans, 1990).

The mechanisms responsible for the relatively slow outer hair cell shape changes were suggested to be muscle-like and involve the interaction of actin and myosin in a calcium-dependent manner. Actin filaments are

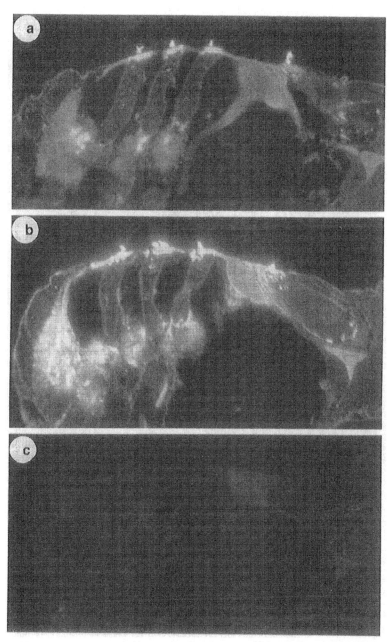

FIG. 14.4.   Tissue sections of the organ of Corti that have been stained with antibodies to the specific isoforms of actin. a. Shows positive staining with antibody P-108, specific for β-cytoplasmic actin. b. Shows positive staining with antibody P-100, which is specific for γ-cytoplasmic actin. c. Staining with antibodies P-87 and P-83, which are specific for muscle isoforms, shows negative results.

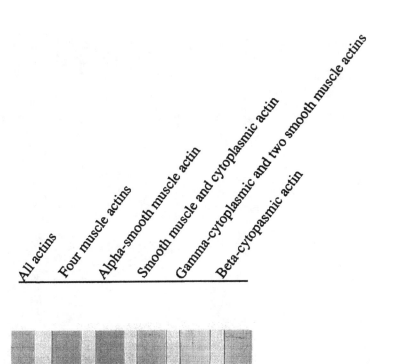

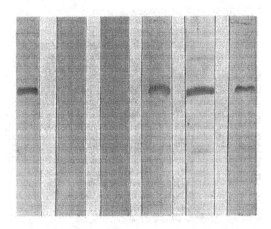

P-72   P-87   P-83   P-7   P-100   P-108

. Organ of Corti

FIG. 14.5. Immunoblots of the organ of Corti to determine if muscle isoforms are present. None of the antibodies that are specific only for muscle isoforms (P-87 and P-83) label the actin band. However, all antibodies that bind to cytoplasmic actin stain positively (P-72, P-7, P-100, and P-108). Based on previous knowledge of the staining pattern of these antibodies it is possible to say that both the β- and the γ-cytoplasmic isoforms are present.

244

present in the cytoplasm of an outer hair cell, and cytoplasmic components are involved in cell shortening (Slepecky, 1989). Actin filaments are also present along the lateral wall of each outer hair cell (Slepecky et al., 1988), and this cortical network is involved in a constriction which results in cell elongation.

A role for calcium in these shape changes is inferred both from work on the isolated cells and from immunocytochemical studies which show that a large number of calcium-binding and regulatory proteins are present in outer hair cells (Slepecky & Ulfendahl, 1993). The effects of calcium are twofold and are manifested in either a shortening or an elongation response. The shortening can be induced in permeabilized cells with calcium and ATP (Flock et al., 1986; Slepecky, 1989; Zenner, 1986) or inositol trisphosphate (Schacht & Zenner, 1987), and in intact cells with caffeine (Slepecky et al., 1988). It is inhibited by pretreatment of the cells with the calmodulin inhibitor trifluoperazine (Zenner, 1988). These results indicate that shortening is coupled with an increase in the levels of intracellular-free calcium, caused by the release of calcium from intracellular storage sites.

The elongation response may result from a calcium-activated constriction of the cell. In addition to a shortening response, permeabilized cells get thinner upon the application of calcium and ATP (Slepecky, 1989), outer hair cell membrane ghosts show a constriction (Slepecky, 1989), and intact cells get longer in the presence of extracellular calcium and the ionophore ionomycin (Dulon et al., 1990). This elongation response is observed only in intact cells, when the increase in calcium ions results from an influx of calcium. These results indicate that a focal increase in the level of free calcium only along the lateral wall of the hair cell could act on the cortical network of actin filaments, causing a cellular response opposite to that seen with a release of calcium from intracellular storage sites.

Because calcium seems to be responsible for both the shortening and the elongation seen in response to chemical stimulation, the two events could occur sequentially in response to local increases in the levels of intracellular-free calcium, and in this manner the cell would be able to modulate its resting length. Through these shortening and elongation processes it would be possible for the outer hair cell to change the micromechanics of the cochlear partition and modulate motion of the basilar membrane.

Other than indicating a role for calcium and actin, the experiments to date have done little to elucidate the actual mechanisms involved in slow shape changes and to test the hypothesis that motility is muscle-like. In fact, more recent results from this lab argue against this similarity. Because actin plays such a prominent role in maintaining cell shape and participating in cell motility, we have further investigated this protein in hair cells.

Actin is one of the most abundant and highly conserved proteins in nature, comprising almost 10% of the total cellular proteins in some cells.

Its role in the contractile apparatus of muscle cells is well known, and it plays a major role in other activities including maintaining cell shape, cell motility, and cell division. In mammals, at least six different actin isoforms are known (Vandekerckhove & Weber, 1978). Among the four muscle isoforms of actin, there appear to be distinct functional differences based on the tissue in which they predominate and on the organization of the filaments within different cell types.

The α-skeletal and α-cardiac forms are present as filaments only in striated muscle, in which they are arranged in well-organized sarcomeric structures and interact with myosin in the presence of calcium and ATP, in a manner regulated by troponin and tropomyosin. The α-smooth and γ-smooth isoforms are found in smooth muscle cells of the vascular system and gut. In these cells, the filaments are present in a less well-organized sarcomeric arrangement and interact with a phosphorylated form of myosin in a manner regulated by caldesmon and tropomyosin. The cytoplasmic forms — β-cytoplasmic and γ-cytoplasmic — predominate in nonmuscle cells such as the brain, testes, and red blood cells, but can be found to some extent in all cells. The cytoplasmic actins have a less precise organization, with filaments arranged in bundles and networks (DeNofrio, Hoock, & Herman, 1989; Otey et al., 1987; Pardo, Pittinger, & Craig, 1983).

In the current study, antibodies specific for the different isoforms of actin were used to probe the sensory and supporting cells in the guinea pig organ of Corti. On immunoblots of control tissue, all antibodies stained one band of protein with a molecular weight of approximately 43 kDa, demonstrating specificity of all the antibodies only for actin. Isoform specificity was demonstrated by the pattern of staining of the antibodies on immunoblots of control tissue homogenates and on immunocytochemical preparations in which specific cells in tissue sections were stained. When these antibodies were used on homogenates and sections of the organ of Corti, none of the four muscle isoforms of actin were detected. The finding that muscle isoforms of actin are not abundant proteins in the cochlea is supported by anatomical as well as biochemical evidence. Outer hair cells are unlike muscle cells in that they lack an organized contractile apparatus (Slepecky, Hozza, & Cefaratti, 1989); lack caldesmon (Slepecky & Ulfendahl, 1993), a major regulatory protein for smooth muscle; and lack muscle-type myosins in the cytoplasm, although myosin has been found in the cuticular plate and along the lateral wall (Slepecky & Ulfendahl, 1992).

If the mechanisms involved in outer hair cell motility are more similar to those occurring in nonmuscle cells, this leaves open to investigation the role that cytoplasmic actins play. It becomes of interest to determine if there exists a differential distribution of the two cytoplasmic actins within the cells of the ear. At present, few cells are used as model systems for the study of cytoplasmic actin. It will be increasingly important to study the subcellular organization of the filaments to determine if motility occurs as a result of sol/gel transformations or depolymerization/polymerization. Moreover, the role of other cytoskeletal elements such as microtubules in motility and in remodeling the cytoplasm of the hair cells during and following the motile event becomes important. The presence and pattern of actin synthesis following mechanical or acoustic trauma, also remains to be determined along with which of the isoforms might be involved in recovery and repair.

REFERENCES

Brownell, W. E. (1986). Outer hair cell motility and cochlear frequency selectivity. In B. Moore & R. Patterson (Eds.), *Auditory frequency selectivity* (pp. 109–118. New York: Plenum.

DeNofrio, D., Hoock, T. C., & Herman, I. M. (1989). Functional sorting of actin isoforms in microvascular pericytes. *Journal of Cell Biology, 109*, 191–202.

Dulon, D., Zajic, G. J., & Schacht, J. (1990). Increasing intracellular free calcium induces circumferential contractions in isolated outer hair cells. *Journal of Neuroscience, 10*, 1388–1397.

Evans, B. N. (1990). Fatal contractions: Ultrastructural and electromechanical changes in outer hair cells following transmembraneous electrical stimulation. *Hearing Research, 45*, 265–282.

Flock, A., Flock, B., & Ulfendahl, M. (1986). Mechanisms of movement in outer hair cells and a possible structural basis. *Archives of Otorhinolaryngology, 243*, 83–90.

Garrels, J. I., & Gibson, W. (1976). Identification and characterization of multiple forms of actin. *Cell, 9*, 793–805.

Laemmli, U. K. (1970). Cleavage of structural proteins during the assembly of the head of bacteriophage T4. *Nature, 227*, 680–685.

Otey, C. A., Kalnoski, M. H., & Bulinski, J. C. (1987). Identification and quantification of actin isoforms in vertebrate cells and tissues. *Journal of Cellular Biochemistry, 34*, 113–124.

Pardo, J. V., Pittinger, M., & Craig, S. W. (1983). Subcellular sorting of isoactins: Selective association of γ-actin with skeletal muscle mitochondria. *Cell, 32*, 1093–1103.

Pinder, J. C., & Gratzer, W. B. (1983). Structural and dynamic states of actin in the erythrocyte. *Journal of Cell Biology, 96*, 768–775.

Rubenstein, P. A., & Spudich, J. A. (1977). Actin microheterogeneity in chick embryo fibroblasts. *Proceedings of the National Academy of Sciences, 74*, 120–124.

Schacht, J., & Zenner, H. P (1987). Evidence that phosphoinositides mediate motility in cochlear outer hair cells. *Hearing Research, 31*, 155–160.

Slepecky, N. B. (1989). Cytoplasmic actin and cochlear outer hair cell motility. *Cell and Tissue Research, 257*, 69–75.

Slepecky, N. B., Hozza, M. J., & Cefaratti, L. K. (1989). Intracellular distribution of actin in the cells of the organ of Corti—A structural basis for cell shape and motility. *Journal Electron Microscopy Techniques, 15*, 280–292.

Slepecky, N. B., & Ulfendahl, M. (1992). Actin-binding and microtubule associated proteins in the organ of Corti. *Hearing Research, 57*, 201–215.

Slepecky, N. B., & Ulfendahl, M. (1993). Evidence for calcium-binding proteins and calcium-dependent regulatory mechanisms in sensory cells of the inner ear. *Hearing Research.*

Slepecky, N. B., Ulfendahl, M., & Flock, A. (1988). Effects of caffeine and tetracaine on outer hair cell shortening suggest intracellular calcium involvement. *Hearing Research, 32*, 11–22.

Ulfendahl, M. (1987). Motility in auditory sensory cells. *Acta Physiologicia Scandinavica, 130,* 521–527.

Vandekerckhove, J., & Weber, K. (1981). Actin typing on total cellular extracts. *European Journal of Biochemistry, 113,* 595–603.

Vandekerckhove, J., & Weber, K. (1978). At least six different actins are expressed in higher mammals: An analysis based on the amino acid sequence of the amino-terminal tryptic peptide. *Journal of Molecular Biology, 126,* 783–802.

Wolosewick, J., & deMey, J. (1982). Localization of tubulin and actin in polyethylene glycol embedded rat seminiferous epithelium. *Biology of the Cell, 44,* 85–88.

Zenner, H. P. (1986). Motile responses in outer hair cells. *Hearing Research, 22,* 83–90.

Zenner, H. P. (1988). Motility of outer hair cells as an active, actin mediated process. *Acta Otolaryngologica, 105,* 39–44.

15 Physiology and Functional Implications of a Unique Vertebrate Visual System

Gustav A. Engbretson
Eduardo Solessio
Syracuse University

INTRODUCTION

Around the beginning of the 20th century anatomists brought the light microscope to bear on a small organ located on the dorsal midline of the cranium of some lizards (de Graaf, 1886 Dendy, 1899; Leydig, 1890; Nowikoff, 1910; Spencer, 1887; Studnicka, 1905). Their work clearly revealed the existence of another eye, a second photoreceptive system in vertebrates. This parietal, or third, eye was seen to possess a lens, photoreceptor cells, and neurons (Fig. 15.1). The neurons were found to project axons to the brain, and several targets there were reported (Kappers, 1967). Homologous photoreceptive pineal systems have been found in agnathans, fish, and amphibians (Oksche, 1965). The subsequent development of the electron microscope stimulated a study of the ultrastructural and ontogenetic aspects of this eye.

A series of electron-microscopic investigations conclusively showed that the parietal eye contained the ultrastructural elements characteristic of a vertebrate eye (Eakin, 1960; Eakin & Westfall, 1959; 1960; Petit, 1968; Steyn, 1959; 1960). The photoreceptors were shown to be derived from ciliated cells and to resemble retinal cones with their extradiscal space in communication with extracellular space, oil droplets, and synaptic ribbons.

Developmentally, the parietal eye derives from an outpocketing of the roof of the diencephalon and is related to the pineal complex (Eakin, 1964). At maturity the parietal eye consists of a neuroepithelial lens and retina separated by a lumen that is analogous to the subretinal space in the vertebrate lateral eye (Fig. 15.1). The retina consists of a layer of photoreceptors with outer segments projecting into the lumen. Photoreceptor basal

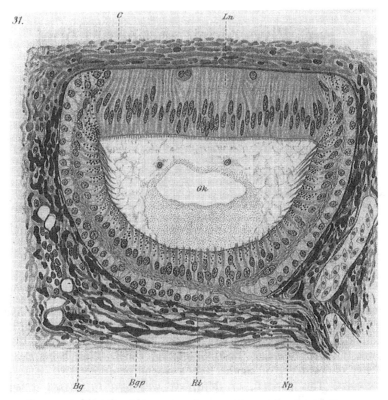

FIG. 15.1.   Midsagittal section of the parietal eye of *Lacerta agilis* reproduced from the original hand-colored plate (Fig. 31) of Nowikoff (1910) illustrates general structure. A transparent corneal dermis (*C*) overlies the lens (*Ln*), beneath which is the lumen (*Gk*). Ganglion cells of the retina (*Rt*) are found in a peripheral layer that also includes glial cell somata. The plexiform layer consists of glial, photoreceptor, and ganglion-cell processes. Ganglion-cell axons form the parietal-eye nerve (*Np*) that projects to the brain. Somata of other glial cells and the photoreceptors are seen between the plexiform layer and the lumen. Glial cells span the entire retina much like retinal Müller cells. *Bg*, meningeal tissue; *Bgp*, pigmented meningeal tissue. Magnification is not stated in the original, but the diameter is probably 200–250 μm.

processes extend into a plexiform layer in which they make synaptic contact with the dendrites and somata of two populations of ganglion cells (Engbretson & Anderson, 1990; Jenison & Nolte, 1979). Axons of the ganglion cells project primarily to two fields in the left medial habenular nucleus (Engbretson, Reiner, & Brecha, 1981), though other small projections have been noted (Korf & Wagner, 1981). About 50 centrifugal fibers project from the dorsal sac (Engbretson et al., 1981) and scattered central nervous system (CNS) centers (Korf & Wagner, 1981), and they influence the photoresponsiveness of the ganglion cells (Engbretson & Lent, 1976). There is no clear evidence of interneurons in this eye. Despite the absence of interneurons, the parietal eye extracts and encodes from incident light information about intensity and wavelength (Dodt & Scherer, 1968; Hamasaki, 1969).

Nothing is known of the biochemical aspects of phototransduction in the third eye. Because its photoreceptors are of the vertebrate type, we have assumed that the transduction mechanism for the vertebrate rod holds also for the receptors of the parietal eye. When vertebrate retinal photoreceptors capture a photon, an enzymatic cascade beginning with rhodopsin activation is initiated (review by Pugh & Lamb, 1990). Activated rhodopsin in turn activates a G-protein which activates cGMP phosphodiesterase and ultimately decreases the intracellular concentration of cGMP, the molecule responsible for maintaining the open state of the light-sensitive cation channel in the outer segment membrane. The membrane potential responds to light with a hyperpolarization accompanied with a resistance increase as the light-sensitive channels close. Our recent electrophysiological experimentation revealed that although the parietal eye photoreceptors structurally resemble retinal cones, they likely are not biochemically identical from the standpoint of transduction.

EXPERIMENTAL WORK

We used glass or quartz (kindly supplied by Sutter Instrument Co., San Rafael, CA) micropipettes (impedance = 60–100 MΩ) to impale cells in the parietal eye and record their responses to light (Solessio & Engbretson 1993). Light from an arc source was focused on isolated parietal-eye preparations after passing through interference and neutral density filters. Organ culture medium was superfused over the preparation, and standard electrophysiological recording techniques were used. Figure 15.2A shows a typical response of a dark-adapted preparation to 524-nm stimuli of increasing intensity. Note that the intensity-graded responses are depolarizations from a dark membrane potential of about − 50 mV. Responses of up to 20 mV were recorded.

With shorter wavelength stimulation (here 452 nm) the dark-adapted organ responds similarly (Fig 15.2B), though the waveform is slightly altered. The rapid onset transient, characteristic of the green response, is truncated, and an additional depolarizing transient appears at stimulus off. When a blue stimulus is delivered to a green-adapted organ the response polarity is reversed (Fig. 15.2C). The green-adapting field depolarizes the cell, and an intense blue stimulus can hyperpolarize the cell back to its dark resting potential. Chromatic adaptation experiments confirmed the existence of depolarizing and hyperpolarizing mechanisms with maximal response at 495 nm and 440 nm, respectively. The green mechanism is sufficiently more sensitive, and its spectral sensitivity curve overlaps that of the blue mechanism, such that blue stimulation of dark-adapted eyes preferentially stimulates the green mechanism, causing depolarization.

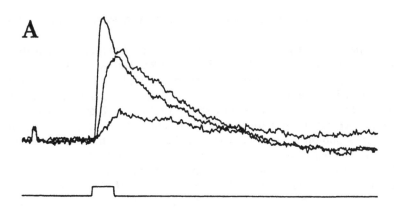

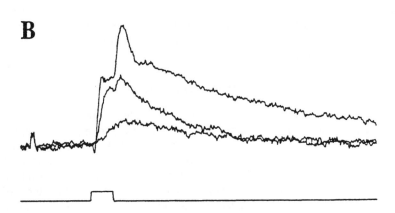

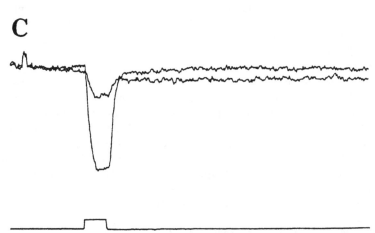

FIG. 15.2.

The depolarization and hyperpolarization are accompanied by a resistance decrease and increase, respectively (Fig 15.3). Input resistance values measured for these cells ranged between 120 and 250 MΩ. A bridge circuit was used to measure changes in input impedance during light stimulation. Green flashes initiated a resistance decrease of 20–30 MΩ. Blue flashes produced similar, though somewhat smaller, resistance changes in dark-adapted eyes. In the presence of a green-adapting field, however, blue flashes caused an increased input impedance. Thus, short-wavelength stimuli appear to be closing conductance channels, while longer-wavelength stimuli open channels.

Ion substitution and current clamp experiments suggest that a single, rather nonspecific, cation conductance is being modulated by the blue and green mechanisms. In Na^+-free superfusate both the blue and green photoresponses are nearly abolished, though not completely. When $[Ca^{2+}]_o$ is buffered to 10^{-8} M the amplitudes of the photoresponses decay with time, however, the relative degree of blue–green antagonism remains constant. We believe the photoresponses are due to the modulation of a rather nonspecific cation channel through which Na^+ normally flows. We also observed an increase in extracellular K^+ in response to light (Solessio & Engbretson, 1991).

THEORETICAL WORK

Figure 15.4 shows intensity response curves for the steady-state response of the blue and green mechanisms. We find that the green mechanism can be well fit with Zwislocki's generalized function for sensory receptors (Zwislocki, 1973):

$$E(S) = E_D(S) + E_0 = E_m \left(1 - e^{-(E_0/E_m)(1 + S/N_1)^\theta}\right)$$

where: $E(S)$ = Total average receptor potential
$E_D(S)$ = Total average receptor potential less average noise
E_0 = Average noise
E_m = Maximum average receptor potential
S = Stimulus energy
N_I = Intrinsic noise energy.

FIG. 15.2. (Opposite page) Intracellularly recorded responses of parietal-eye photoreceptors to increasing intensities of monochromatic light stimuli. A. Depolarizing responses of a dark-adapted cell to 524 nm stimuli show a prominent "ON" transient at high intensity. B. The response of a dark-adapted cell to 452-nm flashes is also a depolarization but shows a prominent "OFF" transient at high intensity. Also, the return to dark membrane potential ($\approx$ 55 mV) is more gradual with intense short wavelength flashes than with longer wavelength flashes. C. Here the cell is depolarized by a green-adapting field, and the response to intense 452-nm flashes is a hyperpolarization which very rapidly returns to prestimulus levels. Stimulus duration = 1 sec; preresponse calibration pulse = 1 mV.

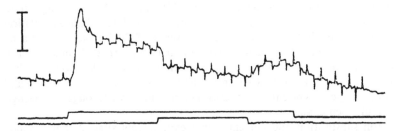

FIG. 15.3. Intracellularly measured input resistance changes of a parietal-eye photoreceptor due to chromatic stimulation. Upper stimulus trace shows time course of green stimulus, lower trace is blue stimulus. A bridge circuit was balanced in the dark-adapted state such that current pulses across the membrane elicited no steady-state voltage deflection. Green stimulation depolarized the cell, inducing voltage deflections indicative of reduced membrane resistance. The superimposed blue stimulus hyperpolarized the cell and returned the bridge circuit to balanced state indicating return to near-dark membrane resistance level. At blue stimulus off, the cell again depolarized and decreased membrane resistance. Cessation of green stimulus returned voltage and resistance to prestimulus levels.

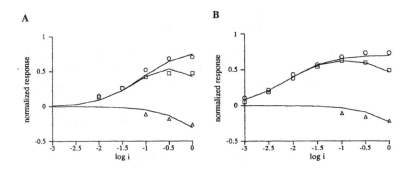

FIG. 15.4. Intracellularly recorded steady-state response versus intensity functions for two (A & B) parietal-eye photoreceptor cells. They are normalized to the peak amplitude of the depolarizing onset transient. The symbols indicate recorded data; ○, dark-adapted, 524-nm stimulus; □, dark-adapted, 452-nm stimulus; △, cell adapted to 547-nm field, 452-nm stimulus. Note that the hyperpolarizations elicited in the green-adapted state begin at the same intensity where the dark-adapted blue and green responses begin to diverge. At higher intensities the amplitude of the dark-adapted blue response actually decreases, suggesting that as stimulus intensity increases and the more sensitive green response nears saturation, the blue mechanism contributes a larger portion of the response voltage. The solid lines are response versus intensity functions calculated using the model described in the text.

The function fits well with an exponent (θ) of 0.95, suggestive of linear energy summation (Fig. 15.5). According to Professor Zwislocki (personal communication, 1992), this high value of θ is typical of primitive receptor types, such as olfactory or gustatory, and somewhat above the average value of 0.7 for hyperpolarizing vertebrate photoreceptors.

It remains to be tested whether Zwislocki's generalized function for sensory receptors predicts ganglion-cell discharge in the parietal eye, but evidence in the literature supports that hypothesis. Hamasaki and Brooks (1971) showed that in the frog frontal organ (the amphibian homolog of the parietal eye) the rate of ganglion-cell discharge was proportional to the amplitude of the ERG recorded simultaneously (Fig. 15.6A). We find that the amplitude of the ERG in the parietal eye is proportional to the amplitude of the intracellularly recorded photoreceptor response (Fig. 15.6B). Assuming that these homologous photoreceptive systems operate similarly, we predict that the parietal-eye ganglion-cell discharge is proportional to photoreceptor response, at least in the steady-state condition. Preliminary evidence from our lab (see further on in chapter) supports our prediction, though a strict analysis is not yet completed.

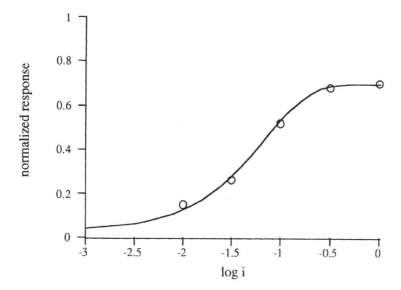

FIG. 15.5. Intensity response function for the steady state of the green response mechanism of the parietal eye. The data points are those (O) in Fig. 15.4B. The solid line is the response predicted by Zwislocki's generalized function for sensory receptors (Zwislocki, 1973) with an exponent (θ) of 0.95. This value suggests that the green mechanism is essentially summing intensity in a linear fashion. The predicted function closely matches the actual data.

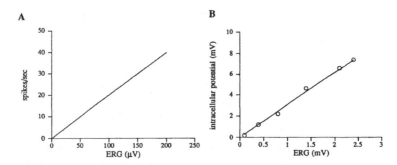

FIG. 15.6. The relationship between ERG amplitude and (A) ganglion-cell discharge rate, and (B) intracellularly recorded photoreceptor-response amplitude. Data for A were replotted from Hamasaki and Brooks (1971) for frog frontal organ. In B we recorded photoreceptor responses and ERGs in the same preparation. Note that ERG amplitude is linearly related to both photoreceptor response and ganglion-cell discharge. Therefore, we suggest that ganglion-cell discharge in the parietal eye is probably linearly related to photoreceptor-response amplitude.

Response Model

We have developed a model that predicts the recorded intensity-response relation with a reasonable degree of accuracy, and we will use the results of that model to speculate further on the heretofore unproven function of the parietal eye. This model does not take into account any elements of light or dark adaptation. The model is a modification of that introduced by Naka and Rushton (1966) for the retina and assumes that the observed responses originate in a system of three states (Figure 15.7): G, a green-sensitive state; B, the blue-sensitive state that drives the electrical response; and X, an inactive state that is neither light sensitive nor does it have an effect on the receptor potential. The three states are related by transition rates (light-driven G to B ($\sigma_g I_g$) and B to X ($\sigma_b I_b$) and thermally driven B to X (K_{bx}), X to B (K_{xb}), and B to G (K_{bg})).

The system can be described by a set of differential equations:

$$\frac{dG}{dt} = -\sigma_g I_g G + K_{bg} B \tag{1}$$

$$\frac{dB}{dt} = \sigma_g I_g G - (\sigma_b I_b + K_{bx} + K_{bg}) B + K_{xb} X \tag{2}$$

$$\frac{dX}{dt} = (\sigma_b I_b + K_{bx}) B - K_{xb} X \tag{3}$$

with the restriction that:

$$G + B + X = 1 \tag{4}$$

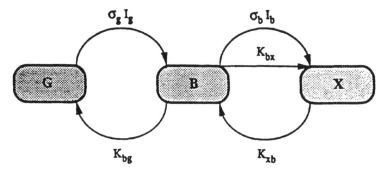

FIG. 15.7. The model employed to describe parietal-eye photoresponses consists of three states (G, B, & X) with 5 transition rates. State G is a green-sensitive state, B is blue-sensitive and drives the electrical response, and X is an inactive state having no effect on the receptor potential. G, B, and X are related by light-driven transition rates ($\sigma_g I_g$) and ($\sigma_b I_b$), and thermally driven rates (K_{bx}), (K_{xb}), and (K_{bg}). The system is described by a set of differential equations as noted in the text.

The equations were solved for B—the active state driving the electrical response—under steady-state conditions:

$$B = \frac{\sigma_g I_g}{\sigma_g I_g + \sigma_g I_g \left(\dfrac{\sigma_b I_g + K_{bx}}{K_{xb}} \right) + K_{bg}} \tag{5}$$

Equation 5 can be rewritten in the form:

$$B = \frac{I_g}{I_g \left(1 + \dfrac{K_{bx}}{K_{xb}} \right) + \dfrac{I_g I_b}{m_b} + m_b} \tag{6}$$

where m_g and m_b represent the intensity values required to drive the response to half saturation when stimulating with green or blue light, respectively, in the presence of a green background. The values of m_g and m_b are obtained experimentally. The ratio K_{bx}/K_{xb} is the only free parameter in the model and is adjusted to provide the best fit. We tested the model by comparing the predicted intensity-response curves with values measured by intracellular recording. The results are presented as the solid lines in Fig. 15.4, and one can see that the model predicts the actual responses of the dark- and green-adapted preparations quite well.

We then made the assumption that the output of the ganglion cell is proportional to the photoreceptor potential. We already established that the ERG is proportional to the receptor potential. We recently recorded several parietal-eye ganglion-cell responses in the dark-adapted and green-adapted states (data not shown). We find that the envelope of the post-stimulus-time (PST) histogram of spike discharge follows the time course of the slow potential quite well under dark- and green-adapted conditions. Therefore, for the purpose of this chapter we will make the assumption that the train of action potentials sent to the brain is proportional to the photoreceptor membrane potential fluctuations that we record.

Functional Implications

Previous investigators have put forth a variety of possible functions for the parietal eye (review by Eakin, 1973). The most popular idea is that the parietal-eye output is a Zeitegber used to synchronize bodily function with time of day and year, acting essentially like a dosimeter for solar radiation (Glaser, 1958; Stebbins & Eakin, 1958). This would be especially important for lizards with temperate-zone centers of distribution as day length in these regions is a better indicator of time of year than are some other environmental variables such as daily mean temperature or rainfall. These hypotheses about function have been based largely on behavioral experiments with control and parietalectomized animals. There is no consensus on what sort of information the parietal eye sends to the brain. We reasoned that knowing the output of the parietal eye to the brain might shed light on function.

Given the position of the parietal eye on the top of the head, it seemed logical to use the spectral distribution of skylight as the normal stimulus to which the eye responds. We used the program SOLRAD (Porter, 1989) to calculate the photic input to the eye. SOLRAD computes the energy of the solar spectrum in 5-nm bandwidths for any location on Earth, for any day of the year, at hourly intervals. Altitude and environmental conditions are variables for the program. We examined the solar input to the parietal eye on cloudless days for January 1 and July 1 in the Joshua Tree National Monument, near where our animals were collected. Figures 15.8A & 15.8B illustrate the spectral energy for visible wavelengths from sunrise to noon (the noon to sunset spectra are symmetrical) for those two days.

The measured spectral sensitivities of the green and blue mechanisms (Figure 15.8C) describe the sampling by the photoreceptor of the incident solar energy. These spectral sensitivities were measured by plotting criterion responses in the linear ranges of monochromatic intensity-response curves and using chromatic adaptation to uncover the blue response from the more sensitive and overlapping green response.

To allow an analytic rather than a numerical solution, the spectral composition of the solar spectrum was approximated using a piecewise-linear approach (illustrated by the dotted lines in Fig. 15.8A and Fig. 15.8B), and the spectral sensitivity curves of the two chromatic mechanisms

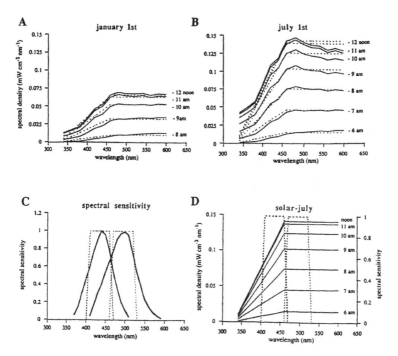

FIG. 15.8. Solar input and spectral sampling by the *Xantusia* parietal eye. A. Solid lines, spectral energy at visible wavelengths for the morning of January 1 in the vicinity of Joshua Tree National Monument. These data were calculated using SOLRAD (Porter, 1989). Spectra for the afternoon hours are symmetrical about 12:00 noon. Dotted lines are piecewise linear approximations of the energy spectra. B. Same as A but for July 1. Note the increased energy level and day length. C. Electrophysiologically measured spectral sensitivities for the blue and green mechanisms of parietal-eye photoreceptors (solid lines). We approximated the spectral sensitivity curves with ideal filters of appropriate bandwidth (dotted lines) for the purpose of numerical analysis. D. Photoreceptors sample the incident solar spectrum. Here the piecewise linear approximations of the hourly solar spectra (from B) are overlaid by the ideal filters representing photoreceptor spectral sensitivity (from C) for the purpose of deriving stimulus intensities to the two photoreceptor mechanisms throughout the day. Note that the knees of the curves for solar spectra fall between the maximal sensitivities of the two spectral components. The calculated values for stimulus intensity to the two mechanisms were used as input to our photoreceptor-response model (Fig. 15.7).

were approximated by ideal filters (dotted lines in Fig. 15.8C). These assumptions are illustrated in Fig. 15.8D.

The energies of the hourly incident photic spectra as sampled by the ideal filters were used as stimulus intensities and Equation 5 was used to predict the output of the photoreceptors (and by assumption, the ganglion cells). Figure 15.9 illustrates the estimated responses of photoreceptors on January and July 1. Note that there are peaks in the response shortly after sunrise

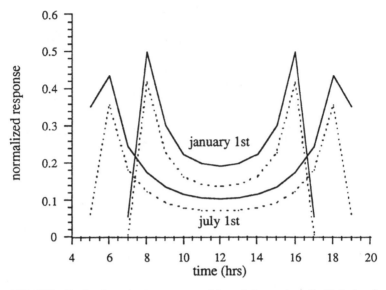

FIG. 15.9. Predicted steady-state response of two photoreceptor cells (dashed and solid lines) for January 1 and July 1. We believe the photoreceptor response is linearly related to ganglion-cell output to the brain (see text). The phasic nature of this predicted response emphasizes intensity transitions and would increase the reliability of the parietal eye as a monitor of day length. Unexpectedly, the total area under the curves for both midwinter and midsummer days is nearly the same. Any functional significance of this predicted output pattern is unclear.

and before sunset in both winter and summer. This is due to the decreased inhibitory drive of the blue-sensitive mechanism at low stimulus intensities and the dominance of the green-sensitive mechanism. With the increased light intensities in midday the blue mechanism makes a larger contribution and parietal-eye output decreases. Interestingly, the areas under the two curves differ by less than 10%. This suggests that, in the absence of adaptational or seasonal effects, the total daily activity of the eye would remain relatively constant throughout the year, despite seasonal changes in photophase length and light intensity.

The striking thing about the predicted output of the eye is the increased level of activity in the early morning and late afternoon. The eye does more than simply monitor light intensity. It may actually emphasize the transitions between the light and dark phases of the animal's daily cycle. In this regard, our predicted neural output of the parietal eye seems optimal for signaling the length of the photophase and supports the notion that this simple vertebrate eye may play a role in synchronizing the animal with its environment. We do not understand the predicted constant total daily activity of the eye, but it may be indicative of some aspect of photostasis.

A first step toward authenticating the model will be to record ganglion cell activity over the period of a day with the animal exposed to a natural lighting regimen.

In closing, we should caution that the inferences resulting from our model should be regarded with healthy skepticism. The model is an oversimplification of the processes involved and has not been tested on a large number of units. While the basic assumptions seem like common sense, their validity remains untested. Nevertheless, we feel that our results support the notion that the parietal eye is involved in the maintenance of circadian and circannual rhythms.

REFERENCES

de Graaf, H. W. (1886). Zur anatomie und Entwicklung der Epiphyse bei Amphibien und Reptilien. *Zoologische Anzeige, 9,* 191-194.

Dendy, A. (1899). On the development of the parietal eye and adjacent organs in *Sphenodon* (Hatteria). *Quarterly Journal of Microscopical Science, 51,* 1-29.

Dodt, E., & Scherer, E. (1968). Photic responses from the parietal eye of the lizard *Lacerta sicula campestris* (De Betta). *Vision Research, 8,* 61-72.

Eakin, R. M. (1960). Number of photoreceptors and melanocytes in the third eye of the lizard, *Sceloporus occidentalis. Anatomical Record, 138,* 345.

Eakin, R. M., (1964). Development of the third eye in the lizard, *Sceloporus occidentalis. Revue Suisse de Zoologie, 71,* 267-285.

Eakin, R., M. (1973). *The third eye.* Berkeley: University of California Press.

Eakin, R. M., & Westfall, J. A. (1959). Fine structure of the retina in the reptilian third eye. *Journal of Biophysical and Biochemical Cytology, 6,* 133-134.

Eakin, R. M., & Westfall, J. A. (1960). Further observations on the fine structure of the parietal eye of lizards. *Journal of Biophysical and Biochemical Cytology, 8,* 483-499.

Engbretson, G. A., & Anderson, K. J. (1990). Neuronal structure of the lacertilian parietal eye, I: A retrograde label and electron-microscopic study of the ganglion cells in the photoreceptor layer. *Visual Neuroscience, 5* 395-404.

Engbretson, G. A., & Lent, C. M. (1976). Parietal eye of the lizard: Neuronal photoresponses and feedback from the pineal gland. *Proceedings of the National Academy of Sciences, 73,* 654-657.

Engbretson, G. A., Reiner, A., & Brecha, N. (1981). Habenular asymmetry and the central connections of the parietal eye of the lizard. *Journal of Comparative Neurology, 198,* 155-165.

Glaser, R. (1958). Increase in locomotor activity following shielding of the parietal eye in night lizards. *Science, 128,* 1577-1578.

Hamasaki, D. I. (1969). Spectral sensitivity of the parietal eye of the green iguana. *Vision Research, 9,* 515-523.

Hamasaki, D. I., & Brooks, B. (1971). Quantitative analysis of excitation and inhibition in the stirnorgan of the frog. *Vision Research, 11,* 1125-1134.

Jenison, G., & Nolte, J. (1979). A second class of neurons within the retinas of the parietal eyes of *Anolis carolinensis* and *Iguana iguana. Brain Research, 168,* 615-618.

Kappers, J. A. (1967). The sensory innervation of the pineal organ in the lizard, *Lacerta viridis,* with remarks on its position in the trend of pineal phylogenetic structural and functional significance. *Zeitschriff für Zellforschung, 81,* 581-618.

Korf, H., W., & Wagner, U. (1981). Nervous connections of the parietal eye in adult *Lacerta s. sicula*, Rafinesque, as demonstrated by anterograde and retrograde transport of horseradish peroxidase. *Cell and Tissue Research, 219*, 567–583.

Leydig, F. (1890). Das Parietalorgan der Amphibien und Reptilien. *Abhandlungen der Senckenberger naturforschung Gesellschaft, 16*, 441–550.

Naka, K. -I., & Rushton, W. A. H., (1966). S-potentials from colour units in the retina of fish (Cyprinidae). *Journal of Physiology, 185*, 587–599.

Nowikoff, M. (1910). Untersuchungen über den Bau, die Entwicklung und die Bedeutung des Parietalauges von Sauriern. *Zeitschrift für Wissenschlaftliche Zoologie, 96*, 118–207.

Oksche, A. (1965). Survey of the development and comparative morphology of the pineal organ. *Progress in Brain Research, 10*, 3–28.

Petit, A. (1968). Ultrastructure de la rétine de l'oeil pariétal d'un Lacertilien, *Anguis fragilis*. *Zeitschrift für Zellforschung, 92*, 70–93.

Porter, W. P. (1989). *SOLRAD*. Madison, WI: University of Wisconsin.

Pugh, E. N. J., & Lamb, T. D. (1990). Cyclic GMP and calcium: The internal messengers of excitation and adaptation in vertebrate photoreceptors. *Vision Research, 30*, 1923–1948.

Solessio, E., & Engbretson, G. A. (1991). Local ERG, extracellular potassium changes and glial cell responses in a two-neuron vertebrate retina. *Investigative Ophthalmology & Visual Science, 32*, (Suppl. 4), 904.

Solessio E., & Engbretson, G. A. (in press) *Antagonistic chromatic mechanisms in photoreceptors of the parietal eye of lizards. Nature.*

Spencer, W. B. (1887). On the presence and structure of the pineal eye in Lacertilia. *Quarterly Journal of Microscopical Science, 27*, 165–238.

Stebbins, R. C., & Eakin, R. M. (1958). The role of the "third eye" in reptilian behavior. *American Museum Novitates, 1870*, 1–40.

Steyn, W. (1959). Ultrastructure of pineal eye sensory cells. *Nature, 183*, 764–765.

Steyn, W. (1960). Observations on the ultrastructure of the pineal eye. *Journal of the Royal Microscopy Society, 79*, 47–58.

Studnicka, F. K. (1905). Die parietalorgane. In A. Oppel (Ed.), *Lehrbuch der vergleichenden Mikroskopischen Anatomie der Wirbeltiere* (pp. 1–254). Jena: Gustav Fischer.

Zwislocki, J. J. (1973). On intensity characteristics of sensory receptors: A generalized function. *Kybernetik, 12*, 169–183.

16
Process and Mechanism: Mechanoreceptors in the Mouth as the Primary Modulators of Rhythmic Behavior in Feeding?

Karen M. Hiiemae
Syracuse University

INTRODUCTION

"We are what we eat" may have been, originally, social comment. It also reflects biological reality. Without adequate intake of essential nutrients, no living organism grows, matures, or reproduces. Complex multicellular organisms have developed processes by which sources of nutrients are *ingested* (enter the body) and *digested* in the gastrointestinal tract (mechanically and chemically reduced to absorbable nutrients). In mammals, that process has come to involve a set of highly integrated behaviors relying on sensory information from the visual and auditory systems. Not only does sensory information lead to a locomotor response, it also activates the autonomic nervous system preparing the mouth and stomach for food intake. The special senses play a vitally important role in the acquisition of food: in identifying food sources, in facilitating food acquisition, and in evaluating its edibility. More than a century ago, Pavlov showed that the conditioned anticipation of food would trigger reflex mechanisms which, by producing saliva, facilitate the conversion of a food source into "digestible material." As human society has developed, the "sight," "sound" and "smell/taste" of food has assumed social significance. The psychosociology and psychophysics of sight, sound, and touch, as well as the intraoral perception of taste and texture have, and are, playing a major role in the production of secondary (processed) food sources for consumption by most "developed" populations. While sensory "choices" may be a greater determinant of behavior (selectivity of acquisition) in a "supermarket society," it appears that the processes and mechanisms by which food is rendered digestible have changed little as mammals have evolved, despite the morphological specializations of jaws and teeth associated with differences in their primary food sources.

Further, while it is clear that the elderly, and especially those suffering from the onset of the senile dementias, lose their "enthusiasm" for food; it is by no means clear that this is simply a function of the failure of higher centers in the central nervous system (CNS). There is empirical evidence (M. R. Heath, personal communication, July 1992) that the problem may be, at least in part, a failure of intraoral stimulation coupled with the response of caregivers to those failure(s). If it is "difficult" to process food intraorally, "difficult" foods are avoided, or are not supplied by caregivers. The extent to which degenerative changes in higher centers, in the coordination of hand-eye movements for the simple mechanics of ingesting food, in taste perception, and/or a failure or difficulty in the process of moving and processing food within the mouth is not at all well understood. Clearly all these factors, and probably others, contribute to a distressing, and for its victims, a demoralizing, downward spiral. The result does, however, have serious consequences for those affected, which extend beyond the purely psychophysical and very much into the arena of "perceived quality of life." Many of us tend to think that elucidating the fundamental mechanisms of feeding is a biomechanical, neurophysiological, or psychophysical problem: It is also a very human problem.

This chapter is not only intended to honor Josef Zwislocki, but to show how his pervasive influence extends into areas far beyond the psychophysics of hearing. If a familiar food "sounds wrong" but "looks right," and certainly if it "feels wrong," defensive mechanisms are triggered. The complex mechanisms of feeding have an auditory as well as a visual, olfactory, and gustatory base. The *mechanisms* involved in feeding have been extensively studied in man, especially jaw movement patterns, given clinical concerns for the maintenance or enhancement of feeding and speech when morphology falls outside "normal range" or when behavior impairs normal function.

There is also a very large literature on aspects of the feeding process in other mammals and on the neurophysiology of their jaws and teeth. However, my purpose in this chapter is to *briefly* address the issues associated with the identification and description of the mechanisms by which sensory information might regulate the CNS control of food processing. We know a great deal about the "special senses." They play, unequivocally, the dominant role in food selection and acceptance. Thereafter, a process is triggered: Food is reduced, rendered "fit" to swallow, and so enters the digestive tract, but the role of sensory information in the regulation of that process continues to be a matter for discussion.

THE CENTRAL CONTROL OF MASTICATION

Once triggered by higher centers, mastication is a rhythmic activity: The jaws are opened and closed repeatedly. Sherrington (1917) postulated that this behavior could be produced by the alternating reflexes he had demonstrated, that is, the "jaw closing reflex" producing jaw closing, and the sensory response to that action producing reflex "jaw opening" (Fig. 16.1). Bremer (1923) demonstrated that masticatory behavior was regulated by a *pattern generator* in the pontine-medullary area of the CNS. Since then it has been shown that the rhythmic patterns of jaw movement can be elicited

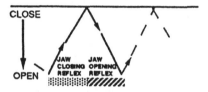

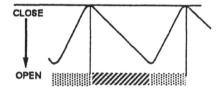

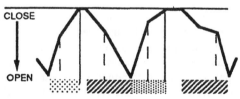

FIG. 16.1. Jaw movement profiles (diagrammatic). *Top*: Sherrington (1917) postulated that the oscillating "open–close" pattern of jaw movement in feeding was produced by reciprocating reflexes. *Middle*: Bremer (1923) demonstrated in rabbit that the rhythmic movement was generated by a *pattern generator* (Centre de Correlation) in the hindbrain, an observation confirmed by Dellow and Lund (1971). *Bottom*: When mammals are actively processing food, rate changes appear in both Closing and Opening Strokes. Rate change in Closing is associated with tooth-food-tooth contact (Hiiemae, 1976; Van der Bilt et al., 1991). Rate change in Opening is associated with changes in the direction of tongue movement relative to palate (see text and Fig. 16.4).

by stimulation of the motor cortex (Lund, Sasamoto, Murakami, & Olson, 1984), by stimulating the hindbrain (Dellow & Lund, 1971), or by triggering a response with chemical stimulation (Lambert, Goldberg, & Chandler, 1986). These and other studies have shown that the pontine-medullary area of the hindbrain (in which many of the cranial nerves involved have both their sensory and motor nuclei) can generate a rhythmic motorneuron output which results in a repeated pattern of jaw opening and closing (Fig. 16.1). Centrally stimulated patterns of jaw movement in neurophysiological preparations show a high degree of homogeneity and reproducibility. However, the behaviors of intact animals, actually feeding on "bites" of food (delivered intraorally or ingested by the animal), show modified patterns: Jaw movement is rhythmic, but the details of the rhythm change depending on the food and the stage in sequence (Fig. 16.1, see also further in the chapter and Fig. 16.3 later in the chapter).

Mastication differs from the similarly rhythmic processes of respiration and locomotion in that it is designed to *change* the substrate, that is, to render ingested food "swallowable." One would therefore reasonably expect that the pattern of jaw movement responsible for effecting change to change during the process. Clearly, some food sources such as liquids are swallowed without any form of intraoral processing. However, it follows that the state of solid or semisolid food when ingested has to be sensed and, thereafter, a determination made that it has reached a condition suitable for bolus formation. The question also arises as to whether, in order to regulate the process, the state of the food in the oral cavity is continuously monitored, and if so, through what sensory mechanisms.

APPROACHES TO THE PROBLEM

Figure 16.2 shows, with one important exception, the components of the effector system now known to be involved in preparing food for bolus formation. The diagram does not include the salivary glands: Saliva plays a major part in facilitating the process by lubricating the oral cavity, by softening food particles, and in "binding" those particles into a deformable mass which can be transported to the oropharynx for swallowing (Lucas & Luke, 1986). In a series of elegant experiments, Hector (1985) and Hector and Linden (1987) showed that salivary flow is correlated not only with the hardness of the food (the more resistant to chewing, the greater the salivary flow), but also with the side of the mouth on which the food is chewed. Even with this omission, the complexity of the system is evident.

To date, neurophysiological studies of the jaws and teeth have focused primarily on characterizing the pattern generator (see prior discussion), exploring the regulation of jaw muscle activity with a special emphasis on

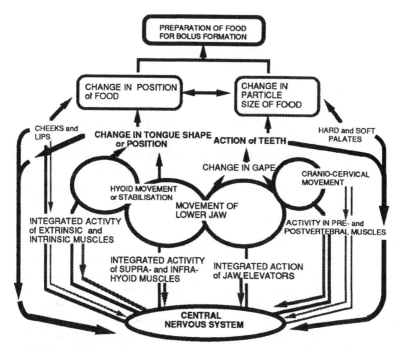

FIG. 16.2. The components of the orofacial complex involved in the ingestion, transport, and reduction of food exclusive of the salivary glands (see text) showing the sequence of activities involved in producing jaw and tongue movement (efferent arrows) and the sources of possible proprioceptive input to the CNS (pale afferent arrows). The very dark afferent arrows indicate the possible sources of sensory input from mechanoreceptors which could play a significant role in modifying the efferent output from the CNS pattern generator (see text).

the characteristics of the muscle spindles found in the elevators, their central connections, and reflex behavior (reviews by Appenteng, 1990; Taylor, 1990), on the jaw reflexes (Lund, 1990), and on the organization, structure, and projections of the trigeminal nuclei (reviews by Elias, 1990; Goldberg & Chandler, 1990; Olsson & Landgren, 1990). In addition, the characteristics of the mechanoreceptors in the periodontal ligament have been studied (Linden, 1990). Although some reports of the anatomy and performance characteristics of sensory receptors within the orofacial complex antedate Sherrington, almost all experimental studies have, perforce, used decerebrate or anaesthetized animals, usually cats, rats, or rabbits. Luschei and Goodwin (1974) were an exception when they recorded the jaw movement pattern with the elevator and digastric EMG in intact macaques to establish a baseline for studying the effect of ablation of parts of the trigeminal mesencephalic nucleus on the proprioceptive control of jaw movement (Goodwin & Luschei, 1975). While we now know a great deal about the behavior of both peripheral and central components of the system, we know comparatively little about the way they are integrated to produce normal functions in the intact orofacial complex.

An alternative approach is to record and analyze normal feeding behavior in the intact animal and then to develop hypotheses based on changes in that behavior and the associated condition of the substrate to explain how those changes might be produced with the expectation that those hypotheses can be tested using a more tightly controlled experimental method. Not only is this difficult, involving the analysis of very large volumes of data, it is also less satisfactory, because "cause and effect" are more difficult to demonstrate. Effector behavior can be documented, but the role (and source) of sensory information modifying that behavior has to be deduced. However, such behavioral studies led to our knowledge of the way tongue and jaw movements are integrated (Franks, German & German, & Crompton, 1984; Franks, 1991; Hayenga, Hiiemae, Reese, Crompton, & Thexton 1992; Hiiemae, Thexton, & Crompton, 1978; Thexton, & McGarrick, 1988, 1989) and the discovery that the swallow is a behavior intercalated into the normal chewing cycle (Crompton, Hylander, Kong, Palmer & German, in preparation; Crompton, Hylander, Weiss & German, in preparation; Hiiemae, et al., 1978; Palmer, Rudin, Lara, & Crompton, 1992) as well as the way jaw movement profiles change between initial ingestion and terminal swallow.

A third approach has been used with human subjects: Jaw movements, often with synchronous jaw muscle EMG, have been recorded using a variety of electromagnetic, optoelectronic, and mechanical devices when subjects were feeding on natural or synthetic test foods. The focus in these experiments has been on either the differential behavior of dentate, partially dentate, and edentulous subjects (Kazazoglu, 1991) or on the relationship between food type, numbers of chews, and resultant particle size (Lucas, Ow, Ritchie, Chew, & Keng, 1986). More recently the relationship of rate change in closing to the size of the food between the teeth and the dimensions of the maximum gape between successive cycles has been examined in normal human subjects as a method of exploring motor-control mechanisms (Van der Bilt, Van der Glas, Olthoff, & Bosman, 1991). All these studies show that the type of food and the way it breaks down under load affects the pattern of jaw movement.

JAW MOVEMENTS IN NORMAL FEEDING

The simple rhythmic movements of the jaws elicited by stimulation of the CNS in rabbits (Dellow & Lund, 1971; Lund et al., 1984) or guinea pigs (Lambert et al., 1986) show the output of the pattern generator under those experimental conditions and in the absence of solid food in the mouth. Cinefluorographic studies on intact nonhuman mammals including the American opossum (Crompton, Thexton, Hiiemae, & Parker, 1977; Hiiemae & Crompton, 1971; Hiiemae et al., 1978), the hyrax (Franks, German, Crompton, & Hiiemae, 1985; German & Franks, 1991), the cat (Thexton, Hiiemae, & Crompton, 1980; Thexton & McGarrick, 1988, 1989) and the macaque (Franks et al., 1985; German, Saxe, Crompton, & Hiiemae, 1989; Hylander, Johnson, & Crompton, 1987) have all shown that the shape of the masticatory cycle changes as food is moved into and within the mouth, chewed, and moved posteriorly for bolus formation. In contrast to the optoelectronic techniques used for recording jaw movement by other authors (e.g., Byrd, Milberg, & Luschei, 1978; Luschei & Goodwin, 1974; Schwartz, Enomoto, Valiquette, & Lund, 1989) or the cinephotographic or video techniques used, for example, by De Vree and Gans (1975) and Herring and Scapino (1973), cineradiography allows the gross position of the food in the mouth to be visualized and the movements of the tongue measured. Although all these studies showed differences in jaw movement profile as between the stage in sequence and food type, their focus was primarily on the *mechanisms* of chewing, that is, on the correlation between the EMG of the jaw musculature and the movement pattern (e.g., De Vree & Gans, 1975), on the forces acting on the jaws (e.g., Hylander et al., 1987), or on the linkage between jaw, tongue, and hyoid movement (e.g., Crompton et al., 1977; German & Franks, 1991; Hiiemae, Thexton & Crompton, 1981; Thexton & McGarrick, 1988, 1989). Few studies have attempted to investigate the effect of initial food type on the total *process* from ingestion to mouth clearance and, by extension, the way in which sensory input from the oral cavity might change the outflow from the pattern generator and thus the jaw movement profile. In 1980, Thexton et al. showed, in cats, that both initial size and consistency affected the number of cycles and their profile in each sequence. A more recent study in which macaques were fed similar volumes of three different foods (apple, banana, and chow) also showed that the initial state of the food affects subsequent sequence behavior (Hiiemae, Thexton, & Crompton, 1992; Hiiemae et al., in preparation).

If behavioral data are to be used as an index of the possible effect of sensory input from the orofacial complex on the output of the CNS pattern generator, several related questions have to be addressed: First, does the pattern change with the stage in process? Second, does the pattern change within stage? And third, how are those changes correlated with the state of the substrate at any point in the sequence? All these questions are based on the assumption that the "output data" measured by movement profile (and, usually, associated EMG) is at least fairly tightly related to a stream of afferent information. Such a relationship has been demonstrated in parts of the orofacial complex, for example, between muscle spindles and the contractile behavior of the jaw muscles in which they are situated (Taylor, 1990) and between receptors in the periodontal ligament and load on the teeth (Linden, 1990). Moreover, there is accumulating evidence that, with the exception of anthropoid primates and man in which the mechanism of Stage II transport is different from other mammals so far studied (Crompton et al., in preparation; Palmer et al., 1992) and can be correlated with the anatomy of the oropharynx, the relationship between initial food consistency and the changes in the morphology of jaw movement during the sequence are very similar. This suggests that the same basic regulatory mechanisms may operate in all but the most specialized mammals (e.g., anteaters) until the food reaches a threshold acceptable for swallowing.

BEHAVIOR IN PROCESS

Based on our earlier cinefluorographic studies of the opossum (Hiiemae et al., 1978), we identified three intraoral stages in the process from ingestion to deglutition: *Stage I transport* in which food is moved by the tongue from the incisal region to the premolar-molar area of the mouth; *chewing* in which food is reduced; and *Stage II transport* in which food is moved by the tongue posteriorly to the oropharynx for deglutition. Figure 16.3 (upper trace) shows a single sequence of jaw movement for a rabbit chewing small pellets of chow. Although Schwartz and his coauthors had no tongue data, the similarity between the jaw movement profiles in their "preparatory series" and those seen in Stage I transport in macaques (see German et al., 1989) warrants the conclusion that transport is occurring. Similarly, the profiles of the last two cycles of the "preswallowing series" have morphologies consistent with those found for Stage II transport cycles in cats and other mammals (see Thexton & McGarrick, 1989). The 16 cycles of the "reduction series" are typical "chewing cycles," although numbers 1–4 show closing profiles consistent with the compression and fracture of lumps of hard material as does number 10 (Hiiemae, 1976).

The rabbit data in Fig. 16.3 could be interpreted, using the criteria and descriptions in the original paper, as evidence for either: (a) three patterns or "subpatterns" of motorneuron output from the pattern generator (for initial transport; for 'food reduction' and the third for bolus collection and transport); (b) a single pattern which is continuously modified by sensory input from the orofacial complex; or (c) by sensory modulation acting on each pattern or subpattern. The hypothesis that the pattern generator can produce more than one variation on a basic output "pattern," given appropriate sensory "signals," is not unreasonable: It could be argued as analogous to the different patterns in locomotion associated with "walk,"

RABBIT, feeding on small pellets of Chow (after Schwartz et al., 1989)

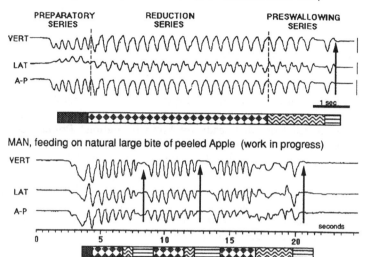

MAN, feeding on natural large bite of peeled Apple (work in progress)

FIG. 16.3. Jaw movement profiles (vertical: open down, close up) for complete sequences of rabbit and human feeding. The rabbit data (modified from Fig. 3 in Schwartz et al., 1989) were obtained from an optoelectronic system, the human from an electromagnetic system. Baselines for all traces are shown at the beginning and end of each trace. The arrows indicate cycles in which a swallow is initiated. The bars below the experimental records indicate the type of activity (see text) occurring in each part of the sequence and are shaded to show Stage I transport, chewing, and Stage II transport. The same shading conventions are used in Figs. 16.5 and 16.6. The time scale for the two records is very different: the whole sequence for the rabbit lasts about 7 secs, that for the human subject about 19.5 secs. It is important to note that the greater the compression of the time axis, the greater the loss of resolution in the jaw movement profile.

"trot," and "run," in which the proportions of time spent in the "swing" and "stance" phase change with rate (see MacMahon, 1984, Fig. 7.6, citing Grillner, 1975). Neither does it exclude the possibility that each "pattern" can be modified during the process. In contrast to locomotion, in which the focus of most studies has been on behavior at specific and different rates, the focus in feeding, given the changes the process induces in the substrate, should be on the transitions between rates and changes in cycles at each specific "rate."

Most of the data available on sequence behavior, such as that described by Schwartz, Enomoto, Valiquette, and Lund (1989), has involved feeding *small* volumes of food to experimental animals. Work in progress, in which human subjects were instructed to take a large *natural* bite, shows that even for a soft food, there are multiple transitions between behaviors (Fig. 16.3). Instead of a single terminal swallow, there are several swallows (two "in sequence" and one "terminal" in the example shown). This observation suggests that under these circumstances, the process involved a Stage I transport mechanism (which may take only one cycle given the anatomy of the human oral cavity), followed by the repetition of subsequences with a few chews, possibly one preswallow cycle, and a swallow. Given the occurrence of multiple swallows, it can be inferred that some component/ volume of material in the mouth is rendered "acceptable for swallowing" before the remainder. This raises the questions: How is that determined, so that preswallowing behavior is triggered? and how is inadequately triturated food segregated from that ready for bolus formation? *Prima facie* both must involve a response to sensory input from the oral cavity. Logically, one would expect that input to be at least partly derived from the tongue, and possibly the hard palate, because the gustatory surface of the tongue is moving against the palate for much of each cycle. It could also come in part from the mucosa of the cheeks, because they act with the tongue to reposition inadequately chewed material on the occlusal surfaces of the postcanine teeth for further triturition.

TONGUE-JAW LINKAGES

There is now a substantial body of evidence which shows that movements of the tongue are highly integrated with those of the jaws. Furthermore, there is evidence that the movements of the tongue can directly affect jaw movement profile. The most obvious examples are suckling in infants (e.g., German, Crompton, Levitch, & Thexton, 1992) in which jaw movement is negligible, but tongue movements are pivotal, and drinking or lapping in adult nonhuman mammals (see Hiiemae et al., 1978; Thexton & McGarrick, 1988). In both cases, the food has a texture well below the threshold for swallowing, flows, and is transported directly into and through the mouth. More recent work in which the relationship between tongue and jaw movement patterns was intensively analyzed in the macaque has not only confirmed the linkage between tongue and jaw behavior described in opossums and cats, but has shown that changes in jaw movement profile may be predictive of tongue behavior, at least in that anthropoid primate (Hayenga et al., 1992). Figure 16.4 summarizes the results of that analysis and illustrates the relationship of tongue movement to jaw movement profile. The important finding is that the amplitude and duration of tongue forward travel relative to the palate (the component of the tongue movement cycle which positions the tongue to move food distally in Stage I transport or actually moves it distally in Stage II transport in macaques) is highly variable, but the reversal to backwards travel is tightly, to within 20-30 ms, correlated with the onset of rapid jaw opening (Hiiemae et al., in

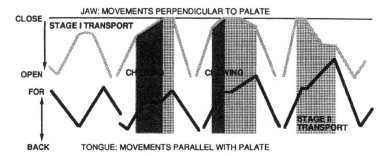

FIG. 16.4. Jaw–tongue linkages in macaque (diagrammatic). Four types of jaw movement cycle are shown with the corresponding pattern of tongue movement (represented by the change in position of a marker in the anterior part of the tongue, ATM). The reversal of ATM from forward to backward movement occurs within 30 msecs of the initial or last rate change in opening. The proportions of each chewing cycle spent in (a) food reduction (stippled bar), and (b) in food transport or manipulation (hatched bar) are shown. Overall cycle durations are shown as very similar. Statistical analysis shows that modal frequency in macaques is in the range of 450–550 msecs, but the data have a wide range (Hiiemae et al., in preparation).

preparation). When food is not transportable, the amplitude of forward tongue movement is minimal and has no, or a very small, effect on jaw-opening movement profile.

It is therefore reasonable to infer that not only are the movements of the tongue responsive to the condition of that part of the food in the mouth with which it is in physical contact, but that those movements directly affect the expressed output of the jaw movement pattern generator. The alternative interpretation, that sensory information from the jaw muscles, the temporomandibular (squamo-dentary) joint, and the periodontal ligaments controls tongue movement patterns, is a little hard to swallow (*pun intended*) given the ontogeny of this system and its behavior in adults lapping liquids or semisolids such as ice cream, in which the first physical contact between the material and a part of the orofacial complex occurs outside the mouth.

A MODEL FOR PROCESS CONTROL

Based on our studies of feeding behavior in the American opossum, representative of early mammals, we developed a model for the mechanisms by which the feeding process might be controlled (Hiiemae & Crompton, 1985); Hiiemae et al., 1978). That model (Fig. 16.5) postulates the existence of two intraoral "sensory gates." The first operates at the point food is actually in the anterior oral cavity and serves as a check on the decision to

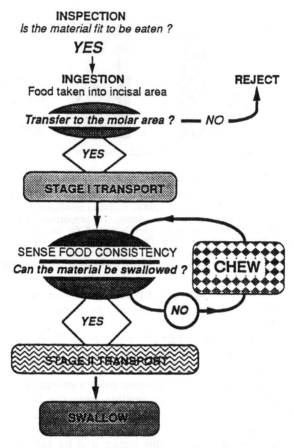

FIG. 16.5.   The "Process Model." The stage in the process at which the two postulated "Sensory Gates" operate, and the criteria are shown in the dark ovals (modified from Hiiemae & Crompton, 1985). Shading corresponds to that in Figs. 16.3 and 16.6.

ingest that material. If the sensory input from the oral cavity confirms that the food is edible, then it is transferred to the postcanine area. If, however, the sensory input from the oral cavity (for example, taste, texture) indicates that it is not fit to eat, it is promptly rejected. Gate I involves very complex mechanisms, including associative memory, and the special senses in that context. Anecdotal, but not irrelevant, is the common experience of seeing a child rejecting a food item, because, once in the mouth, he or she found it different from expectation based on visual, auditory, or gustatory memory, although the item might be perfectly eatable and edible—even nutritionally valuable. Notwithstanding the vagaries of human behavior, Gate I clearly has a protective function for mammals in the feral state.

It is Gate II that is of particular interest in terms of the intraoral sensory input to the pattern generator. The model postulates that the state of the food within the postcanine area of the mouth is assessed to determine whether it is fit to be swallowed. Despite the many studies examining the physical state of chewed food, usually particle size (see above), as well as sophisticated modeling of the selection functions of the tongue (e.g., Van der Bilt, Olthoff, Van der Glas, Van der Weelen, & Bosman, 1987), these shed limited light on the mechanism(s) by which the process is controlled largely because their focus continues to be on tooth-food-tooth relations, that is, chewing *sensu strictu*, rather than on the mechanisms involved in the totality of the process by which food is delivered from the mouth to the oropharynx and hence to the stomach for chemical digestion.

Is there such a physiological Gate? If so, the fundamental questions are: (a) How is the determination that food is not acceptable for swallowing made? (b) How is that determination acting to regulate the effector output? (c) Is that determination made on a continuing or an intermittent basis? and (d) What receptors, located where, are responsible? Or, to rephrase the question, is the transition between chewing and preswallowing in masticatory behavior based on a set of thresholds such as volume/particle size/flow properties of food material collected by the tongue, and how are those thresholds determined?

The model is difficult to test directly given the complexity of the system. However, like a more formal hypothesis, it predicts certain outcomes given specific input conditions. Those predictions are illustrated in Figure 16.6 This second, behavioral, model was originally developed as the framework within which the process model could be tested and underlays the design of an experiment on the effect of initial food consistency and particle size in the cat (Thexton et al., 1980). The results confirmed the core predictions of the model. They have now been confirmed in the macaque (Hiiemae et al., in preparation), but with an important difference: The process occurs in stages with intermittent swallows, rather than a single terminal swallow when a large bite is supplied (Fig. 16.6: Solids, Large lumps/volumes).

It has to be recognized that this approach incorporates, but does not specifically acknowledge, a series of second-order questions. For example, because the teeth are the medium through which both compressive and shear forces generated by the jaw-closing muscles are applied to the food, the reaction to those forces will be a function of the specific mechanical properties of each food type. A highly fibrous material (grass, woody leaves) will behave differently under load from a highly compressible vegetable or fruit (e.g., apple, orange). Some foods (chow, biscuit, most nuts) fracture into pieces, others (banana) may simply deform and spread as they are squashed and mixed with saliva. The physical properties of individual foods notwithstanding, the model argues that the difficulty of

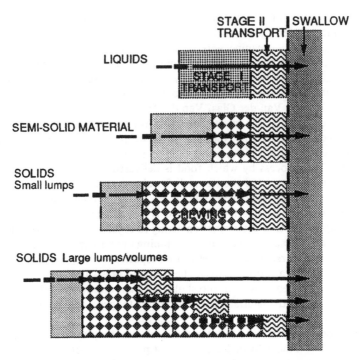

FIG. 16.6. The "Behavioral Model." The shading corresponds to that in Figs. 16.3 and 16.5. The heavy arrow indicates the process, breaks in the arrow indicate the times at which Gates I and II are postulated to operate. In the case of liquids, which have a consistency below the threshold for swallowing, Stage I transport and Stage II transport become a continuum (Hiiemae et al., 1978; Thexton & McGarrick, 1988). In this case "Gate I" could subsume the role of "Gate II." The predictions for liquids, semisolids, and solids (small lumps) were confirmed, even for large lumps (1.5 cm cubes), in cats (Thexton et al., 1980). The predictions for solids (large lumps/ volumes) is based on data for macaque (see text) and has been confirmed in man (work in progress). See also Fig. 16.7.

reducing that material to a consistency suitable for swallowing can be measured by the time spent in its reduction after Stage I transport and before Stage II transport. Similarly, the model, by addressing *total net effect* based on initial differences in food type, incorporates the role played by saliva and the different solubilities of food in saliva. The primary question remains: Is there a physiological "Gate II," and how does it operate, especially if there are multiple subsequences each terminating in a swallow?

EVIDENCE FOR GATE II

The cat study showed that initial food size and consistency did influence behavior in feeding, and by inference, that those behavioral differences reflected the response of the effector mechanism to the state of the food as ingested and during the process in a highly evolved carnivore which does not normally chew for more than a few cycles. In contrast, herbivores such as rabbits and hyraces normatively feed on highly fibrous material which is relatively difficult to reduce to shreds or particles small enough for bolus formation and so have long series of almost completely homogeneous jaw movement cycles (German & Franks, 1991). The differences between cats and hyraces may accurately reflect the mechanical problems afforded by their preferred foods. Clearly, a more convincing case for a physiological "Gate II" would be made were the predictions of the behavioral and process models to be confirmed in an omnivore feeding on foods of demonstrably different consistency and, preferably, also in man under similar experimental conditions.

A recent study of masticatory behavior in macaques feeding on bananas, apples, and chow (Hiiemae et al., 1992, in preparation) and a study in progress using the same foods (but hard ginger biscuits rather than proprietary monkey chow) in man (Hiiemae, Heath, & Kazazoglu, 1993) show that there are very distinct differences in behavior when foods of different initial consistency are either supplied in volumes judged consistent with a "natural bite" (macaques) or the subjects take "natural but large" bites (human subjects). Preliminary raw data for one human subject feeding on three different foods are given in Fig. 16.7. The results hold for all five subjects so far studied and show that the predictions of the behavioral model hold in man, that is, the harder the food, the larger the number of cycles before the first swallow. [The subjects also reported that the first swallow, especially when eating an apple (peeled or unpeeled), was a "juice swallow" which strongly suggests that one effect of "chewing" may be to dramatically and rapidly change the physical nature of some substrates.]

Given the totality of the data available for opossum, cat, and hyrax, and now macaque and man, it is not unreasonable to suggest that not only does "Gate II" exist, but it may have similar properties in all mammals. However, the problem of how it operates remains.

POSSIBLE GATE II MECHANISMS

As shown in Fig. 16.2, there are three possible sources of sensory information from which the orofacial complex, exclusive of taste, could act to operate this "Gate." They are (a) proprioceptors in muscle, tendons, and the temporomandibular joint; (b) mechanoreceptors in the periodontium, specifically the periodontal ligament; and (c) receptors in the mucosal surfaces of the oral cavity (cheeks, lips, and tongue) which come into contact with material in the mouth.

The distribution of spindles in the muscles of the orofacial complex is

RH. Apple (no peel) 11.20.91

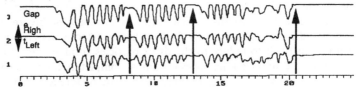

RH. Banana 11.20.91

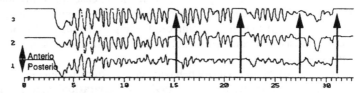

RH. Hard Biscuit 11.20.91

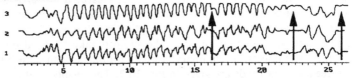

FIG. 16.7. Sequence behavior in man (work in progress) from raw data computer printouts. Arrows indicate swallows. The irregular cycle pattern preceding the last (top and middle records) or last two swallows (bottom record) were associated with extensive tongue movement as particles in the cheeks and floor of the mouth were collected for mouth clearance. The number of cycles before the first swallow increased with food " hardness," although in the case of the banana, the correct descriptor might be "stickiness."

very uneven (Taylor, 1990). They are found in significant numbers in parts of the masseter, temporalis, and medial pterygoid muscles, all elevators of the jaw, but not in the digastric, long considered the primary jaw-opening muscle. Whether they are found in the other muscles now known to play an important role in jaw opening (geniohyoid, sternohyoid, stylohyoid) appears not to have been investigated. The muscles of the tongue had long been thought to lack spindles. A scrupulous study of the tongue by Smith (1989) showed that they are present in small numbers. There is no question that spindles, where present, fulfill functions in the jaw muscles comparable to those in other skeletal muscles. However, while they act to regulate muscle behavior in the elevators, their afferent contribution clearly cannot account for the sensory input required to produce the integration of jaw and tongue movement seen in normal feeding. Even more significant may be the results obtained by Goodwin and Luschei (1975) who showed that selective destruction of jaw-elevator spindle afferents had little lasting effect on jaw movement or EMG patterns in macaques.

As Taylor (1990, p. 237) observes, "temporomandibular joint receptors are potentially significant sources of information but little is known of their central connections." While that is certainly the case, it remains difficult to envisage tongue behavior as dependent to any significant degree on information from that joint. Tendon organs are present in the system, although far fewer than in the limb muscles, and, again, little is known about their central connections (Taylor, 1990). When the nature of the mechanisms required to operate a "Gate II" are carefully considered in terms of the performance of the tongue–jaw system as now known, it becomes clear that the proprioceptors responsible for the regulation of muscle behavior and movement in activities such as locomotion cannot account for the totality of changes in the behavior of the jaw apparatus during normal function.

In contrast, afferent information from the mechanoreceptors in the periodontal ligament is indisputably linked to the regulation of food reduction in feeding. As Linden and others have shown (see Linden, 1990), receptors in the periodontal ligament are responsive to forces applied to the teeth and to the direction of those forces (as a function of the differential pattern of response by receptors in the ligament surrounding the loaded tooth). Sensory information from these mechanoreceptors certainly influences the behavior of jaw-closing muscles and their activity in food reduction. Because rate change in closing has long been argued to be a function of tooth-food-tooth contact and the resistance of the food to the compressive forces of jaw closure (Hiiemae, 1976), the behavioral data obtained by Van der Bilt et al. (1991) coupled with the work of Linden and others lend credence to the view that mechanoreceptors in the periodontal ligament play a major role in regulating the profile in *jaw closing*. Conversely, it is possible, but inherently unlikely, that information from periodontal mechanoreceptors serves to quantify the state of food particles on the tongue or in the vestibules of the cheeks and thus patterns of movement during *jaw opening* (see Fig. 16.4). This would be less unlikely if all, or the vast majority, of those particles were repositioned on the occlusal surfaces for each chewing cycle. Although, given the behavioral data, it is doubtful that this is the case, the possibility remains.

The neurophysiological literature (see Linden, 1990; Taylor, 1990) makes allusions to "other receptors in the periodontium" or, inferentially, to the possibility that there are receptors in the oral mucosa. The tongue is barely mentioned, except in the context of swallowing. "Although the tongue is involved in a number of precisely defined movements, current neurophysiological knowledge does not permit one to describe definitively the mechanisms involved in the co-ordinated events which occur" (Lowe, 1990, p. 322). Almost no attention has been paid to the possibility that the tongue is a major source of general afferent information in *normal feeding*, since the linkage between jaw and tongue movement in jaw opening was first described. An exception is a study by Thexton and Crompton (1989). Even without the use of "Occam's Razor," it is difficult to escape the conclusion that afferents from the tongue must play a substantial part in the regulation of its own behavior and therefore, given the tongue–jaw linkages thus described, in the pattern of jaw movement once the masticatory sequence is triggered.

What type of sensory information might be involved? The terms *consistency* and *hardness* have been used in this chapter, as have physical descriptions such as *liquid*, *semisolid*, and *solid*. Clearly, as mammals are weaned and learn to eat solid food, visual and auditory stimuli coupled with associative memory will have established an expectation or "standard" for its edibility and for its behavior in the mouth. Discontinuities in the process (the proverbial bite on the lead shot in the pheasant) trigger a dramatic reflex response. Such protective mechanisms notwithstanding, normal feeding involves the primarily unconscious completion of a process in which food is physically changed and one in which the tongue has a continuous and vital role.

For food to be swallowed, it has to have a particle size below threshold and/or be aggregated into a soft deformable mass (see Lucas & Luke, 1986). This suggests that at least three interrelated determinations have to be made in relation to the food: particle size, volume, and distribution. Both, by analogy with skin, involve spatial discrimination. Both also involve pressure or a response to the resistance they offer to apposing mucosal surfaces. Almost all the mucosa covering the palate, cheeks, and intraoral surface of the lips is derived from ectoderm and could be expected to have at least some of the sensory properties of glabrous skin. The mucosa of the tongue is embryologically endoderm (Williams & Warwick, 1980, p. 197). However, the tongue moves relative to the palate and the lips in complex patterns in activities such as speech as well as in feeding. We can "feel" the rugae, small as they are, on the hard palate. This suggests, and the effects of local anesthesia confirm, that the tongue subserves a conscious sensation of touch. It is not unreasonable to postulate that that mechanism, probably coupled with an as yet unidentified proprioceptive system regulating the behavior of its musculature, plays a pivotal role in regulating the output of the pattern generator(s) producing the rhythmic movements of both the jaw and the tongue in feeding. The challenge is to identify the receptors involved and demonstrate their behavior and CNS connections.

ACKNOWLEDGMENTS

In addition to my undergraduate research students, Andrew Reese and Shawne Hayenga, who did much of the work involved in analyzing tongue behavior in the macaque, I want to thank Robin Heath, Ender Kazazoglu, and Tony Ferman of the Biometrics Laboratory at the Dental Institute of the Royal London Hospital Medical College who have spent much effort and time working with me to start to test whether humans are like macaques (or vice versa) if fed the same foods. The contributions of my coworkers and friends, especially A.W. Crompton, A.J. Thexton, and Rebecca German to the body of work that made this review possible is evident in the text. My colleagues at the Institute for Sensory Research, especially Joe Zwislocki, Ron Verrillo, Sandy Bolanowski, and Steve Chamberlain have stimulated my interest in the problems outlined here. Last, but by no means least, the effort Professor A. Taylor, Sherrington Professor of Physiology in the United Medical and Dental Schools, University of London, put into organizing the Symposium and producing the volume on *The Neurophysiology of the Teeth and Jaws* cannot go unremarked. Without that volume, life would be much harder for all of us!

The macaque experiments described here were supported by USPHS DE 05738. Data reduction and analysis and the pilot studies in London were in part supported by Syracuse University intramural research funds provided by the Vice President for Research.

REFERENCES

Appenteng, K. (1990). Jaw muscle spindles and their central connections. In A. Taylor (Ed.), *Neurophysiology of the jaws and teeth* (pp. 97–141). London: Macmillan.

Bremer, F. (1923). Physiologie nerveuse de la mastication chez le chat et le lapin. *Archives internationale de Physiologie, 21,* 309–352.

Byrd, K. E., Milberg, D. J., & Luschei, E. S. (1978). Human and macaque mastication: A quantitative study. *Journal of Dental Research, 57,* 834–843.

Crompton, A. W., Thexton, A. J., Hiiemae, K. M., & Parker, P. (1977). The activity of the hyoid and jaw muscles during chewing of soft food in the American opossum. In. D. Gilmore & B. Stonehouse (Eds.), *Biology and environment, Vol. 2, No. 17, The biology of marsupials* (pp. 287–305). London: Macmillan.

Crompton, A. W., Hylander, W. L., Weiss, J. & German R. Z. (in preparation). Swallowing in the American Opossum *Didelphis virginiana.*

Crompton, A. W., Hylander, W. L, Kong, G. Palmer, J. B., German R, Z, (in preparation). Swallowing in the crab-eating macaque, *Macaca fascicularis.*

Dellow, P. G., & Lund, J. P. (1971). Evidence for the central timing of rhythmical mastication. *Journal of Physiology, 215,* 1–13.

De Vree, F., & Gans, C. (1975). Mastication in pygmy goats 'Capra hircus.' *Annales Societe Royale Zoologique Belgique, 105,* 255–306.

Elias, S. A. (1990). Trigeminal projections to the cerebellum. In A. Taylor (Ed.), *Neurophysiology of the jaws and teeth* (pp. 192–236). London: Macmillan.

Franks, H. A., German, R. Z., & Crompton, A. W. (1984). Mechanism of intra-oral transport in Macaques. *American Journal of Physical Anthropology, 58,* 275–282.

Franks, H. A., German, R. Z., Crompton, A. W., & Hiiemae K. M. (1985). Mechanisms of intraoral transport in an herbivore, the hyrax. *Archives of Oral Biology, 30,* 539–544.

German, R. Z., Crompton, A. W., Levitch, L. C., & Thexton, A. J. (1992). The mechanism of suckling in two species of infant mammal: Miniature pigs and longtailed macaques. *Journal of Experimental Zoology, 260,* 322–330.

German, R. Z., & Franks, H. A. (1991). Timing in the movement of jaws, tongue and hyoid during feeding in the Hyrax, *Procavia syriacus*. *Journal of Experimental Zoology, 257,* 34–42.

German, R. Z., Saxe, S., Crompton, A. W., & Hiiemae, K. M. (1989). Mechanism of food movement through the anterior oral cavity in anthropoid primates. *American Journal of Physical Anthropology, 80,* 369–377.

Goldberg, L. J., & Chandler, S. H. (1990). Central mechanisms of rhythmical trigeminal activity. In A. Taylor (Ed.), *Neurophysiology of the jaws and teeth* (pp. 268–293). London: Macmillan.

Goodwin, G. M., & Luschei, E. S. (1975). Discharge of spindle afferents from jaw closing muscles during chewing in alert monkeys. *Journal of Neurophysiology, 38,* 560–571.

Grillner, S. (1975). Locomotion in vertebrates: Central mechanisms and reflex interaction. *Physiological Reviews, 55,* 247–304.

Hayenga, S., Hiiemae, K. M., Reese, A., Crompton, A. W., & Thexton, A. J. (1992). Linkage between jaw opening and tongue movements in Macaque [Special Issue] *Journal of Dental Research, 72* (1826), 744. [Abstract]

Hector, M. P. (1985). The masticatory-salivary reflex. In S. Lisney & B. Matthews (Eds), *Current topics in oral biology* (pp. 311–320). Bristol: University of Bristol Press.

Hector M. P., & Linden, R. W. A. (1987). The possible role of periodontal mechanoreceptors in the control of parotid secretion in man. *Quarterly Journal of Experimental Physiology, 72,* 285–301.

Herring, S. W., & Scapino, R. P. (1973). Physiology of feeding in miniature pigs. *Journal of Morphology, 141,* 427–460.

Hiiemae, K. M. (1976). Masticatory movements in primitive mammals. In D. J. Anderson & B. Matthews (Eds.), *Mastication* (pp. 105–118). Bristol: John Wright & Sons.

Hiiemae, K. M. (1978). Mammalian mastication: A review of the activity of the jaw muscles and the movements they produce in chewing. In P. M. Butler & K. A. Joysey (Eds.), *Development, function, and evolution of teeth* (pp. 359–398). London: Academic Press.

Hiiemae, K. M., & Crompton, A. W. (1971). A cinefluorographic study of feeding in the American opposum (*Didelphis marsupialis* L.). In A.A. Dahlberg (Ed.), *Dental morphology and evolution* (pp. 299–334). Chicago: University of Chicago Press.

Hiiemae, K. M. & Crompton, A. W. (1985). Mastication, food transport, and swallowing. In M. Hildebrand, D. M. Bramble, K. F. Liem, & D. B. Wake (Eds.), *Functional verterbrate morphology* (pp. 262–290). Cambridge: The Belknap Press of Harvard University Press.

Hiiemae, K. M., Thexton, A. J., & Crompton, A. W. (1978). Intra-oral food transport—A fundamental mechanism in feeding? In D. Carlson & J. McNamara (Eds.), *Muscle adaptation in the cranio-facial region, Monograph No. 8, Craniofacial growth series* (pp. 181–208). Ann Arbor: University of Michigan.

Hiiemae, K. M., Thexton, A. J., & Crompton, A. W. (1981). The movement of the cat hyoid during feeding. *Archives of Oral Biology, 26,* 65–181.

Hiiemae, K. M., Thexton, A. J., & Crompton, A. W. (1992). The effect of food consistency on jaw profile in Macaques [Special Issue]. *Journal of Dental Research, 72,* Abstract No. 1824 p. 744. [Abstract]

Hiiemae, K. M., Heath, M. R., Kazazoglu E. (1993), Natural bites, food consistency and insequence feeding behavior in man. *Journal of Dental Research* (Special Issue 72:267 No. 1311 [Abstract].

Hiiemae, K. M., Hayenga, S., Reese, A., Crompton, A. W., Thexton A. J. (in preparation) Correlations between tongue and jaw movements during feeding in the macaque.

Hiiemae, K. M., Thexton, A. J., Crompton A. W., (in preparation). Food consistency and jaw movement profile in macaques: A cineradiographic study.

Hylander, W. L., Johnson, K. R., Crompton, A. W. (1987). Loading patterns and jaw movements during mastication in *Macaca Fascicularis;* A bone-strain, electromyographic and cineradiographic analysis. *American Journal of Physical Anthropology, 72,* 287-314.

Kazazoglu, E. (1991). *The functional analysis of mandibular movements during mastication related to dental state and food texture.* Unpublished doctoral thesis, Faculty of Medicine, University of London.

Lambert, R. W., Goldberg, L. J., & Chandler, S. H. (1986). Comparison of mandibular movement trajectories and associated patterns of oral muscle electromyographic activity during spontaneous and apomorphine induced rhythmic movements in the guinea pig. *Journal of Neurophysiology, 55,* 301-319.

Linden, R. W. A. (1990). Periodontal mechanoreceptors and their functions. In A. Taylor (Ed.), *Neurophysiology of the jaws and teeth,* (pp. 52-96). London: Macmillan.

Lowe, A. R. (1990). Neural control of tongue posture. In A. Taylor (Ed.), *Neurophysiology of the jaws and teeth* (pp. 322-368). London: Macmillan.

Lucas, P. W., & Luke, D. A. (1986). Is food particle size a criterion for the initiation of swallowing? *Journal of Oral Rehabilitation, 13,* 127-136.

Lucas, P. W., Ow, R. K. K., Ritchie, G. M., Chew, C. L., & Keng, S. B. (1986). Relationship between jaw movement and food breakdown in human mastication. *Journal of Dental Research, 65,* 400-404.

Lund, J. P. (1990). Specialization of the reflexes of the jaws. In A. Taylor (Ed.), *Neurophysiology of the jaws and teeth* (pp. 142-161). London: Macmillan.

Lund, J. P., Sasamoto, K., Murakami, T., & Olson, K. A. (1984). Analysis of rhythmical jaw movements produced by electrical stimulation of the motor-sensory cortex of rabbits. *Journal of Neurophysiology, 52,* 1014-1029.

Luschei, E. S., & Goodwin, G. M. (1974). Patterns of mandibular movement and jaw muscle activity during mastication in the monkey. *Journal of Neurophysiology, 37,* 954-966.

MacMahon, T. A. (1984). *Muscles, reflexes and locomotion.* Princeton:Princeton University Press.

Olsson, K. A., & Landgren, S. (1990). Primary afferent and descending cortical convergence on the interneurons in the border zone of the trigeminal motor necleu: A comparison between spinal and trigeminal interneurons. In A. Taylor (Ed.), *Neurophysiology of the jaws and teeth* (pp. 161-191). London:Macmillan.

Palmer, J. B., Rudin, N. J., Lara, G., & Crompton, A. W. (1992). Coordination of mastication, oral transport and swallowing. *Dysphagia,7,* 187-200.

Schwartz, G., Enomoto, S., Valiquette, C., & Lund, J. P. (1989). Mastication in the rabbit: A description of movement and muscle activity. *Journal of Neurophysiology, 62,* 273-287.

Sherrington, C. S. (1917). Reflexes elicitable from pinna, vibrissae and jaws. *Journal of Physiology, 51,* 404-451.

Smith, K. (1989). Muscle spindles are present in the tongue of the rat. *Archives of Oral Biology, 34,* 529-534.

Taylor, A. (1990). Proprioceptive control of jaw movement. In A. Taylor (Ed.), *Neurophysiology of the jaws and teeth* (pp. 237-267). London:Macmillan.

Thexton, A. J., & Crompton, A. W. (1989). Effect of sensory input from the tongue on jaw movement in normal feeding in the opossum. *Journal of Experimental Zoology, 250,* 233-243.

Thexton, A. J., Hiiemae, K. M., & Crompton, A. W. (1980). Food consistency and particle size as regulators of masticatory behavior in the cat. *Journal of Neurophysiology, 44,* 456-474.

Thexton, A. J., & McGarrick, J. D. (1988). Tongue movements in the cat during lapping. *Archives of Oral Biology, 33,* 331-339.

Thexton, A. J., & McGarrick, J. D. (1989). Tongue moovements in the cat during the intake of solid food. *Archives of Oral Biology, 34,* 239-248.

Van der Bilt, A., Olthoff, L. W., Van der Glas, H. W., Van der Weelen, K., & Bosman, F. (1987). A mechanical description of the comminution of food during mastication in man. *Archives of Oral Biology, 32*, 579–586.

Van der Bilt, A., Van der Glas, H. W., Olthoff, L. W., & Bosman, F. (1991). The effect of particle size reduction on jaw gape in human mastication. *Journal of Dental Research, 70*, 931–937.

Williams, P. J., & Warwick, R. (1980). *Gray's Anatomy* (36th ed). Philadelphia: W. B. Saunders; London: Churchill Livingstone.

17 The Effects of Aging on the Sense of Touch

Ronald T. Verrillo
Syracuse University

INTRODUCTION

As life expectancy increases, the physical problems associated with advancing age are becoming more prevalent in our society. Life expectancy has more than doubled in the past 200 years, from 35 years in 1776 to 75 years in 1989. In 1989 there were 30 million people in the United States over 65 years of age, 12% of the population, and this figure is increasing by approximately 6 million each decade. From 1970 to 1990 the rate of increase of persons over 65 years of age was twice that of the remainder of the population. In 1900 about 3% of the total life span was spent in retirement (1.2 years), and in 1980 that figure increased to 13.6% (10.2 years). These changes toward an increased life span have resulted in a multiplication of the personal hardships often associated with old age as well as an enormous increase in the obligations of society towards its elderly citizens.

Many changes in sensory capacity accompany growing older. In fact, *all* sensory systems, with the possible exception of taste, suffer deficits as a consequence of aging. It is considered "normal" to need reading glasses by the mid-to late 40s, and hearing sensitivity, especially above 2,000 Hz, decreases from age 20 onward with rather severe losses in evidence after age 70. Tactile sensation is no exception, which is the topic of this chapter. The impact of sensory deficits that accompany the aging process is felt financially, both to the individual and to society, and the elderly often experience personal hardships because of changes in the quality of life that can sometimes be dramatic.

Compared to the volume of research on vision and hearing, studies on the sense of touch run a very poor third. This is due in part to the fact that tactile deficits lack the dramatic quality of blindness and deafness. However, in recent years there has been a surge of interest in tactile sensation which may be attributed to a very practical reason: the sense of touch is being revisited seriously as a surrogate channel of communication to compensate for deficits in vision and hearing.

Many devices have been developed to accomplish this task, some marketed, but so far there can be no substantial claim for success of any of these devices, even among younger persons. As you might suspect, the effects of aging on tactile sensitivity have been virtually ignored by the developers of these devices.

The skin is a complex sense organ, unique in size and in the number of sensations it mediates. The largest sensory system, it is approximately 1.75 m^2 in surface area in the adult and accounts for about 6% of total body weight. It conveys not only sensations of touch, but also of warmth, cold, and pain, all mediated by receptors distributed beneath its entire surface and in rather close proximity to each other.

In this chapter I describe what is known about the sense of touch as a function of life-span development. The experimental results will be presented under three major categories: (a) absolute thresholds for the detection of vibration, (b) responses to suprathreshold vibratory stimulation, and (c) thresholds for the detection of temporally spaced stimuli.

THRESHOLD

Studies that report a loss of sensitivity to mechanical distortion of the skin go back over 60 years to an investigation by Pearson in 1928 (Axelrod & Cohen, 1961; Cosh, 1953; Pearson, 1928; Rosenberg, 1958; Whanger & Wang, 1974). There has been a small but steady trickle of studies from both the clinic and from laboratories to register the finding that as we grow older our ability to detect vibrations on the skin is diminished. (There have been a few exceptions, but there has been no serious challenge to the general trend in the data.) I do not consider the more primitive studies using von Frey hairs and cotton swabs that abound in the early literature, but rather concentrate on systematic, scientific investigations in which controlled stimuli were used. The first carefully performed studies using modern equipment were reported by Plumb and Meigs (1961) and Goff, Rosner, Detre, and Kennard (1965), who both found a general loss of vibrotactile sensitivity with age.

Our first study (Verrillo, 1977) was concerned only with changes in sensitivity measured on the thenar eminence between the ages of 10 and 20 years. There was a loss of sensitivity at frequencies that activate primarily the Pacinian receptor system (40 to 600 Hz), but not at 25 Hz, at which the response is determined by non-Pacinian receptors. The same result was obtained by Frisina and Gescheider (1977) who replicated the experiment. These preliminary experiments were extended to include the range of ages between 10 and 65 years, with subjects grouped at mean ages of 10, 20, 35, 50, and 65 years, in an attempt to track the changes in vibrotactile sensitivity over many years (Verrillo, 1979, 1980). Figure 17.1 shows the dramatic loss of sensitivity between the ages of 20 and 65 years at frequencies above 40 Hz, but with no changes at 25 and 40 Hz. The next figure (Fig. 17.2) shows that the drama is softened by a gradual loss of sensitivity in the upper frequencies that starts to manifest itself somewhere between 20 and 35 years of age. Again, thresholds at the lower frequencies tended to remain stable with advancing age. Similar results were reported recently by Muijser (1990). The same data are replotted in Fig. 17.3 as a function of age in years. There, it is clearly apparent that at the higher frequencies, at which the Pacinian-corpuscle system is optimally excited, there is a steady decline in sensitivity. At the two lowest frequencies tested (25 and 40 Hz), which optimally activates non-Pacinian receptors, sensitivity does not appear to change with age. In general, lumping together all frequencies, vibrotactile sensitivity is shown to decrease with age, but it is the Pacinian system that causes the lion's share of this decline.

We were fortunate in being able to retest 13 years later six subjects in the

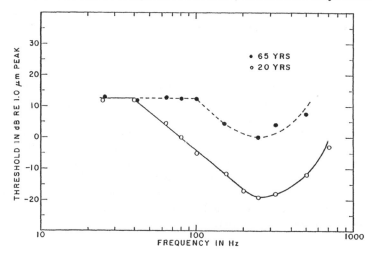

FIG. 17.1. Vibrotactile detection thresholds on the thenar eminence plotted as a function of sinusoidal frequency. The results show a substantial loss in sensitivity in the older group at frequencies (above 40 Hz) that optimally activate the Pacinian receptor system. Age does not appear to have an effect in the lower frequencies (non-Pacinian). (From Verrillo, 1982. Reprinted with permission from Perception & Psychophysics.)

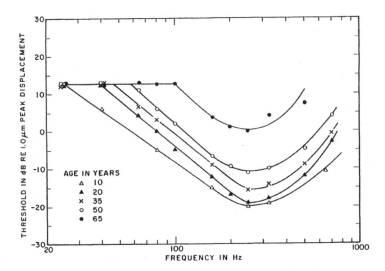

FIG. 17.2. Detection thresholds as a function of sinusoidal frequency measured in five age groups. The data show that there is a progressive loss of vibrotactile sensitivity over the age span of 10 to 65 years in the Pacinian systems whereas the non-Pacinian systems appear to be unaffected. (From Verrillo, 1979; 1980. Reprinted with permission from Journal of Gerontology.)

10-year-old group from our original study (Verrillo, 1980). This longitudinal experiment confirmed the results of the earlier cross-section design showing sensitivity losses at higher frequencies and none at lower frequencies.

The reason for the considerable changes of sensitivity with age in the Pacinian system is not known. Our most educated guess at this time is that the loss of sensitivity is the result of the gradual loss of Pacinian corpuscles with age (Cauna, 1965). Another factor that may be involved is the temperature at the surface of the skin. Lowered skin temperature decreases the sensitivity of the Pacinian system, but not that of the non-Pacinian systems (Bolanowski & Verrillo, 1982). In a national survey of over 1,000 persons in Britain, those over 65 years of age had significantly lower skin (hand) and core body temperatures than did those who were younger. It is possible that skin temperature and core body temperature could be a factor in lowered vibrotactile sensitivity.

SUPRATHRESHOLD

The previous section considered only the effects of aging on the absolute threshold for the detection of vibrotactile stimuli. But, we live in a world

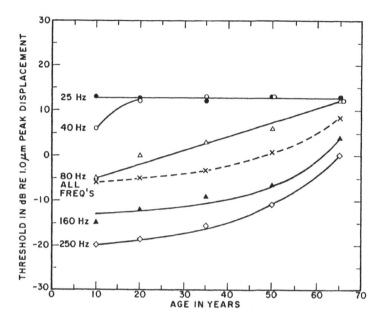

FIG. 17.3.   The data shown in Fig. 17.2 replotted as a function of age. It is clear that sensitivity is lost in the aging Pacinian system, but not in non-Pacinian systems. Across all frequencies (x) there is a gradual, overall loss with age. (From Verrillo, 1980. Reprinted with permission from Journal of Gerontology.)

that constantly bombards us with stimuli at suprathreshold magnitudes. It is imperative for many theoretical and practical reasons that we know what changes take place in sensations produced by stimulus intensities above threshold.

The method of choice that we have used for studying the growth of sensation as a function of stimulus intensity has been magnitude estimation, pioneered by Stevens (1957) and refined by Zwislocki and Hellman (Hellman & Zwislocki, 1961; Zwislocki & Goodman, 1980). Earlier studies had shown that this direct-scaling method could be used successfully to measure suprathreshold responses to vibration (Stevens, 1959; Verrillo, 1974; Verrillo, Fraioli, & Smith, 1969). We subsequently studied the effect of age on the growth of vibrotactile sensation magnitude.

In auditory research, it is from the loudness power functions, which are the form of the results of magnitude estimation, that the phenomenon of recruitment is clearly visible. Recruitment refers to the abnormal rate of increase in loudness with stimulus intensity that accompanies some hearing losses. These data provide evidence to the clinician concerning the locus of the malfunction in the auditory system that is causing a hearing loss. The sensation-growth curves of a group of 25-year-olds and a group of

66-year-olds were compared at two frequencies: 25 Hz to assess the effect of age on non-Pacinian receptors, and 250 Hz to assess the effect on the Pacinian population (Verrillo, 1982). The resultant curves were double-linked power functions at both frequencies and in both age groups. From the results shown in Fig. 17.4, it is apparent that the growth of subjective magnitude at 25 Hz is not affected by age. However, when subjects were tested at 250 Hz an age difference did surface. The results in Fig. 17.5 show the loss of sensitivity in the older subjects found at this frequency in earlier studies. At intensities near threshold there is no difference in the slope values of the young and older subjects, which is consistent with the results of Knight and Margolis (1984) who found no recruitment of hearing in presbycusic subjects. However, at higher intensities the vibrotactile curve was significantly steeper in the older group, in agreement with results reported by Goetzinger, Proud, Dirks, and Embrey (1961) for hearing in elderly subjects. Lindblom and Verrillo (1979) found vibrotactile recruitment in middle-aged subjects suffering from chronic neuralgia in the presence of both "normal" and elevated thresholds. At this point in time we must concede that the question of recruitment as a function of age does not have a definitive answer for vibrotaction. Much more research is needed, and we are now in the process of doing a more detailed study of the problem.

TEMPORAL EFFECTS

Investigations of the effects of age on the capacity of individuals to make sensory discriminations of tactile stimuli varying in the time domain are very sparse, indeed. We have concentrated on the phenomenon of "persistence," gap detection, and forward masking.

Persistence refers to interference in the detection of a signal by the presence of another stimulus preceding it by a short period of time. It was first reported in vision experiments, then in hearing, and finally in vibrotaction. Botwinick (1978) and Coltheart (1980) have provided reviews of the literature as well as hypotheses about its mechanism. The explanation generally given is that in the elderly nervous system the activity of neurons generated by external stimuli tends to persist for a longer period of time than it does in the young nervous system; thus sequentially presented stimuli are able to interact, usually to the detriment of sensory perception. There is no direct evidence that this working hypothesis is valid.

Tactile sensory persistence was studied as a function of age by a matching procedure that measured the effect of a conditioning stimulus on a test stimulus that followed it by a short, variable time interval (Verrillo, 1982). Subjects were required to adjust the intensity of a short vibratory burst to match the perceived magnitude of another short burst (test) that preceded it

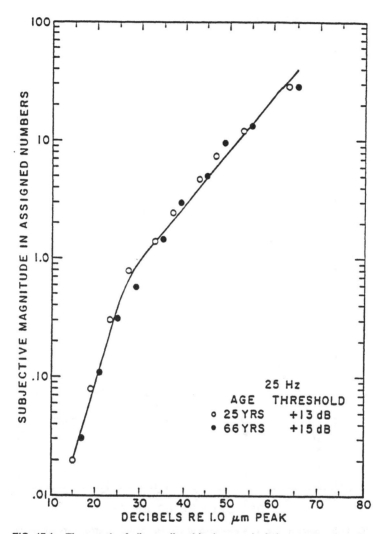

FIG. 17.4.   The growth of vibrotactile subjective magnitude in two age groups as a function of displacement amplitude of a 25-Hz sinusoid. There is no difference between the ages of 25 and 66 years in threshold or in the growth of sensation in the non-Pacinian systems. (From Verrillo, 1982. Reprinted with permission from Perception & Psychophysics.)

by a fixed period of time. A conditioning burst was set prior to the test burst at varying time intervals. The effect of the conditioning stimulus on the subjective intensity of the test stimulus is to make it appear to be greater than when the test stimulus is experienced alone. This phenomenon is known as *enhancement* (Verrillo & Gescheider, 1975; Zwislocki & Ketkar, 1972).

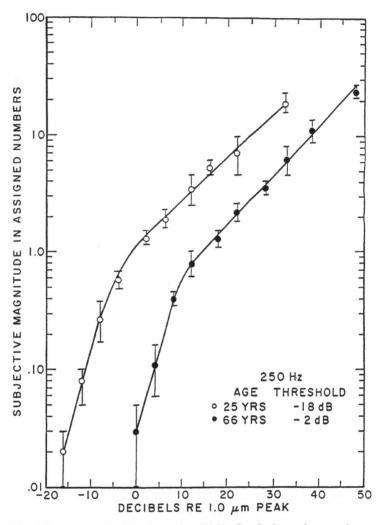

FIG. 17.5. Same as Fig. 17.4 measured at 250 Hz. Standard error bars are shown. Near threshold there is no recruitment effect, but the upper portion of the curves is significantly steeper in the older group. (From Verrillo, 1982. Reprinted with permission from Perception & psychophysics.

The older of two age groups (22 and 66 years) was unable to distinguish two short vibratory bursts separated by any time interval less than 150 ms in duration. They experienced the two bursts as a single event. The younger group, on the other hand, was easily able to distinguish the two bursts as separate events at separations of 50 ms or less. The older subjects also showed more enhancement. The effect of the first (conditioning) pulse on the subjective intensity of the second (test) at time intervals of 150 ms or longer appears to increase with age (Fig. 17.6). It is possible that both of these findings are manifestations of persistence in the elderly nervous system.

In another study, subjects were asked to detect a silent interval (gap detection) between two short vibrotactile bursts (Van Doren, Gescheider, & Verrillo, 1990). As expected, the ability to detect the gap improved as the gap duration was increased, regardless of the age of the subject, and gap detection was not affected by increasing age when sinusoidal bursts were used. However, when the sinusoids were replaced by bandpass noise, the older subjects performed significantly poorer than did the younger group (Fig. 17.7). We concluded that what is being measured and called *persistence* in the literature may not be a simple, single process, but may reflect multiple processes, including persistence of neural activity, slower recovery from stimulation (adaptation), and the use of differing strategies for stimulus detection.

A forward-masking paradigm was used to test a group of young (mean age of 19.4 years) and a group of older (mean age 64.6 years) subjects in another approach to the persistence phenomenon (Gescheider, Valettuti, Padula, & Verrillo, 1992). Detection thresholds of 50-ms signals were measured as a function of the time interval (Δt) between the offset of a 500-ms masker and the onset of the test stimulus. The amount of forward masking, which in this context may be considered a persistence effect, was expressed as the threshold shift, due to presentation of the masker, as a function of Δt. As expected, the threshold shift decreased in both groups as Δt increased, but at all values of Δt the older subjects exhibited significantly more masking (or if you will, persistence) than did the younger subjects (Fig. 17.8). Furthermore, the effect of age was more pronounced for stimuli that primarily affect the Pacinian receptor system (250 Hz) than it was for those that affect the non-Pacinian systems (25 Hz).

Another method used in our exploration of sensory persistence required the subject to adjust the temporal position of a short auditory click to match either the onset or offset of a vibrotactile stimulus (25 and 250 Hz) of long duration (500 ms) (Gescheider et al., 1992). All subjects could adjust the click to the stimulus onset with near-perfect accuracy. However, when the match was made to the offset of vibration, delays of up to 200 ms were observed in the older subjects (72 years) and the delays were significantly longer than those of the younger (21 years) subjects. Measurements of the effects of varying actual durations, temporal summation, yielded two kinds of responses. Half of the elderly subjects showed the same summation curve as the young subjects, and in the other half there was a substantial reduction in the amount of temporal summation. It appears that there are large individual differences in the effects of aging on the neural mechanisms

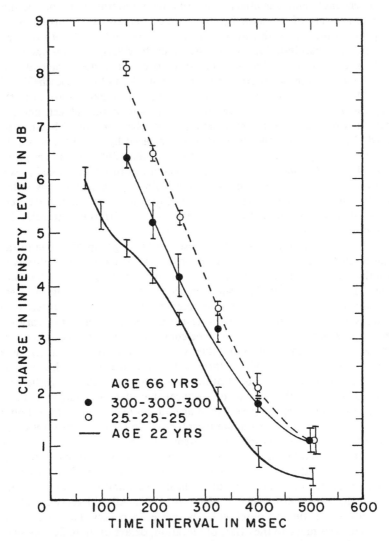

FIG. 17.6. Effect of the conditioning stimulus on the subjective intensity of the test stimulus, plotted as a function of the interstimulus time interval. There was no frequency (25 and 300 Hz) difference in the younger group, so their data are represented by a single line. Standard error bars are shown. (From Verrillo, 1982. Reprinted with permission from Perception & Psychophysics.)

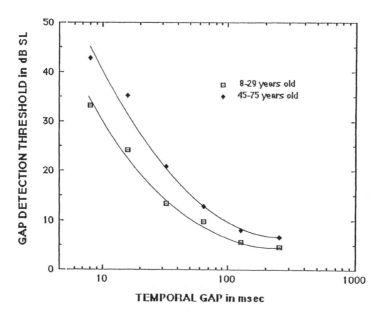

FIG. 17.7.   Detection thresholds for two age groups (means = 20 and 60 years) plotted as a function of the temporal gap between two bursts of band-limited noise. Detection thresholds are significantly higher in the older group.

responsible for temporal summation. Experiments showed that raised levels of internal noise in the elderly is probably not a contributing factor. The fact that there is a dramatic reduction of temporal-summation effects in the Pacinian system, however, is a significant finding.

The measurements of actual and apparent duration suggest that both sensory persistence and adaptation are profoundly affected by aging. Because adaptation appeared to be the more dominant factor for stimuli having durations as long as 500 ms, it was concluded that the effects on forward masking are due mainly to increased amounts of adaptation produced by the masker. Because all of the effects that we measured were substantially more pronounced in the Pacinian system, we may suggest that changes in this system associated with the aging process may be found at central levels of the nervous system as well as those found in the peripheral end organ by Cauna (1965).

Our most recent results of frequency functions from 0.4 to 500 Hz, using controlled skin-surface temperature, suggest that the loss of sensitivity does not occur in all four vibrotactile channels (Bolanowski, Gescheider, Verrillo, & Checkosky, 1988) at the same time in the life span of the individual. Just as the loss of hearing does not occur simultaneously across all frequencies, the loss of sensitivity among vibrotactile channels appears to be selective.

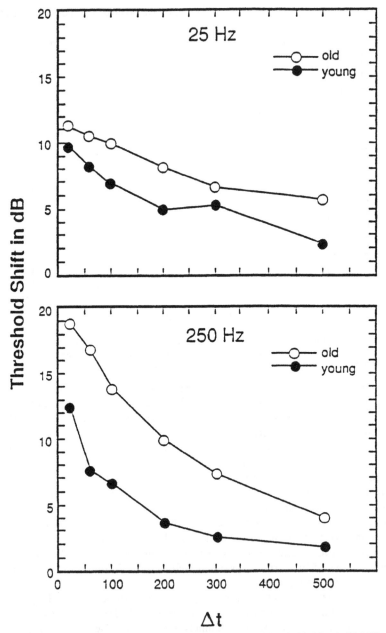

FIG. 17.8. The difference between masked and unmasked thresholds (threshold shift) as a function of the time between the offset of a masking stimulus and the onset of a test stimulus Δt). Old and young subjects were tested at 25 and 250 Hz. (From Gescheider, Valetutti, Padula & Verrillo, 1992. Reprinted with permission by the Journal of the Acoustical Society of America.

SUMMARY

Although it is a gradual process, one of the early signs of advancing age is an awareness of a failing in sensation, usually starting in vision followed closely by losses in hearing and touch. The loss of touch sensitivity often goes unnoticed. It is important that we understand the nature of these losses because of the importance of sensations to the quality and safety in the everyday lives of aging individuals. The tactile sense is important not only because of its role in the quality of life of the elderly (numbness of hands and feet is annoying and can be dangerous), but in a practical way it is important particularly to those who suffer a loss of hearing. Sensory aids for those with hearing losses have been designed to utilize residual hearing (hearing aids), lip reading, and the sense of touch (tactile vocoders). However, most of our knowledge about the sense of touch is based on research in which the subjects were young, mostly of college age. Our research is an approach to understanding the effects of aging on vibration sensitivity for the purpose, in part, of optimizing speech-communication aids for hearing-impaired listeners of all ages, but with a special consideration for those of advanced age.

ACKNOWLEDGMENT

The author gratefully acknowledges the research support from Grant DC 01243, National Institutes of Health, U.S. Department of Health and Human Services.

REFERENCES

Axelrod, S., & Cohen, L. D. (1961). Senescence and embedded-figure performance in vision and touch. *Perception & Motor Skills, 12,* 283–288.

Bolanowski, J. J., Jr., Gescheider, G. A., Verrillo, R. T., & Checkosky, C. M. (1988). Four channels mediate the mechanical aspects of touch. *Journal of the Acoustical Society of America, 84,* 1680–1694.

Bolanowski, S. J., Jr., & Verrillo, R. T. (1982). Temperature and criterion effects in the somatosensory system: A neurophysiological and psychological study. *Journal of Neurophysiology, 48,* 837–856.

Botwinick, J. (1978). *Aging and behavior* (2nd ed.) New York: Springer-Verlag.

Cauna, N. (1965). The effects of aging on the receptor organs of the human dermis. In W. Montagna (Ed.), *Advances in biology of skin-aging, VI* (Vol. VI, pp. 63–96). New York: Pergamon Press.

Coltheart, M. (1980). Iconic memory and visible persistence. *Perception & Psychophysics, 27,* 183–228.

Cosh, J. A. (1953). Studies in the nature of vibration sensation. *Clinical Science, 12,* 131–151.

Frisina, R. D., & Gescheider, G. A. (1977). Comparison of child and adult vibrotactile thresholds as a function of frequency and duration. *Perception & Psychophysics, 22,* 100–103.

Gescheider, G. A., Valettuti, A. A., Jr., Padula, M., & Verrillo, R. T. (1992). Vibrotactile forward masking as a function of age. *Journal of the Acoustical Society of America, 91*, 1690–1696.

Goetzinger, C., Proud, G., Dirks, D., & Embrey, J. (1961). A study of hearing in advanced age. *Archives of Otolaryngology, 73*, 662–674.

Goff, G. D., Rosner, B. S., Detre, T., & Kennard, D. (1965). Vibration perception in normal man and medical patients. *Journal of Neurology, Neurosurgery, & Psychiatry, 18*, 503–509.

Hellman, R. P., & Zwislocki, J. J. (1961). Some factors affecting the estimation of loudness. *Journal of the Acoustical Society of America, 33*, 683–694.

Knight, K. K., & Margolis, R. H. (1984). Magnitude estimation of loudness: II. Loudness perception in prebycusic listeners. *Journal of Speech & Hearing Research, 27*, 28–32.

Lindblom, U., & Verrillo, R. T. (1979). Sensory function in chronic neuralgia. *Journal of Neurology, Neurosurgery, & Psychiatry, 42*, 422–435.

Muijser, H. (1990). The influence of spatial contrast on the frequency-dependent nature of vibration sensitivity. *Perception & Psychophysics, 48*, 431–435.

Pearson, G. H. J. (1928). Effect of age on vibratory sensibility. *Archives of Neurology & Psychiatry, 20*, 482–496.

Plumb, C. S., & Meigs, J. W. (1961). Human vibration perception: Part 1. Vibration perception at different ages. *Archives of General Psychiatry, 4*, 611–614.

Rosenberg, G. (1958). Effect of age on peripheral vibratory perception. *Journal of the American Geriatrics Society, 6*, 471–481.

Stevens, S. S. (1957). On the psychophysical law. *Psychological Review, 64*, 153–181.

Stevens, S. S. (1959). Tactile vibration: Dynamics of sensory intensity. *Journal of Experimental Psychology, 57*, 210–218.

Van Doren, C. L., Gescheider, G. A., & Verrillo, R. T. (1990). Vibrotactile temporal gap detection as a function of age. *Journal of the Acoustical Society of American, 876*, 2201–2206.

Verrillo, R. T. (1974). Vibrotactile intensity scaling at several body sites. In F. A. Geldard (Ed.), *Cutaneous communication systems and devices* (pp. 9–14). Austin, TX: The Psychonomic Society.

Verrillo, R. T. (1977). Comparison of child and adult vibrotactile thresholds. *Bulletin of the Psychonomic Society, 9*, 197–200.

Verrillo, R. T. (1979). Change in vibrotactile thresholds as a function of age. *Sensory Processes, 3*, 49–59.

Verrillo, R. T. (1980). Age-related changes in the sensitivity to vibration. *Journal of Gerontology, 35*, 185–193.

Verrillo, R. T. (1982). Effect of aging on suprathreshold responses to vibration. *Perception & Psychophysics, 32*, 61–68.

Verrillo, R. T., Fraioli, A. J., & Smith, R. L. (1969). Sensation magnitude of vibrotactile stimuli. *Perception & Psychophysics, 6*, 366–372.

Verrillo, R. T., & Gescheider, G. A. (1975). Enhancement and summation in the perception of two successive vibrotactile stimuli. *Perception & Psychophysics, 18*, 128–136.

Whanger, A. D., & Wang, H. S. (1974). Clinical correlates of the vibratory sense in elderly psychiatric patients. *Journal of Gerontology, 29*, 39–45.

Zwislocki, J. J., & Goodman, D. A. (1980). Absolute scaling of sensory magnitudes: A validation. *Perception & Psychophysics, 28*, 28–38.

Zwislocki, J. J., & Ketkar, I. (1972). Loudness enhancement and summation in pairs of short sound bursts. *Journal of the Acoustical Society of America, 51*, 140(A).

18 Does Efferent Input Improve the Detection of Tones in Monaural Noise?

Bertram Scharf
Northeastern University and
Laboratoire de Mécanique et
d'Acoustique, Marseille

Joseph Nadol
Massachusetts Eye
and Ear Infirmary

Jacques Magnan
Hôpital Nord, Marseille

André Chays
Hôpital Nord

Alain Marchioni
Laboratoire de Mécanique
et d'Acoustique, Marseille

INTRODUCTION

The auditory system contains a large number of efferent fibers that terminate via the olivocochlear bundle at the hair cells of the cochlea. Two distinct groups of fibers have been identified—the *lateral* and *medial* efferents (Guinan, Warr, & Norris, 1983; Warr, Guinan, & White, 1986). The lateral fibers originate near the lateral superior olivary nucleus and innervate afferent dendrites at the inner hair cells, mostly in the ipsilateral cochlea; the medial fibers originate in the medial superior olivary nucleus and end directly on outer hair cells, mostly in the contralateral cochlea. Neurophysiological studies (cf. Wiederhold, 1986) have shown that activation of the efferents, usually by electrical stimulation, inhibits afferent activity in the eighth nerve. When the stimulus is tone plus noise, this inhibition may reduce the response to the noise, especially at higher stimulus levels, such that the tone evokes a relatively stronger response; accordingly, the effective neural signal-to-noise ratio would be greater than without efferent stimulation (Winslow & Sachs, 1987). Of course, electrical stimulation is not necessary to activate the efferents, and Liberman (1988) has shown that efferent discharge increases in the presence of broadband noise. These results suggested to Liberman (1988) "a potent role of the olivocochlear bundle in increasing the rate-response of auditory-nerve afferents to narrow-band stimuli embedded in broadband noise" (p. 1797), thereby possibly increasing "the detectability of narrow-band stimuli embedded in noise" (p. 1779). However, animal behavioral studies have not revealed a significant impairment of the ability to detect tones in noise after sectioning of the olivocochlear bundle (Igarashi, Alford, Nakai, & Gordon, 1972; Trahiotis & Elliot, 1970). This chapter suggests similar negative findings for human listeners whose vestibular nerve (which contains the olivocochlear bundle) had been sectioned to relieve severe vertigo, usually caused by Ménière's disease.

Ideally, we should compare signal detection in such patients before and after the operation. This was possible for three patients. In those three and in the rest of our sample we also compare detection in the operated ear with that in the healthy ear and with that reported in the literature for normally hearing subjects.

PROCEDURE

A two-interval, forced-choice method was employed to measure the detection of tones in continuous noise. Both an adaptive and a single-stimulus version were used. The adaptive procedure followed a 5-down, 1-up rule to estimate an 87% asymptote except in a few runs when a 2-down, 1-up rule yielding a 71% asymptote was followed. The masking noise was on continuously throughout a block. Feedback was provided on each trial. At the beginning of a run, the level decreased by 5 dB after five correct responses (after two by the 2-down rule) and increased by 5 dB after one incorrect response; after two inversions in the direction of level change, the 5-dB step was reduced to 2 dB. A threshold estimate was based on the last four of a total of six inversions; the thresholds reported are based on four estimates obtained by the 2-down rule and on two or three obtained by the 5-down rule. The single-stimulus procedure was part of a larger study of the ability to focus attention on a particular frequency region. In many blocks, signals could be at one of two or more frequencies. However, reported values in this chapter are based on those blocks of trials in which the signal was always at the same frequency. A trial began with a 350-ms tone burst set 5 dB above the 87% detection level. After 1 sec, two 350-ms observation intervals separated by 450 ms were indicated by the numbers 1 and 2 on a terminal screen. The tone burst was presented in one of the intervals at 1 dB above the assumed 87% detection level. No feedback was provided.

For two of the subjects, a Békésy tracking method was also employed. A 300-ms tone was repeated every 700 ms until the listener had changed the direction of attenuation 16 times. Threshold was based on the midpoints of the last 12 inversions. Attenuation was at the rate of 1 dB per 700 ms. Signal frequency was fixed at 1 kHz. The masking noise was 800-Hz wide at 60 or 70 dB SPL.

STIMULI

All stimuli were presented monaurally through a Yamaha or AKG (K340) earphone. Signal frequencies were chosen from the region in which a subject's thresholds in the quiet were closest to normal. Rise-fall times were 10 ms. The bandwidth and overall sound-pressure level of the masking noise was set to appropriate values for each subject, depending mainly on the degree of hearing loss. The overall level varied from 55 dB to around 80 dB.

SUBJECTS

Eight subjects, four women and four men from 30 to 50 years old, served in these experiments. All underwent an operation to relieve severe vertigo caused by Méinère's disease, except for AM whose diagnosis is uncertain. This operation involves the sectioning of the vestibular nerve. The olivo-cochlear bundle, which almost surely contains all the efferent fibers going to the hair cells, runs within the vestibular nerve before leaving it to enter the cochlea. Three subjects—CA, CF, and IP—were operated on by Dr. Nadol at the Massachusetts Eye and Ear Infirmary in Boston. The section was made at a point just before the olivocochlear bundle leaves the vestibular nerve. The other five subjects were operated on by Drs. Magnan and Chays at the Hôpital Nord in Marseille. The section was made retrosigmoidally, somewhat farther back from the cochlea than in Boston. Hearing levels were near normal over the region of measurement for four subjects, was around 25–35 dB for three others, and was close to 55 dB for one (see Table 18.1).

TABLE 18.1
Comparison of Masked Thresholds Within Subjects (Differences in dB are given between masked thresholds in operated and unoperated ears.)

Subject	Sex	Age	Frequency Region	HL	Before/After 2IFC	Healthy/Operated	
						2IFC	Békésy
SB	M	30 y	.4-1.85 kHz	15 dB	− 1.1 dB	− 0.8 dB	0.3 dB
AM	M	50	.6-1.4	25	− 1.3	−	
JO	M	39	.8-1.2	20	− 0.4	− 0.5	0.9
CA	F	39	.3-2.0	35		10.5	
JA	M	35	.8-1.2	30		0.3	
CF	F	30	1.0-4.0	20		0.2	
JM	F	39	.7-1.0	10		0.0	
IP	F	50	1.5-3.9	55		2.4	

In three subjects, masked thresholds were measured before and after the operation; in five, measurements were made only afterwards.

RESULTS

First we present the differences in masked thresholds between unoperated and operated ears. Then we present the signal-to-noise ratios required in operated ears for signal detection and compare them to published values.

Table 18.1 presents comparisons within subjects. The frequency region refers to the lowest and highest signal frequencies used. The hearing loss is based on ANSI standard S3.6 (American National Standard Institute, 1969) dB. Before/after refers to a comparison of signal detection in noise before and after the olivocochlear bundle was severed; healthy-ear/operated-ear refers to a comparison of detection in a subject's healthy ear and in his or her operated ear. Each decibel value given is the increase in signal level required for detection after the operation as compared to before, or in the operated ear as compared to the healthy ear. A negative value means the required signal level was lower in the operated ear. In measurements made by 2-interval forced choice (2IFC) under the adaptive procedure and by Békésy tracking, decibel differences could be obtained directly, because thresholds were measured in decibels and almost always in the same masking noise. Under 2IFC with constant signal and noise levels, performance was measured as percentage correct. Differences in percentage correct could be transformed to decibels by assuming that performance improved at the rate of 5% per 1-dB increase in signal level (assumed slope of the psychometric function as per Buus, Schorer, Florentine, & Zwicker, 1986). Thus, if under identical stimulus conditions, performance was at 90% in the healthy ear and at 80% in the operated ear, it was assumed that the operated ear would require a 2-dB higher signal level to reach the same 90% performance as the healthy ear.

Decibel values obtained directly from the adaptive 2IFC procedure and by transformation from the single-stimulus procedure were very close. For example, under the adaptive procedure the mean dB difference for subject CA was 9 dB and under the single-stimulus procedure, it was 11 dB. For IP, the mean difference was near 2 dB measured both ways.

Before/after differences, which were obtained for three subjects, are all negative, meaning that the subjects detected signals at lower signal-to-noise ratios after the operation than before. However, this apparent improvement cannot be considered significant. Not only is the size of the change small, between 0.4 and 1.3 dB, but the before measurements were made under stressful conditions, the day before the scheduled operation. The comparison of the healthy to the operated ears suggests no difference between

TABLE 18.2

Critical Ratios in Operated and in Normal Ears (Signal/noise spectrum level for 87% correct on 2IFC task.)

Sub-ject	Signal Fre-quency	HL	Noise Spectrum Level	Operated Ear		Normal Ears (Hawkins & Stevens)
				Adaptive	Single Stimulus	
SB	1,000 Hz	15 dB	28.2 dB	20.2 dB	20.7 dB	20.5 dB
AM	1,000	25	28.2	20.8	20.9	20.5
JO	1,000	20	28.2	18.3	18.8	20.5
CA	500	35	43.6	29.0	30.4	19.2
JA	1,000	30	38.2	20.3	20.2	20.5
CF	2,150	20	32.8	20.2	20.2	22.5
JM	1,000	10	23.2	18.7	18.1	20.5
IP	3,000	55	47.0	23.0	23.0	23.8

them, except for CA and IP who had higher masked thresholds in the operated ear. (It is probably coincidental that SB and JO show small negative differences here as well as in the before/after comparison.)

Table 18.2 presents the critical ratios measured in the operated ear of each subject and those published by Hawkins and Stevens (1950). The critical ratio is the ratio of the signal, at masked threshold, to the spectrum level of a masking noise wider than the critical band (Scharf, 1970). For each subject the signal frequency, hearing level, and masking noise spectrum level are given in addition to the critical ratios calculated from measurements by the adaptive 2IFC procedure and by the single-stimulus procedure. (The signal level at threshold is the sum of the critical ratio and corresponding noise spectrum level; thus for SB his average 87% threshold for the 1000-Hz signal in the adaptive procedure was 48.4 dB.) The critical ratios listed are based on 1 to 2 blocks of trials for the adaptive procedure and from 1 to 11 blocks (52 to 64 trials per block) for the single-stimulus procedure (mean of 5.1 blocks per subject). All values are based on signal levels required for 87% correct judgements after adjustments based on the 5%-per-dB rule described previously. For five of the subjects, the signal frequency was 1000 Hz and the noise spectrum level was between 23.2 and 38.2 dB. Although the literature contains a number of studies since that of Hawkins and Stevens (1950) that report critical ratios (e.g., Bilger & Hirsh, 1956; Green, McKey, & Licklidker, 1959; Reed & Bilger, 1973), we have limited our comparison to Hawkins and Stevens, because they provide the most extensive set of data. Although their four experienced subjects made judgments by a method of adjustment, their measured critical ratio of 18.5 dB at 1000 Hz is very close to that reported by Buus et al. (1986) who used a constant-stimulus 2IFC procedure very similar to our single-stimulus procedure. At 1100 Hz against a noise spectrum level of 25 dB, their critical ratio from eight subjects for 75% correct is 18.1 dB. Critical ratios from other studies are generally similar, varying by only 1 or 2 dB owing largely to differences in procedure or stimulus parameters.

The critical ratios listed for Hawkins and Stevens (1950) are 2 dB higher than the data points from their Fig. 6. This adjustment was made on the assumption that their subjects were setting signal levels to a value that would have led to 77% correct in a 2IFC task like ours. The 77% value comes from a comparison between their critical ratio of 18.5 dB at 1000 Hz and the 18.1 dB measured by Buus et al. (1986) at 1100 Hz. A 0.4-dB increase in level is equivalent to a 2% increase in performance. Another 2-dB increase is needed to bring performance up to our 87% level. (We have chosen not to correct for the frequency difference of 100 Hz.)

Of the eight subjects, four have critical ratios within 0.8 dB of those culled from Hawkins and Stevens (1950), three have ratios about 2 dB lower, and only one, CA, has a clearly higher ratio.

DISCUSSION

The results are strikingly clear. None of the three subjects for whom before and after measurements were available shows a deterioration in the ability to detect a tone in monaural noise after the vestibular neurotomy. Moreover, these three had normal critical ratios despite the presence of Ménière's or other pathology. Of the other five, only CA required an unusually large signal-to-noise ratio for detection. It is reasonable to assume on the basis of the results from the rest of the subjects that CA already had this large critical ratio before her operation, a result of her Ménière's. Moreover, she reported no change in her hearing after the operation. Also subject IP who suffers a 55-dB loss appears to have an inflated critical ratio, at least with respect to her own healthy ear (Table 18.1).

Given that all but two of the eight operated subjects showed as good a detection of tones in noise in their healthy as in their operated ear and that most critical ratios were normal, we see no evidence that this type of signal detection deteriorates after vestibular neurotomy. We also point out that in the majority of subjects, thresholds in quiet did not change after the operation.

Despite the clarity of the psychoacoustical data, we cannot be sure that efferent input is entirely absent in the operated ears. Although all the patients, except AM, were nearly free of vertigo after the operation, the entire vestibular nerve need not be severed to achieve that clinical outcome. We have no independent confirmation of the surgeon's visual observations which do suggest very strongly that the whole nerve was sectioned.

Consequently, although the inferior vestibular nerve appears to contain all the fibers of the olivocochlear bundle (cf. Arnesen, 1984), we cannot be sure that some of them may not have been spared in some patients.

As indicated in our introduction, the hypothesis that the efferent nerve may serve to improve the detection of tones in noise was based on neurophysiological data. Our results yield no evidence for such an improvement for the detection of *monaural* tone bursts in *monaural* noise. Even though we cannot be sure that all efferent input was eliminated in our patients, it is almost certain that a good portion of it was. Consequently, unless the vestibular neurotomy spares just that subset of efferent fibers that are involved in monaural signal detection, some deterioration in performance should have been uncovered by our psychoacoustical procedures.

Our conclusion must be limited to monaural signals, at levels not exceeding about 65-dB SPL. We did not use any binaural or dichotic stimuli. Liberman (1988) has shown that most efferent units respond better to binaural stimuli than to monaural stimuli. Whereas it seems unlikely that simple binaural stimulation would yield results different from those for monaural stimulation in our operated subjects, it would not be unreasonable for dichotic stimulation to reveal an important role for the olivocochlear bundle. In particular, our operated patients may do poorly in detecting a signal to the operated ear when a binaural noise is lateralized to the healthy ear, that is, they would show a smaller masking-level difference than normal. The lack of efferent input to the ear receiving the signal would mean that the neural signal-to-noise ratio would not be enhanced in the manner suggested by Liberman (1988). On the other hand, central masking, the masking of a signal in one ear by a monaural masker to the other, a type of masking studied extensively by Zwislocki (1972), might be reduced when the signal goes to the operated ear, because the contralateral noise could not increase efferent response in that ear and thereby reduce afferent output. These various possibilities are currently under study. Owing to a lack of independent confirmation that the whole olivocochlear bundle was cut in our patients, we can only conclude tentatively that the olivocochlear bundle does not appear to play a role in monaural masking of a tone by noise. Furthermore, it remains to be seen how it affects masking under dichotic listening.

ACKNOWLEDGMENTS

We thank Georges Canévet, Carol Meiselman, and Thierry Voinier for their aid in carrying out this research which was supported in part by a grant from NIDCD (DC00084-16), National Institutes of Health, and U.S. Department of Health and Human Services. We thank John Guinan for helpful comments about an earlier version of the manuscript.

REFERENCES

American National Standards Institute. (1969). *American national standard specifications for audiometers S3.6.* New York: American National Standards Institute.

Arnesen, A. R. (1984). Fibre population of the vestibulocochlear anastomosis in humans. *Acta Oto-Laryngologica, 98,* 501–518.

Bilger, R. C., & Hirsh I. J. (1956). Masking of tones by bands of noise. *Journal of the Acoustical Society of America, 28,* 623–630.

Buus, S., Schorer, E., Florentine, M., & Zwicker, E. (1986). Decision rules in detection of simple and complex tones. *Journal of the Acoustical Society of America, 80,* 1646–1657.

Green, D. M., McKey, M. J., & Licklider, J. C. R. (1959). Detection of a pulsed sinusoid as a function of frequency. *Journal of the Acoustical Society of America, 31,* 1446–1452.

Guinan, J. J., Jr., Warr, W. B., & Norris, B. E. (1983). Differential olivocochlear projections from lateral versus medial zones of the superior olivary complex. *Journal of Comparative Neurology, 221,* 358–370.

Hawkins, J. E., & Stevens, S. S. (1950). The masking of pure tones and of speech by white noise. *Journal of the Acoustical Society of America, 22,* 6–13.

Igarashi, M., Alford, B. R., Nakai, Y., & Gordon, W. P. (1972). Behavioral auditory function after transection of crossed olivo-cochlear bundle in the cat. I. Pure-tone threshold and perceptual signal-to-noise ratio. *Acta Oto-Laryngologica, 73,* 455–466.

Liberman, M. C. (1988). Response properties of cochlear efferent neurons: Monaural vs. binaural stimulation and the effects of noise. *Journal of Neurophysiology, 60,* 1779–1798.

Reed, C. M., & Bilger, R. C. (1973). A comparative study of S/N and E/N. *Journal of the Acoustical Society of America, 53,* 1039–1044.

Scharf, B. (1970). Critical bands. In J. V. Tobias (Ed.), *Foundations of modern auditory theory,* (Vol. 1, pp. 157–202). New York: Academic Press.

Trahiotis, C., & Elliot, D. N. (1970). Behavioral investigation of some possible effects of sectioning the crossed olivocochlear bundle. *Journal of the Acoustical Society of America, 47,* 592–596.

Warr, W. B., Guinan, J. J., Jr., & White, J. S. (1986). Organization of the efferent fibers: The lateral and medial olivocochlear systems. In R. A. Altschuler, D. W. Hoffman, & R. P. Bobbin (Eds.), *Neurobiology of hearing: The cochlea,* (pp. 333–348). New York: Raven Press.

Wiederhold, M. L. (1986). Physiology of the olivocochlear system. In R. A. Altschuler, R. P. Bobbin, & D. W. Hoffman (Eds.), *Neurobiology of hearing: The cochlea* (pp. 349–370). New York: Raven Press.

Winslow, R. L., & Sachs, M. B. (1987). Effect of electrical stimulation of the crossed olivocochlear bundle on auditory nerve response to tones in noise. *Journal of Neurophysiology, 57,* 1002–1021.

Zwislocki, J. J. (1972). A theory of central auditory masking and its partial validation. *Journal of the Acoustical Society of America, 52,* 644–659.

Author Index

---

*Page numbers that are underlined refer to references.
**Page numbers that are italicized refer to Figure legends.

Subject Index